Injury & Trauma Sourcebook

Learning Disabilities Sourcebook, 4th Edition

Leukemia Sourcebook

Liver Disorders Sourcebook

Medical Tests Sourcebook, 4th Edition

Men's Health Concerns Sourcebook, 4th Edition

Mental Health Disorders Sourcebook, 5th Edition

Mental Retardation Sourcebook

Movement Disorders Sourcebook, 2nd Edition

Multiple Sclerosis Sourcebook

Muscular Dystrophy Sourcebook

Obesity Sourcebook

Osteoporosis Sourcebook

Pain Sourcebook, 4th Edition

Pediatric Cancer Sourcebook

Physical & Mental Issues in Aging Sourcebook

Podiatry Sourcebook, 2nd Edition

Pregnancy & Birth Sourcebook, 3rd Edition

Prostate & Urological Disorders Sourcebook

Prostate Cancer Sourcebook

Rehabilitation Sourcebook

Respiratory Disorders Sourcebook, 3rd Edition

Sexually Transmitted Diseases Sourcebook,
    5th Edition

Sleep Disorders Sourcebook, 3rd Edition

Smoking Concerns Sourcebook

Sports Injuries Sourcebook, 4th Edition

Stress-Related Disorders Sourcebook, 3rd Edition

Stroke Sourcebook, 3rd Edition

Surgery Sourcebook, 3rd Edition

Thyroid Disorders Sourcebook

Transplantation Sourcebook

Traveler's Health Sourcebook

Urinary Tract & Kidney Diseases & Disorders
    Sourcebook, 2nd Edition

Vegetarian Sourcebook

Women's Health Concerns Sourcebook, 4th Edition

Workplace Health & Safety Sourcebook

Worldwide Health Sourcebook

Teen Health Series

Abuse & Violence Information for Teens

Accident & Safety Information for Teens

Alcohol Information for Teens,
    3rd Edition

Allergy Information for Teens,
    2nd Edition

Asthma Information for Teens,
    2nd Edition

Body Information for Teens

Cancer Information for Teens,
    3rd Edition

Complementary & Alternative
    Medicine Information for Teens,
    2nd Edition

Diabetes Information for Teens,
    2nd Edition

Diet Information for Teens, 3rd Edition

Drug Information for Teens, 3rd Edition

Eating Disorders Information for Teens,
    3rd Edition

Fitness Information for Teens,
    3rd Edition

Learning Disabilities Information for
    Teens

Mental Health Information for Teens,
    4th Edition

Pregnancy Information for Teens,
    2nd Edition

Sexual Health Information for Teens,
    3rd Edition

Skin Health Information for Teens,
    3rd Edition

Sleep Information for Teens

Sports Injuries Information for Teens,
    3rd Edition

Stress Information for Teens,
    2nd Edition

Suicide Information for Teens,
    2nd Edition

Tobacco Information for Teens,
    2nd Edition

Surgery

SOURCEBOOK

Third Edition

Health Reference Series

Third Edition

Surgery
SOURCEBOOK

*Basic Consumer Health Information about Common
Surgical Techniques and Procedures, Including Appendectomy,
Breast Biopsy, Carotid Endarterectomy, Cataract Removal,
Cesarean Section, Coronary Artery Bypass, Cosmetic Surgery,
Dilation and Curettage, Gallbladder Surgery, Hemorrhoid-
ectomy, Hysterectomy, Hernia Repair, Low Back Surgery,
Mastectomy, Prostatectomy, Tonsillectomy, and
Weight-Loss (Bariatric) Surgery*

*Along with Facts about Emergency Surgery and Critical
Care and Tips on Preparing for Surgery, Getting a Second
Opinion, Managing Pain and Surgical Complications, and
Recovering from Surgery, a Glossary of Related Terms,
and a Directory of Resources for More Information*

Edited by
Amy L. Sutton

Omnigraphics

155 W. Congress, Suite 200, Detroit, MI 48226

Bibliographic Note

Because this page cannot legibly accommodate all the copyright notices, the Bibliographic Note portion of the Preface constitutes an extension of the copyright notice.

Edited by Amy L. Sutton

Health Reference Series

Karen Bellenir, *Managing Editor*

David A. Cooke, MD, FACP, *Medical Consultant*

Elizabeth Collins, *Research and Permissions Coordinator*

EdIndex, Services for Publishers, *Indexers*

* * *

Omnigraphics, Inc.

Matthew P. Barbour, *Senior Vice President*

Kevin M. Hayes, *Operations Manager*

* * *

Peter E. Ruffner, *Publisher*

Copyright © 2013 Omnigraphics, Inc.

ISBN 978-0-7808-1291-8

E-ISBN 978-0-7808-1292-5

Library of Congress Cataloging-in-Publication Data

Surgery sourcebook : basic consumer health information about common surgical techniques and procedures, including appendectomy, breast biopsy, carotid endarterectomy, cataract removal, cesarean section, coronary artery bypass, cosmetic surgery ... / edited by Amy L. Sutton. -- Third edition.
  pages cm. -- (Health reference series)
 Includes bibliographical references and index.
 Summary: "Provides basic consumer health information about common surgical procedures, potential risks and complications, pain control options, and recovery issues. Includes index, glossary of related terms, and other resources"-- Provided by publisher.
  ISBN 978-0-7808-1291-8 (hardcover : alk. paper) 1. Surgery--Popular works. 2. Consumer education--Popular works. I. Sutton, Amy L., editor.
 RD31.3.S87 2013
 617--dc23

                                                                  2012044721

∞

Table of Contents

Visit www.healthreferenceseries.com to view *A Contents Guide to the Health Reference Series*, a listing of more than 16,000 topics and the volumes in which they are covered.

Part II: Preparing for Surgery

Part III: Common Types of Surgery and Surgical Procedures

Part IV: Managing Pain and Surgical Complications

Part V: Recovering from Surgery

Part VI: Additional Help and Information

Preface

About This Book

According to the Agency for Healthcare Research and Quality, more than 15 million people undergo surgery each year at hospitals or same-day surgery centers in the U.S. Whether it is done to relieve pain, prevent or treat a serious health condition, or repair trauma, surgery carries significant risks, such as infection, anesthesia reactions, and bleeding. Fortunately, new developments in surgical techniques, including cryotherapy, lasers, and laparoscopic surgery, have enabled surgeons to better control surgical complications and minimize patient risks.

Surgery Sourcebook, Third Edition, describes the most common surgical procedures, including appendectomy, breast surgery, carotid endarterectomy, cataract removal, cesarean section, coronary artery bypass, cosmetic surgery, dilation and curettage, gallbladder surgery, hemorrhoidectomy, hysterectomy, hernia repair, low back surgery, prostatectomy, tonsillectomy, and weight-loss (bariatric) surgery. The book discusses preparations patients may want to make prior to undergoing surgery, including choosing a surgeon, getting a second opinion, and donating blood, as well as postsurgical physical discomforts, nutrition and exercise considerations, and strategies for facilitating recovery. The book concludes with a glossary of related terms and a directory of resources for additional help and information.

How to Use This Book

This book is divided into parts and chapters. Parts focus on broad areas of interest. Chapters are devoted to single topics within a part.

Part I: Introduction to Surgery provides basic information about surgical specialties, including general surgery, neurosurgery, obstetrics and gynecology, ophthalmology, orthopedic surgery, otolaryngology, plastic surgery, and urology. It discusses specific types of surgical techniques—including cryosurgery, laparoscopic surgery, laser surgery, natural orifice surgery, and stereotactic radiosurgery—and special surgical considerations with pediatric and geriatric patients. The part concludes with an examination of trends in surgical mortality rates and facts about medical tourism.

Part II: Preparing for Surgery offers patients information on finding a qualified surgeon, obtaining a second opinion, preparing for surgery, choosing ambulatory care, and dealing with preoperative anxiety. The part also discusses blood donation prior to surgery, tips on ensuring patient safety and preventing medical errors, financial planning facts, and the use of advance directives.

Part III: Common Types of Surgery and Surgical Procedures provides details about head and neck, eye, dental and endodontic, breast, lung, heart and vascular, joint and spine, gastrointestinal, weight-loss (bariatric), gynecologic and obstetric, and urological surgeries. The part also highlights cosmetic and reconstructive surgical procedures, such as abdominoplasty, blepharoplasty, body contouring surgery, liposuction, rhinoplasty, and surgery for skin cancer. The part concludes with information about organ transplants and emergency and critical care surgery.

Part IV: Managing Pain and Surgical Complications focuses on the postoperative period and discusses methods for controlling pain, managing blood loss, and preventing surgical site and healthcare-associated infections that may develop during hospitalization, such as catheter-associated urinary tract infections and methicillin-resistant *Staphylococcus aureus* (MRSA). The part also identifies other complications that may affect surgical patients, including abdominal adhesions, deep vein thrombosis, pneumonia, sepsis, and shock.

Part V: Recovering from Surgery offers insight into the process of recovering from surgery. Hospital discharge planning, postsurgical nutrition and exercise recommendations, and strategies for caring for incisions, surgical drains, and ostomy bags are discussed, along with information about safety concerns when driving and traveling after surgery.

Part VI: Additional Help and Information provides a glossary of important terms related to surgery and a directory of organizations that offer information to people undergoing surgery or their caregivers.

Bibliographic Note

This volume contains documents and excerpts from publications issued by the following U.S. government agencies: Agency for Healthcare Research and Quality (AHRQ); Centers for Medicare and Medicaid Services (CMS); Centers for Disease Control and Prevention (CDC); National Cancer Institute (NCI); National Center for Complementary and Alternative Medicine (NCCAM); National Eye Institute (NEI); National Heart, Lung, and Blood Institute (NHLBI); National Highway Traffic Safety Administration (NHTSA); National Institute of Arthritis and Musculoskeletal and Skin Diseases (NIAMS); National Institute of Diabetes and Digestive and Kidney Diseases (NIDDK); National Institute of Neurological Disorders and Stroke (NINDS); National Institute on Aging (NIA); National Institute on Deafness and Other Communication Disorders (NIDCD); National Institutes of Health (NIH): Office on Women's Health (OWH); and the U.S. Food and Drug Administration (FDA).

In addition, this volume contains copyrighted documents from the following organizations: A.D.A.M., Inc.; American Association of Endodontists; American College of Surgeons; American National Red Cross; American Pregnancy Association; American Psychological Association; American Rhinologic Society; American Society for Laser Medicine and Surgery; American Society for Metabolic and Bariatric Surgery; American Society for Reproductive Medicine; American Society of Anesthesiologists; American Society of PeriAnesthesia Nurses; American Society of Plastic Surgeons; American Thoracic Society; American Thyroid Association; Cleveland Clinic Foundation; Sol Goldman Pancreatic Cancer Research Center; Hormone Health Network; The Joint Commission; McMahon Publishing; National Hospice and Palliative Care Organization; Nemours Foundation; Planned Parenthood Federation of America; Regents of the University of California; United Hospital Fund; United Network for Organ Sharing; United Ostomy Associations of America, Inc.; University of Southern California Center for Pancreatic and Biliary Diseases; University of Wisconsin Hospitals and Clinics Authority; and Zimmer, Inc.

Full citation information is provided on the first page of each chapter or section. Every effort has been made to secure all necessary rights to reprint the copyrighted material. If any omissions have been made, please contact Omnigraphics to make corrections for future editions.

Acknowledgements

Thanks go to the many organizations, agencies, and individuals who have contributed materials for this *Sourcebook* and to medical consultant Dr. David Cooke and prepress service provider WhimsyInk. Special thanks go to managing editor Karen Bellenir and research and permissions coordinator Liz Collins for their help and support.

About the Health Reference Series

The *Health Reference Series* is designed to provide basic medical information for patients, families, caregivers, and the general public. Each volume takes a particular topic and provides comprehensive coverage. This is especially important for people who may be dealing with a newly diagnosed disease or a chronic disorder in themselves or in a family member. People looking for preventive guidance, information about disease warning signs, medical statistics, and risk factors for health problems will also find answers to their questions in the *Health Reference Series*. The *Series*, however, is not intended to serve as a tool for diagnosing illness, in prescribing treatments, or as a substitute for the physician/patient relationship. All people concerned about medical symptoms or the possibility of disease are encouraged to seek professional care from an appropriate health care provider.

A Note about Spelling and Style

Health Reference Series editors use *Stedman's Medical Dictionary* as an authority for questions related to the spelling of medical terms and the *Chicago Manual of Style* for questions related to grammatical structures, punctuation, and other editorial concerns. Consistent adherence is not always possible, however, because the individual volumes within the *Series* include many documents from a wide variety of different producers and copyright holders, and the editor's primary goal is to present material from each source as accurately as is possible following the terms specified by each document's producer. This sometimes means that information in different chapters or sections may follow other guidelines and alternate spelling authorities. For example, occasionally a copyright holder may require that eponymous terms be shown in possessive forms (Crohn's disease *vs.* Crohn disease) or that British spelling norms be retained (leukaemia *vs.* leukemia).

Locating Information within the Health Reference Series

The *Health Reference Series* contains a wealth of information about a wide variety of medical topics. Ensuring easy access to all the fact sheets, research reports, in-depth discussions, and other material contained within the individual books of the *Series* remains one of our highest priorities. As the *Series* continues to grow in size and scope, however, locating the precise information needed by a reader may become more challenging.

A Contents Guide to the Health Reference Series was developed to direct readers to the specific volumes that address their concerns. It presents an extensive list of diseases, treatments, and other topics of general interest compiled from the Tables of Contents and major index headings. To access *A Contents Guide to the Health Reference Series*, visit www.healthreferenceseries.com.

Medical Consultant

Medical consultation services are provided to the *Health Reference Series* editors by David A. Cooke, MD, FACP. Dr. Cooke is a graduate of Brandeis University, and he received his M.D. degree from the University of Michigan. He completed residency training at the University of Wisconsin Hospital and Clinics. He is board-certified in Internal Medicine. Dr. Cooke currently works as part of the University of Michigan Health System and practices in Ann Arbor, MI. In his free time, he enjoys writing, science fiction, and spending time with his family.

Our Advisory Board

We would like to thank the following board members for providing guidance to the development of this *Series*:

- Dr. Lynda Baker, Associate Professor of Library and Information Science, Wayne State University, Detroit, MI

- Nancy Bulgarelli, William Beaumont Hospital Library, Royal Oak, MI

- Karen Imarisio, Bloomfield Township Public Library, Bloomfield Township, MI

- Karen Morgan, Mardigian Library, University of Michigan-Dearborn, Dearborn, MI

- Rosemary Orlando, St. Clair Shores Public Library, St. Clair Shores, MI

Health Reference Series *Update Policy*

The inaugural book in the *Health Reference Series* was the first edition of *Cancer Sourcebook* published in 1989. Since then, the *Series* has been enthusiastically received by librarians and in the medical community. In order to maintain the standard of providing high-quality health information for the layperson the editorial staff at Omnigraphics felt it was necessary to implement a policy of updating volumes when warranted.

Medical researchers have been making tremendous strides, and it is the purpose of the *Health Reference Series* to stay current with the most recent advances. Each decision to update a volume is made on an individual basis. Some of the considerations include how much new information is available and the feedback we receive from people who use the books. If there is a topic you would like to see added to the update list, or an area of medical concern you feel has not been adequately addressed, please write to:

Editor
Health Reference Series
Omnigraphics, Inc.
155 W. Congress, Suite 200
Detroit, MI 48226
E-mail: editorial@omnigraphics.com

Part One

Introduction to Surgery

Chapter 1

Overview of Surgical Specialties

Colon and Rectal Surgery

A colon and rectal surgeon is trained to diagnose and treat patients with various diseases of the intestinal tract, colon, rectum, anal canal, and perianal area through medical and surgical means. This specialist may also deal with the liver, urinary, and female reproductive systems if they are involved with primary intestinal disease. A colon and rectal surgeon has expertise in diagnosing and managing anorectal conditions such as hemorrhoids, fissures (painful tears in the anal lining), abscesses, and fistulae (infections located around the anus and rectum). Training in colon and rectal surgery also provides the specialist with in-depth knowledge of intestinal and anorectal physiology required for the treatment of problems such as constipation and incontinence. They also treat problems of the intestine and colon and perform endoscopic procedures to detect and treat conditions of the bowel lining, such as cancer, polyps (precancerous growths), and inflammatory conditions. A colon and rectal specialist also performs abdominal surgical procedures involving the colon, rectum, and small bowel for the treatment of cancer, diverticulitis, and inflammatory bowel disease (such as chronic ulcerative colitis and Crohn's disease). These operations may be performed with traditional (open) or minimally invasive (laparoscopic) techniques.

General Surgery

A general surgeon is a specialist who is trained to diagnose, treat, and manage patients with a broad spectrum of surgical conditions affecting almost any area of the body. The surgeon establishes the diagnosis and provides the preoperative, operative, and postoperative care to patients and is often responsible for the comprehensive management of the trauma victim and the critically ill patient. The general surgeon has the knowledge and technical skills to manage conditions that relate to the head and neck, breast, skin and soft tissues, abdomen, extremities, and the gastrointestinal, vascular, and endocrine systems.

Surgeons may further specialize in an additional board certification from the American Board of Surgery in the following areas:

Pediatric Surgery

A pediatric surgeon is a specialist who is trained to diagnose, treat, and manage the preoperative, operative, and postoperative care of the child. They care for and operate on children whose development ranges from the newborn through the teenage years. All pediatric surgeons are board certified in general surgery and then complete two years of additional training before they are eligible to be certified in pediatric surgery. As a result of this additional training, pediatric surgeons have expertise in the following areas of responsibility: Neonatal surgery (specialized knowledge in the surgical repair of birth defects in the newborn); prenatal surgery (detect abnormalities and plan for surgical corrections during the fetal stage of development); trauma (knowledge in the surgical care and prevention of traumatic injuries); pediatric surgical oncology (knowledge of the diagnosis and surgical care of children with tumors and growths); and surgical problems of the gastrointestinal tract, such as inflammatory bowel disease, appendicitis, and gastroesophageal reflux (reflux of food from the stomach to the esophagus or trachea). Pediatric surgeons are also trained to care for certain surgical problems of the neck, skin and soft tissues, and vascular and endocrine systems.

Vascular Surgery

A vascular surgeon is a surgical specialist who cares for patients with diseases that affect the arteries, veins, and lymphatic systems exclusive of the heart and intracranial (within the brain) circulations. Hardening of the arteries or atherosclerosis is a common cause of vascular disease. Specialists in this field perform open operations, endovascular catheter-based procedures, and non-invasive vascular testing and interpretations. Common problems treated include stroke prevention by managing arterial blockages in the neck and upper chest, revascularization of upper and lower limbs for poor circulation, management of aneurysms such as those that occur in the abdomen and elsewhere, vascular trauma, and varicose veins. Treatment also includes angioplasty—stenting of arterial blockages, repair of abdominal aneurysms by less invasive endovascular techniques, as well as medical management of vascular disorders. Vascular surgeons are board certified in general surgery and then complete additional training and testing in vascular surgery.

Surgery of the Hand

This specialty focuses on the investigation and treatment of patients with diseases, injuries, or abnormalities affecting the upper extremities. This specialty includes the performance of microvascular surgery, which is necessary for reattachment of amputated fingers or limbs. All hand surgeons are certified in general surgery and then complete additional training and testing in hand surgery.

Critical Care Surgery

This specialty focuses on the surgical and medical diagnosis and treatment of critically ill and injured patients, particularly the trauma victim. Specialists have the knowledge, skills, and compassion to provide timely, safe, effective and efficient patient-centered care and manage the patient with multiple organ problems. They also coordinate the teams of doctors and nurses needed for the care of the critically ill and injured patient. Surgeons in this discipline are board certified in general surgery and then complete additional training and testing in critical care surgery.

Neurologic Surgery

A neurological surgeon provides operative and nonoperative management (prevention, diagnosis, evaluation, treatment, critical care, and rehabilitation) of patients with disorders of the brain, spinal cord, spinal column, and peripheral nerves, including their support structures and blood supply. They also evaluate and manage disorders that affect the function of the nervous system and the operative and non-operative management of certain types of pain. Common conditions managed by neurologic surgeons include disorders of the brain, meninges (membranes covering the brain and spinal cord), skull, spinal cord, and vertebral column. This also includes the carotid and vertebral arteries, the pituitary gland, spinal fusion or instrumentation, and disorders of the cranial and spinal nerves. Pediatric neurosurgeons manage children with head injuries, brain and spinal tumors, vascular malformation, seizure disorders, and hydrocephalus.

Obstetrics and Gynecology

Obstetrician/gynecologists provide medical and surgical care of the female patient. The focus for this specialty is on the female reproductive system, including performing surgical procedures, managing the care of pregnant women, delivering babies, and rendering gynecologic care, oncology care, and primary health care for women.

Specialty certification in obstetrics and gynecology includes [the following]:

- **Gynecology Oncology:** An obstetrician/gynecologist who is certified in ob/gyn and then has an additional three to four years of specialized training in the treatment of gynecologic cancers including special surgical training and has subspecialty certification through the American Board of Obstetrics and Gynecology for the comprehensive management of patients with cancer unique to women. This specialist provides comprehensive management of women with precancerous and cancerous conditions of the female reproductive system. Expertise in surgery, chemotherapy, and indications for radiation therapy supports continuity of care of the gynecologic cancer patient.

- **Maternal Fetal Medicine:** An obstetrician/gynecologist who is certified in ob/gyn and has additional training in obstetrics and has sub-specialty certification through the American Board of Obstetrics and Gynecology. This individual cares for patients with complications of pregnancy and has advanced knowledge of the obstetrical, medical, and surgical complications of pregnancy and their effect on both mother and their fetuses. This specialist has expertise in the current diagnostic techniques and treatments for woman with complicated pregnancies. Special expertise also exists in the use of sonography in pregnancy.

- **Reproductive Endocrinology and Infertility:** An obstetrician/gynecologist who is certified in ob/gyn and has additional training in reproductive medicine and has sub-specialty certification through the American Board of Obstetrics and Gynecology.

This individual manages patients with complex problems related to reproductive medicine, including assisted reproductive technology, in vitro fertilization, reproductive surgery, infertility, menopause, contraception, endometriosis, and other reproductive disorders.

- **Female Pelvic Medicine and Reconstructive Surgery:**
An obstetrician/gynecologist who is certified in ob/gyn and has additional training in the management of the female bladder and pelvic floor. Disorders managed by this sub-specialty include disorders requiring advanced vaginal and laparoscopic surgery, female urinary incontinence, pelvic organ prolapse, vesicovaginal fistula, and female anal incontinence.

Ophthalmologic Surgery

An ophthalmologist specializes in the comprehensive care of patients with disorders of their eyes and vision. Ophthalmologists are medically trained to diagnose and medically and surgically treat all ocular and visual disorders, including prescribing glasses and contact lenses. These specialists also treat problems affecting the eye and its structures, the eyelids, the orbit, the visual pathway, and acquired onset of double vision in adults and children from neurological and endocrine conditions such as stroke with cranial nerve palsies and thyroid-related eye disease. Cataract operations and basic glaucoma procedures are commonly performed by these specialists. Ophthalmologists may also have additional expertise in the following areas: Adult strabismus, cornea and external disease, glaucoma, neuro-ophthalmology, ophthalmic pathology, ophthalmic plastic surgery, pediatric ophthalmology, and vitreoretinal diseases.

Oral and Maxillofacial Surgery

An oral and maxillofacial surgeon specializes in dentistry which includes the diagnosis and surgical and adjunctive treatment of patients with disease, injuries, and defects involving both the function and appearance of the oral and maxillofacial region. This specialty includes care of the oral cavity and face, removal of diseased and impacted teeth, anesthesia for dental procedures, dental implants, facial trauma, pathologic conditions (tumors or cysts), reconstructive and cosmetic surgery, facial pain including temporomandibular joint disorders, and correction of dentofacial (bite) deformities and birth defects. Certification requires completion of training in an accredited

residency program, evidence of post-training experience, and successful completion of written and oral examinations on the entire scope
of the specialty.

Orthopaedic Surgery

An orthopaedic surgeon is trained in the preservation, investigation,
and restoration of the form and function of the extremities, spine, and associated structures by medical, surgical, and physical means. Specialized
care is provided for patients with musculoskeletal problems including
congenital deformities, trauma, infections, tumors, metabolic disturbance
of the musculoskeletal system, deformities, injuries, and degenerative
disease of the spine, hands, feet, knee, hip, shoulder, and elbow in children
and adults. An orthopaedic surgeon also is involved with treatment of
secondary muscular problems in patients who suffer from various central
or peripheral nervous system lesions such as cerebral palsy, paraplegia,
or stroke, as well as conditions that are treated medically or physically
through the use of braces, casts, splints, or physical therapy.

Specialty certification in orthopaedics includes [the following]:

- **Orthopaedic Sports Medicine:** An Orthopaedic Sports Medicine specialist provides care for all structures in the musculoskeletal system directly affected by participating in sporting
  events. The specialist is proficient in the conditioning, training,
  and fitness of the body as it relates to athletic performance and
  the effects of athletic performance and the impact of dietary
  supplements, pharmaceuticals, and nutrition on athletes' short
  and long term health and performance.

- **Surgery of the Hand:** A specialist trained in the investigation,
  preservation, and medical, surgical, and rehabilitation treatment
  of patients with diseases, injuries, or abnormalities affecting the
  upper extremities. This specialty includes the performance of
  microvascular surgery, which is necessary for reattachment of
  amputated fingers or limbs.

Otolaryngology—Head and Neck Surgery

An otolaryngologist—head and neck surgeon—provides medical and
surgical care for patients with diseases and disorders that affect the
ears, nose, throat, the respiratory and upper alimentary systems, and
related structures of the head and neck. They diagnose and provide
medical and surgical treatment of diseases and have skills and knowledge in audiology and speech-language pathology; the chemical senses;

and allergy, endocrinology, and neurology as they relate to the head and neck. Operations are performed on the head and neck and face. Head and neck oncology, facial plastic and reconstructive procedures, and the treatment of disorders of hearing and voice are fundamental areas of expertise for the otolaryngologist.

Specialty certification in otolaryngology—head and neck surgery includes [the following]:

- **Neurotology:** A neurotologist is an otolaryngologist—head and neck surgeon—who treats patients with diseases of the ear and temporal bone, including disorders of hearing and balance.

- **Pediatric Otolaryngology:** An otolaryngologist—head and neck surgeon— has completed specialty training in the management of infants and children with congenital or acquired disorders of the head and neck, nose, paranasal sinuses, ear, and aerodigestive tract.

- **Plastic Surgery within the Head and Neck:** An otolaryngologist—head and neck surgeon—has completed additional training in plastic, cosmetic, and reconstructive procedures within the head, face, and neck. This area includes skin, head, and neck oncology and reconstruction, management of maxillofacial trauma, soft tissue repair, and neural surgery.

Plastic Surgery

Plastic surgeons specialize in the care of patients requiring repair, replacement, and reconstruction of defects of the form and function of the body covering and its underlying musculoskeletal system, with emphasis on the craniofacial structures, the oropharynx, the upper and lower limbs, the breast, and the external genitalia. This surgical specialty also focuses on the aesthetic surgery of structures with undesirable form. Special knowledge and skill in the design and transfer of skin flaps, in the transplantation of tissues, and in the replantation of structures are vital to the performance of plastic surgery.

Specialty certification in plastic surgery includes [the following]:

- **Surgery of the Hand:** This specialty focuses on the investigation and treatment of patients with diseases, injuries, or abnormalities affecting the upper extremities. This specialty includes the performance of microvascular surgery, which is necessary for reattachment of amputated fingers or limbs. All hand surgeons are certified in plastic surgery and then complete additional training and testing in hand surgery.

9

- **Plastic Surgery within the Head and Neck:** A plastic surgeon with additional training in cosmetic and reconstructive procedures within the head, face, and neck. This area includes skin, head, and neck oncology and reconstruction, management of maxillofacial trauma, soft tissue repair, and neural surgery.

Thoracic and Cardiovascular Surgery

Thoracic surgeons specialize in management of patients with conditions of the chest and heart. This specialty includes providing surgical care of patients for coronary artery disease; cancers of the lung, esophagus, and chest wall; abnormalities of the heart, great vessels, and heart valves; congenital anomalies; tumors of the mediastinum; and diseases of the diaphragm. The management of the airway and injuries to the chest are also areas of surgical practice for the thoracic surgeon. They have specialized knowledge of cardiorespiratory physiology and oncology, as well as capability in the use of extracorporeal circulation, cardiac assist devices, management of cardiac dysrhythmias, pleural drainage, respiratory support systems, endoscopy, and other invasive and noninvasive diagnostic technique.

Urology Surgeon

A surgeon who specializes in urology manages patients with benign and malignant (cancerous) medical and surgical disorders of the adrenal gland and of the genitourinary system. Urologists have comprehensive knowledge of, and skills in, endoscopic, percutaneous, and open surgery of congenital and acquired conditions of the reproductive and urinary systems.

Chapter 2

What Is It Like to Have Surgery?

Even if you're a fan of TV hospital dramas, these shows might also make you nervous about what happens in an operating room. Millions of teens are wheeled into operating rooms (ORs) each year, so it can help to find out what to expect before you get to the hospital.

Depending on the type of surgery you need, you may have inpatient surgery or outpatient surgery (also called ambulatory surgery). Inpatient surgery usually requires that you stay in the hospital for a day or more so the doctors and nurses can monitor your recovery carefully. If you have outpatient surgery, you will go home the same day. This type of surgery may be performed in a hospital or an outpatient surgery clinic and you can go home when the doctor decides you're ready.

What to Expect

If your surgery is not an emergency, it will be planned in advance. You will make a visit to the hospital or outpatient surgery location beforehand. Examples of emergency surgery include a broken elbow and appendicitis. When urgent surgery is required, you will go to the operating room after being diagnosed with a surgical problem.

"What's It Like to Have Surgery?" August 2010, reprinted with permission from www.kidshealth.org. This information was provided by KidsHealth®, one of the largest resources online for medically reviewed health information written for parents, kids, and teens. For more articles like this, visit www.KidsHealth.org, or www.TeensHealth.org. Copyright © 1995–2012 The Nemours Foundation. All rights reserved.

When you know about your surgery ahead of time, you will arrive at the hospital and a nurse or other hospital employee will begin the pre-surgical process. He or she will begin by asking questions about your medical history, including any allergies you might have and any symptoms or pain you may be having. Girls may be asked if there is any chance of being pregnant. Nurses will also take your vital signs like your heart rate, temperature, and blood pressure.

Soon after you arrive, you'll be given an identification bracelet— a plastic tape with your name and birthdate on it—to wear around your wrist. You'll also be asked about the time you last ate or drank anything. This might seem strange, but it's actually very important to your safety. Having food or liquids in your stomach can lead to vomiting during or after the surgery and cause harmful complications.

You might need to have other tests, like X-rays and blood tests, before your surgery begins.

Before Surgery

Before your operation takes place, you and your family will have a chance to meet with the anesthesiologist—the doctor or certified registered nurse anesthetist (CRNA) who specializes in giving anesthetics, the medications that will help you fall asleep or numb an area of your body so you don't feel the surgery. The anesthesiology staff will have your medical information so you can be given the amount of anesthetic you need for your age, height, and weight.

There are several types of anesthesia. General anesthesia causes you to become completely unconscious during the operation. If you're having general anesthesia, the anesthesiologist or CRNA will be present during the entire operation to monitor your condition and ensure you constantly receive the right doses of medications.

If surgery is done under local anesthesia, you'll be given an anesthetic that numbs only the area of your body to be operated on. You also might be given a medication that makes you drowsy during the procedure.

Before your operation, the nurse or doctor will clean (and shave, if necessary) the area of your body that will be operated on. You'll be asked to take off any jewelry, including barrettes and hair ties, and you'll need to take out contact lenses if you wear them. You'll be given a hospital gown to wear in the operating room.

A nurse will put an IV (intravenous) line in your arm and attach it to thin plastic tubing that is connected to a soft bag of fluid. This line will probably be used to give you anesthetic (if you're having general anesthesia) or provide you with fluids or medicine that may be needed during the operation.

As you're wheeled into a hospital operating room, you may notice that the nurses and doctors are wearing face masks and plastic eyeglasses, as well as paper caps, gowns, and booties over their shoes. Patients are vulnerable to infection during an operation, so this protective gear lowers the chance of infection while you're in the operating room.

The nurse or technician will then place monitoring equipment (sticker-like patches) on your skin to measure your heart rate and blood pressure at regular intervals.

Sometimes medical and nursing students observe surgeries, so don't be surprised if doctors and nurses aren't the only people in the room.

After Surgery

After your surgery is over, you'll be taken to the recovery room, where nurses will monitor your condition very closely for a few hours. Sometimes this room is also called the post-op (postoperative) room or PACU (post-anesthesia care unit). Your parent may be able to visit you here.

Every person has a different surgical experience, but if you've had general anesthesia, it's common to feel groggy, confused, chilly, nauseated, or even sad when you wake up. When the surgery has been completed, the surgeon will let you and your parents know how the procedure went and answer any questions you have.

Once your anesthesia has worn off and you're fully awake, you'll be taken to a regular hospital room if you're staying overnight. If you're having an outpatient procedure, you'll be monitored by nurses in another room until you're able to go home.

If you feel pain after the surgery, the doctors and nurses will make sure you have pain relievers to keep you more comfortable. You may also need to take other medications, such as antibiotics to prevent infection.

Taking the Worry out of Your Surgery

The thought of having surgery can be scary. If you're worried, try these tips to help feel more at ease:

- Ask questions ahead of time. Your surgeon, anesthesiologist, and nurses will be able to answer your questions about the surgery, how you'll feel afterward, how long it will take to return to your normal activities, what type of scarring you might have, etc.

Don't feel embarrassed about asking lots of questions—the more informed you are, the more comfortable you'll feel about having surgery.

- Be sure you're clear on instructions—and ask if you're not. Your doctor or a nurse will give you instructions on what to do before the surgery (called preoperative instructions) and what you can and can't do afterward (postoperative instructions). For example, your doctor may tell you to stop taking certain medications for a set period of time before surgery. (If you know about your surgery ahead of time, you should let your doctor know well in advance if you are taking any herbal or other non-prescription medications such as ibuprofen as your medical team might instruct you to stop taking them.) And follow your doctor's orders regarding eating before surgery. After surgery, your exercise and activities might be restricted for a while.

- Practice healthy habits. Smoking is never a good idea, but it's especially bad news after surgery when your body is trying to recover. Ditch the cigarettes, get plenty of rest, and eat nutritious foods.

- Try relaxation techniques. If you're nervous or anxious, taking a few slow, deep breaths or focusing on an object in the room can help you to tune out stressful thoughts and cope with your anxiety. Think of your favorite place and what you like to do there.

- Plan ahead. If you have to miss school because of surgery, talk to your teachers ahead of time and arrange to make up any tests or assignments. Get a friend you trust to take notes for you and drop off homework assignments. By planning ahead, you won't have to spend your recovery time stressing about your grades.

- Tell a few people. If you don't feel like sharing the details of your operation, you don't have to—but telling some friends that you'll be out of school for a few days might ensure you'll have some visitors! Your friends might even have some surgery stories of their own to share.

- Pack a few favorites. After you're out of the recovery room, you might want the comfort that some favorite CDs, iTunes, books, magazines, or a journal can bring, so make sure that when you're packing your hospital bag, you throw in a few goodies.

Chapter 3

Specialized Surgical Techniques

Chapter Contents

Section 3.1

Cryosurgery

"Cryosurgery in Cancer Treatment: Questions and Answers," by the National Cancer Institute (NCI, www.cancer.gov), part of the National Institutes of Health, September 10, 2003. Reviewed by David A. Cooke, MD, FACP, October 10, 2012.

What is cryosurgery?

Cryosurgery (also called cryotherapy) is the use of extreme cold produced by liquid nitrogen (or argon gas) to destroy abnormal tissue. Cryosurgery is used to treat external tumors, such as those on the skin. For external tumors, liquid nitrogen is applied directly to the cancer cells with a cotton swab or spraying device.

Cryosurgery is also used to treat tumors inside the body (internal tumors and tumors in the bone). For internal tumors, liquid nitrogen or argon gas is circulated through a hollow instrument called a cryoprobe, which is placed in contact with the tumor. The doctor uses ultrasound or MRI [magnetic resonance imaging] to guide the cryoprobe and monitor the freezing of the cells, thus limiting damage to nearby healthy tissue. (In ultrasound, sound waves are bounced off organs and other tissues to create a picture called a sonogram.) A ball of ice crystals forms around the probe, freezing nearby cells. Sometimes more than one probe is used to deliver the liquid nitrogen to various parts of the tumor. The probes may be put into the tumor during surgery or through the skin (percutaneously). After cryosurgery, the frozen tissue thaws and is either naturally absorbed by the body (for internal tumors), or it dissolves and forms a scab (for external tumors).

What types of cancer can be treated with cryosurgery?

Cryosurgery is used to treat several types of cancer, and some precancerous or noncancerous conditions. In addition to prostate and liver tumors, cryosurgery can be an effective treatment for the following:

- Retinoblastoma, a childhood cancer that affects the retina of the eye (Doctors have found that cryosurgery is most effective when the tumor is small and only in certain parts of the retina.)

- Early-stage skin cancers (both basal cell and squamous cell carcinomas)

- Precancerous skin growths known as actinic keratosis

Precancerous conditions of the cervix known as cervical intraepithelial neoplasia (abnormal cell changes in the cervix that can develop into cervical cancer).

Cryosurgery is also used to treat some types of low-grade cancerous and noncancerous tumors of the bone. It may reduce the risk of joint damage when compared with more extensive surgery, and help lessen the need for amputation. The treatment is also used to treat AIDS [acquired immunodeficiency syndrome]-related Kaposi sarcoma when the skin lesions are small and localized.

Researchers are evaluating cryosurgery as a treatment for a number of cancers, including breast, colon, and kidney cancer. They are also exploring cryotherapy in combination with other cancer treatments, such as hormone therapy, chemotherapy, radiation therapy, or surgery.

In what situations can cryosurgery be used to treat prostate cancer? What are the side effects?

Cryosurgery can be used to treat men who have early-stage prostate cancer that is confined to the prostate gland. It is less well established than standard prostatectomy and various types of radiation therapy. Long-term outcomes are not known. Because it is effective only in small areas, cryosurgery is not used to treat prostate cancer that has spread outside the gland, or to distant parts of the body.

Some advantages of cryosurgery are that the procedure can be repeated, and it can be used to treat men who cannot have surgery or radiation therapy because of their age or other medical problems.

Cryosurgery for the prostate gland can cause side effects. These side effects may occur more often in men who have had radiation to the prostate.

Cryosurgery may obstruct urine flow or cause incontinence (lack of control over urine flow); often, these side effects are temporary.

Many men become impotent (loss of sexual function).

In some cases, the surgery has caused injury to the rectum.

In what situations can cryosurgery be used to treat primary liver cancer or liver metastases (cancer that has spread to the liver from another part of the body)? What are the side effects?

Cryosurgery may be used to treat primary liver cancer that has not spread. It is used especially if surgery is not possible due to factors such as other medical conditions. The treatment also may be used for cancer that has spread to the liver from another site (such as the colon or rectum). In some cases, chemotherapy and/or radiation therapy may be given before or after cryosurgery. Cryosurgery in the liver may cause damage to the bile ducts and/or major blood vessels, which can lead to hemorrhage (heavy bleeding) or infection.

Does cryosurgery have any complications or side effects?

Cryosurgery does have side effects, although they may be less severe than those associated with surgery or radiation therapy. The effects depend on the location of the tumor. Cryosurgery for cervical intraepithelial neoplasia has not been shown to affect a woman's fertility, but it can cause cramping, pain, or bleeding. When used to treat skin cancer (including Kaposi sarcoma), cryosurgery may cause scarring and swelling; if nerves are damaged, loss of sensation may occur, and, rarely, it may cause a loss of pigmentation and loss of hair in the treated area. When used to treat tumors of the bone, cryosurgery may lead to the destruction of nearby bone tissue and result in fractures, but these effects may not be seen for some time after the initial treatment and can often be delayed with other treatments. In rare cases, cryosurgery may interact badly with certain types of chemotherapy. Although the side effects of surgery may be less severe than those associated with conventional surgery or radiation, more studies are needed to determine the long-term effects.

What are the advantages of cryosurgery?

Cryosurgery offers advantages over other methods of cancer treatment. It is less invasive than surgery, involving only a small incision or insertion of the cryoprobe through the skin. Consequently, pain, bleeding, and other complications of surgery are minimized. Cryosurgery is less expensive than other treatments and requires shorter recovery time and a shorter hospital stay, or no hospital stay at all. Sometimes cryosurgery can be done using only local anesthesia.

Because physicians can focus cryosurgical treatment on a limited area, they can avoid the destruction of nearby healthy tissue. The treatment can be safely repeated and may be used along with standard treatments such as surgery, chemotherapy, hormone therapy, and radiation. Cryosurgery may offer an option for treating cancers that are considered inoperable or that do not respond to standard treatments. Furthermore, it can be used for patients who are not good candidates for conventional surgery because of their age or other medical conditions.

What are the disadvantages of cryosurgery?

The major disadvantage of cryosurgery is the uncertainty surrounding its long-term effectiveness. While cryosurgery may be effective in treating tumors the physician can see by using imaging tests (tests that produce pictures of areas inside the body), it can miss microscopic cancer spread. Furthermore, because the effectiveness of the technique is still being assessed, insurance coverage issues may arise.

Where is cryosurgery currently available?

Cryosurgery is widely available in gynecologists' offices for the treatment of cervical neoplasias. A limited number of hospitals and cancer centers throughout the country currently have skilled doctors and the necessary technology to perform cryosurgery for other non-cancerous, precancerous, and cancerous conditions. Individuals can consult with their doctors or contact hospitals and cancer centers in their area to find out where cryosurgery is being used.

Section 3.2

Laparoscopic and Robot-Assisted Surgery

What Is Laparoscopic Surgery?

Laparoscopic surgery, also referred to as minimally invasive surgery, describes the performance of surgical procedures with the assistance of a video camera and several thin instruments. During the surgical procedure, small incisions of up to half an inch are made and plastic tubes called ports are placed through these incisions. The camera and the instruments are then introduced through the ports, which allow access to the inside of the patient.

The camera transmits an image of the organs inside the abdomen onto a television monitor. The surgeon is not able to see directly into the patient without the traditional large incision. The video camera becomes a surgeon's eyes in laparoscopy surgery, since the surgeon uses the image from the video camera positioned inside the patient's body to perform the procedure.

Benefits of Minimally Invasive or Laparoscopic Procedures

Benefits of minimally invasive or laparoscopic procedures are the following:

- Less postoperative discomfort since the incisions are much smaller

- Quicker recovery times

- Shorter hospital stays

- Earlier return to full activities

- Much smaller scars

There may be less internal scarring when the procedures are performed in a minimally invasive fashion compared to standard open surgery.

Advance Laparoscopic Surgery with Hand-Access Devices

The human hand performs many functions during surgery that are difficult to reproduce with laparoscopic instruments. The loss of the ability to place the hand into the abdomen during traditional laparoscopic surgery has limited the use of laparoscopy for complex abdominal surgery on the pancreas, liver, and bile duct.

Hand-access devices are new laparoscopic devices that allow the surgeon to place a hand into the abdomen during laparoscopic surgery and perform many of the different functions with the hand that were previously possible only during open surgery. Dilip Parekh, MD, at University of Southern California has utilized these new devices to develop a variety of laparoscopic pancreatic, liver, and biliary procedures such as the Whipple operation, distal pancreatectomy, and liver resection that were not possible previously by standard laparoscopic techniques.

Laparoscopic surgery for liver, pancreas, and bile duct disease has been considerably successful. Patients with laparoscopic surgery have much shorter hospital stays, less pain, rapid recovery, and early return to work compared to patients with open surgical procedures.

Robot Assisted Surgery

Da Vinci is a computer-assisted robotic system that expands a surgeon's capability to operate within the abdomen in a less invasive way during laparoscopic surgery. The da Vinci system allows greater precision and better visualization compared to standard laparoscopic surgery.

The operations with the da Vinci System are performed with no direct mechanical connection between the surgeon and the patient. The surgeon is remote from the patient, working a few feet from the operating table while seated at a computer console with a three-dimensional view of the operating field.

The physician operates two masters (similar to joysticks) that control the two mechanical arms on the robot. The mechanical arms are armed with specialized instruments with hand-like movements which carry out the surgery through tiny holes in the patient's abdomen. Three small incisions (approximately one half inch) are made in the abdomen, through which a video camera and the robotic arms with the highly-specialized instruments are introduced. The video camera provides high resolution, high magnification, and depth perception.

Section 3.3

Laser Surgery

This chapter contains text from "Introduction to Devices—Lasers," and "General Surgery," © 2012 American Society for Laser Medicine and Surgery (www.aslms.org). Reprinted with permission.

Introduction to Devices—Lasers

Laser is an acronym that denotes Light Amplification by the Stimulated Emission of Radiation. The first laser was created by Theodore Maiman in 1960 of the Hughes Aircraft Research Laboratories. This ruby laser was based on Albert Einstein's 1917 theory of stimulated emission of radiation. Lasers are unique in that they are artificially created beams of energy that possess intense brightness, can travel long distances, and can be harnessed in millions of ways in our everyday life.

There are presently over 1,000 materials that can create a beam of light, but only around a dozen or two that are clinically used in medicine or aesthetic applications. Laser light can be a visible or an invisible form of energy. Lasers can be in the ultraviolet, visible, or infrared bands of light that make up the electromagnetic spectrum of energy. This specialized light is made up of tiny particles of energy know as photons. Photons travel in waves called waveforms and make up the various types of energy that we know of today. Lasers can be created from a variety of sources and are usually named after its components that create this specialized light energy. Common sources or mediums are gases, crystals, liquid, and diodes.

Most common medical lasers are heat driven in nature and are absorbed by a specific entity or target in the body. This absorption of the laser energy by a particular target or chromophore is usually conducted towards blood, water, pigment, or collagen. In the medical and surgical practice, lasers can be used to cut and vaporize tissue and coagulate or seal blood vessels. Lasers can also be pulsed at very high megawatt powers and be emitted at a billionth of a second pulses to create a shock wave effect to break up stones in the bladder and ureters. It also can be used photoacoustically in ophthalmology to open clouded membranes in the eye and also break up tattoo dye for tattoo removal.

In aesthetic and cosmetic practices, the theory of selective photothermolysis is commonly utilized. It is this concept that through the selection of a specific band of light, (time the light is delivered to the tissue), and energy level, various pigmented lesions, acne, scars, unwanted hair, blood vessels, and much more can be treated without thermal injury to the surrounding tissue.

Research and experimental studies are constantly advancing the development of new wavelengths of laser light in the medical and cosmetic field. New laser light delivery systems using fiberoptics are on the nanometer (billionth of a meter) scale and are now being researched in the treatment of a variety of diseases and medical conditions. It is just a matter of time until laser light will become a common tool in the fight against cancer, diabetes, high blood pressure, and heart disease.

General Surgery

Any surgical procedure can be performed using lasers. General surgeons use a variety of laser wavelengths and laser delivery systems to cut, coagulate, vaporize, or remove tissue. The majority of laser surgeries actually use the laser device in place of other tools such as scalpels, electrosurgical units, cryosurgery probes, or microwave devices to accomplish a standard procedure like mastectomy (i.e., breast surgery) or cholecystectomy (i.e., surgical removal of the gallbladder). Lasers allow the surgeon to accomplish more complex tasks, reduce blood loss, decrease postoperative discomfort, reduce the chance of wound infection, decrease the spread of some cancers, minimize the extent of surgery in selected circumstances, and result in better wound healing, if they are used appropriately by a skilled and properly trained surgeon. They are useful in both open and laparoscopic procedures. Common surgical uses include breast surgery, removal of the gallbladder, hernia repair, bowel resection, hemorrhoidectomy, solid organ surgery, and treatment of pilonidal cyst.

Section 3.4

Natural Orifice Surgery

"Natural Orifice Surgery: Is the Thrill Gone?" by Gabriel Miller, *General Surgery News* (www.generalsurgerynews.com), March 2011. © 2011 McMahon Publishing. All rights reserved. Reprinted with permission.

Five years ago, natural orifice translumenal endoscopic surgery® (NOTES®) seemed to be on the tip of everyone's tongue, at least in surgical circles. At that time, the first white paper on the topic had come out. Ambitious surgeons worldwide were publishing case studies. And news outlets were heralding "surgery without scars" as "the next great surgical evolution."

In the original white paper, lead author David Rattner, MD, outlined 12 challenges needed to be overcome for NOTES to be feasible and safe (*Surg Endosc* 2006;20:329–333). However, as surgeons worked out the kinks, interest in NOTES appeared to fade.

"The air has kind of gone out of the balloon for NOTES; at least that's the perception," said Dr. Rattner, chief of gastrointestinal and general surgery at Massachusetts General Hospital in Boston. "But I think that if you look at where we started five years ago, we have hit the milestones of the original white paper and now we are really into the hard work of doing a clinical trial. We are at a pivotal point."

Dr. Rattner was one of several panelists who spoke at the 12th World Congress of Endoscopic Surgery in National Harbor, Maryland, [in 2010] addressing the future of NOTES. This assessment has come at a time when less radical techniques are taking center stage.

"I think the first telltale sign [of the popularity of NOTES] is to look around the room," said Jeffrey Marks, MD, associate professor of surgery at Case Western Reserve University School of Medicine in Cleveland. "We have a big room for this meeting but there are a lot of empty seats. I think four or five years ago, you would have found standing-room only with people lined up out the door. I think a lot of interest in NOTES now is ' . . . well, it had its 15 minutes of fame, but now it's not very interesting.' "

As interest in NOTES cooled, surgeons shifted their gaze to single-port or single-incision surgery, which sidestepped many of the challenges NOTES posed. In the halls at national meetings, surgeons pointed to the fact that single-incision surgery could be done with "off-the-shelf" instruments and that a single-incision through the umbilicus was cosmetically almost as good. It seemed that surgeons collectively had taken a deep breath, stepped back, and realized that they may have gotten ahead of themselves.

"I feel very strongly that the NOTES train was at the station, and everybody was also at the station but afraid to get on board," said Paul Curcillo, MD, vice chairman of surgery at Drexel University School of Medicine in Philadelphia.

NOTES Progress

Although excitement over NOTES appears to be fizzling, by several measures—case series, clinical trials, technological developments, and published complications—NOTES is still progressing.

As of spring 2010, surgeons reported approximately 1,500 to 2,000 NOTES cases in humans worldwide. Groups in Europe and Latin and North America have advanced their NOTES to the clinical trial stage. And in the United States, a major trial was launched comparing NOTES with laparoscopic cholecystectomy with enough power to compare transgastric and transvaginal NOTES approaches.

Surgeons are continuing to make "steady progress in the arena of NOTES," said Eric Hungness, MD, assistant professor of medicine at the Feinberg School of Medicine at Northwestern University in Chicago. "The clearest way of measuring progress is actual human cases. As expected, the transvaginal route has been the most popular, but there have been a surprising number of transgastric cases."

In the United States, NOTES techniques have been pioneered primarily at Ohio State University, where at least 80 patients have undergone transgastric NOTES procedures, primarily for diagnostic purposes such as peritoneoscopy, and at the University of California, San Diego, where investigators are exploring NOTES approaches to sleeve gastrectomy and incisional hernia, as well as cholecystectomy and appendectomy, all through a transvaginal approach. At least a half-dozen other institutions also have performed NOTES procedures, most of which were enrolled in the first U.S. NOTES clinical trial, launched this past summer.

Research in the United States has been driven largely by Natural Orifice Surgery Consortium for Assessment and Research®

(NOSCAR®), a joint working group drawn from the Society of American Gastrointestinal and Endoscopic Surgeons and a group of expert interventional endoscopists representing the American Society for Gastrointestinal Endoscopy.

NOSCAR has taken a more measured approach to developing NOTES techniques, at least in comparison with other organizations and medical centers in Europe and Latin America. For example, the NOTES cholecystectomy trial in the United States requires participating groups to use an extra visualization port for safety and observation.

"The international experience is much broader than what is currently being done in the United States and some of that has been the result of NOSCAR appropriately slowing down some of the progress here in the United States," Dr. Hungness said. But as of last spring, no major complications have been reported in the NOSCAR registry of NOTES procedures.

Two newer NOTES procedures involving transesophageal and transanal techniques are another sign that NOTES is continuing to evolve, Dr. Hungness said. One of them is the NOTES esophagomyotomy pioneered in Japan by Haruhiro Inoue, MD, at Showa University; the other is NOTES transanal rectal cancer resection performed at Massachusetts General Hospital.

"These two areas are really going to lead NOTES where single-incision can't take us," Dr. Hungness said. "It's a little too early to tell, but I think it's very promising."

One other marker of progress—originally perceived as a major limitation—is new technology. There are at least 11 prototype devices currently being used under the FDA's Investigational Device Exemption program, many of which add articulation to common surgical instruments.

"The fundamental barriers [to the success of NOTES] originally identified by the NOSCAR working group were heavily based on technological innovation and we have already met most of those challenges," said Yoav Mintz, MD, director of the Center for Innovative Surgery at Hadassah-Hebrew University Medical Center in Jerusalem.

The next generation of instruments will "separate our eyes from our hands" by placing miniature high-definition cameras—some as small as 2.5 mm—in strategic places around the abdomen, Dr. Mintz said. He added that several multitasking platforms are already in clinical development, with the goal being to one day incorporate robotic assistance into NOTES procedures.

Evolution of Surgery

Although NOTES is most commonly associated with transvaginal or transgastric operations, the development of more minimally invasive surgery may be better viewed as a constellation of separate but interrelated techniques that are driving the evolution of surgery. These procedures may be divided into endoluminal and translumenal techniques, single-port or single-incision surgery, and the full Monty—natural orifice surgery.

"All the [new techniques] you see with endoluminal surgery couldn't have happened without NOTES research," said Dr. Marks.

Endoluminal approaches to gastrointestinal (GI) diseases have a relatively long history and are generally more acceptable to surgeons. "Endoluminal therapies are far less of a paradigm jump. I think we would all agree that the esophagus, stomach, and colon are all easily accessed organs for most of the endoluminal therapies," said Dr. Marks.

The continuing evolution of endoluminal therapies will likely hinge on two developments, Dr. Marks said—a changing view of GI diseases and the available technology to treat them.

"I think we've learned over the last decade that we can change the way we manage GI disease so that it doesn't require a formal resection of major tissue," Dr. Marks said. For example, mucosal-based diseases such as GI cancers now can be removed either by endoscopic mucosal or submucosal dissection. Endoluminal full-thickness resection also will be possible as technology advances, Dr. Marks added.

"Just because it is endoluminal, doesn't mean we can't make a full-thickness hole and fix it, whether it be with staplers or suturing devices," he said. Ultimately, this technology will allow submucosal myotomies as well as endoluminal anastomoses. Japanese surgeons, for example, already have treated more than 40 patients with achalasia via endoscopic myotomy (*Nippon Rinsho* 2010;68:1749–1752).

Among techniques considered NOTES procedures, the endoscopic approaches are probably closest to bridging the gap between academic medicine and community surgery. "Let's be honest, even though we are much more comfortable making holes in organs, the idea of doing it [purposely] is very hard for many people to accept," Dr. Marks said. "I think the endoluminal therapies are more easily accepted by all of us—patients, industry, the FDA [U.S. Food and Drug Administration], and IRBs [institutional review boards]."

Nevertheless, translumenal approaches continue to evolve, primarily in three areas—experience with the most common approaches, development of new techniques, and emergence of new technology, long considered a prerequisite to clinical practice of natural orifice techniques.

27

Cosmetic or Clinical Benefit?

The major question facing NOTES is whether better cosmesis will be enough to drive wider use.

"Probably not," Dr. Mintz said. Instead, NOTES will have to prove it has significant clinical benefits. "Surgery in the next decade not only will be minimally invasive but also minimalistic, meaning it will be more targeted, less extensive, and more organ- and function-preserving," Dr. Mintz added.

The highly toxic systemic therapies used in cancer are ripe for replacement with an arsenal of localized, highly targeted gene therapies that attack tumors directly and prevent the replication of cancer cells. "The major challenge in gene therapy is drug delivery and this is where NOTES comes in," Dr. Mintz said. "Rather than dealing with difficult molecular mechanisms, we will use the NOTES platform to inject directly into tumors capsules of siRNA drugs specific to those tumors."

Similarly, the use of fluorescent antibodies to identify tumor cells combined with vessel mapping may allow surgeons to visualize and locate small metastases and remove them using smaller and smaller segmental resections.

Before these techniques become a reality, however, surgeons will have to come to terms with a fundamental question: Should NOTES replace laparoscopy or is NOTES better suited for completely new procedures not possible with current standard approaches? The elephant in the room with NOTES is whether or not the technique provides measurable benefits in outcomes after clinical trials.

Speaking of the relatively larger body of single-port studies, Dr. Curcillo said, "I'll be the first to say, the only real benefit right now is cosmetic. We are coming out with data showing it's not worse, that we're not hurting anyone, but if someone tells you there's less pain and better recovery you have to ask them to show you the data. It's not out there."

Surgeons who are in favor of NOTES point to the history of laparoscopy. After laparoscopy was widely introduced 20 years ago, within the first three years, 70% of cholecystectomies were done with this approach even though morbidity was higher compared with the open approach.

"The factors that drove the adoption of innovation were patient demand, low cost for the surgeon during the learning period, manufacturers' aggressive promotion, and the benefits perceived by stakeholders," Dr. Mintz said. "And unfortunately, like a slap in the face for the medical profession, patient outcome and patient benefit were not factors, so it's up to us, the physicians who deal with NOTES, to make sure that patients will eventually benefit from the procedure."

This transition will determine whether or not NOTES has 15 minutes of fame or is here to stay.

"Scientific discovery is one thing but translating that from idea to commercialization is quite another," said Dr. Rattner. "That's really what we are struggling with."

Section 3.5

Stereotactic Radiosurgery

"Stereotactic Radiosurgery," © 2012 A.D.A.M., Inc.
Reprinted with permission.

Stereotactic radiosurgery is a form of radiation therapy that focuses high-powered X-rays on a small area of the body. Other types of radiation therapy are more likely to affect nearby healthy tissue. Stereotactic radiosurgery better targets the abnormal area.

Despite its name, radiosurgery is a treatment, not a surgical procedure.

Description

Some types of stereotactic radiosurgery require a specially fitted face mask or a frame attached to your scalp. This may be done using small pins or anchors that go through your skin, to the surface of your skull or bone.

During your treatment, you will lie on a table, which slides into a machine that delivers radiation. The machine may spin around you while it works. The nurses and doctors will be able to see you on cameras, and hear you and talk with you on microphones.

Each treatment takes about 30 minutes to 1 hour. Some patients may receive more than one treatment session, but usually no more than five sessions.

Why the Procedure Is Performed

Stereotactic radiosurgery is often used to slow down the growth of small, deep brain tumors that are hard to remove during surgery. Such therapy may also be used in patients who are unable to have surgery, such as the elderly or those who are very sick. Radiosurgery may also be used after surgery to treat any remaining abnormal tissue.

Stereotactic radiosurgery was once limited to brain tumors, but today it may be used to treat many other diseases and conditions.

Brain and nervous system tumors:

- Brain metastases
- Acoustic neuroma and other head and neck (nasopharyngeal) cancers
- Pituitary tumors
- Spinal cord tumors
- Cancer of the eye (uveal melanoma)

Other conditions:

- Blood vessel problems such as arteriovenous malformations
- Movement disorders
- Parkinson disease
- Some types of epilepsy
- Trigeminal neuralgia, which causes severe face pain

Other cancers for which radiosurgery is either being used or studied include:

- liver cancer;
- lung cancer;
- prostate cancer.

Risks

Radiosurgery may damage tissue around the area being treated. Brain swelling may occur in people who received treatment to the brain. Swelling can go away without treatment, but some people may need medicine to control this swelling.

Before the Procedure

Before the treatment, you will have MRI [magnetic resonance imaging] or CT scans [computed tomography]. Using these images, a computer creates a 3-D (three dimensional) map of the tumor area. This planning process helps your neurosurgeon and radiation oncologist determine the specific treatment area.

The day before your procedure:

- Do not use any hair creams or hair spray.

- Do not eat or drink anything after midnight unless told otherwise by your doctor.

The day of your procedure:

- Wear comfortable clothing.

- Bring your regular prescription medicines with you to the hospital.

- Do not wear jewelry, makeup, nail polish, or a wig or hairpiece.

- You will be asked to remove contact lenses, eyeglasses, and dentures.

- You will change into a hospital gown.

- An intravenous (IV) line will be placed into your arm to deliver contrast material, medicines, and fluids.

After the Procedure

Often, you will be able to go home about an hour after the treatment is finished. You should arrange for someone to drive you home. Most people go back to their regular activities the next day, if there are no complications such as swelling. Some patients are kept in the hospital overnight for monitoring.

Outlook (Prognosis)

The effects of radiosurgery may take weeks or months to be seen. The prognosis depends on the condition being treated. Many times, your health care provider will monitor your progress using imaging tests such as MRI and CT scans.

Chapter 4

Understanding Pediatric Surgery

When your child needs medical treatment, you want him or her to have the very best care available. So it stands to reason that if your child needs an operation, you will want to consult with a surgeon who is qualified and experienced in operating on children. Surgeons who specialize in general surgery often provide surgical care for children, and they are fully qualified to perform many operations on children. In more urbanized areas of the country, another kind of surgeon—the pediatric surgeon—is also available to provide comprehensive surgical care for children.

Pediatric surgeons operate on children whose development ranges from the newborn stage through the teenage years. In addition to completing training and achieving board certification in general surgery, pediatric surgeons complete two additional years of training exclusively in children's surgery. They then receive special certification in the subspecialty of pediatric surgery.

What is the pediatric surgeon's role in treating the child?

Pediatric surgeons are primarily concerned with the diagnosis, preoperative, operative, and postoperative management of surgical problems in children. Some medical conditions in newborns are not compatible with a good quality of life unless these problems are

"What Is a Pediatric Surgeon?," © American College of Surgeons (www.facs.org). All rights reserved. Reprinted with permission. Reviewed by David A. Cooke, MD, FACP, October 10, 2012.

corrected surgically. These conditions must be recognized immediately by neonatologists, pediatricians, and family physicians. Pediatric surgeons cooperate with all of the specialists involved in a child's medical care to determine whether surgery is the best option for the child.

What is the focus of pediatric surgery?

Pediatric surgeons utilize their expertise in providing surgical care for all problems or conditions affecting children that require surgical intervention. They participate in transplantation operations, and like most surgeons today, they use laparoscopic techniques for some operations. They also have particular expertise in the following areas of responsibility:

- **Neonatal:** Pediatric surgeons have specialized knowledge in the surgical repair of birth defects, some of which may be life threatening to premature and full-term infants.

- **Prenatal:** Pediatric surgeons, in cooperation with radiologists, use ultrasound and other technologies during the fetal stage of a child's development to detect any abnormalities. They can then plan corrective surgery and educate and get to know parents before their baby is born. Prenatal diagnosis may lead to fetal surgery, which is a new forefront in the subspecialty of pediatric surgery. Application of most fetal surgical techniques is still in the experimental stage.

- **Trauma:** Because trauma is the number one killer of children in the United States, pediatric surgeons are routinely faced with critical care situations involving traumatic injuries sustained by children that may or may not require surgical intervention. Many pediatric surgeons are involved in accident prevention programs in their communities that are aimed at curbing traumatic injuries in children.

- **Pediatric oncology:** Pediatric surgeons are involved in the diagnosis and surgical care of children with malignant tumors as well as those with benign growths.

Where do pediatric surgeons work?

Pediatric surgeons practice their specialty in a variety of medical institutions, including children's hospitals, university-related medical centers with major pediatric services, and large urban community hospitals.

How are pediatric surgeons trained and certified?

Pediatric surgeons must have graduated from an accredited medical school and must have completed five years of graduate surgical education in an accredited general surgery residency program. Then, they must complete two additional years of full-time education in an approved fellowship program in pediatric surgery. Following completion of their two-year study in the subspecialty of pediatric surgery, they must pass a written examination to ensure that their surgical knowledge is of the highest level and an oral exam to determine their ability to manage a variety of surgical problems in infants and children. In order to take this examination, they must first become board certified in general surgery. After these requirements have been fulfilled, surgeons are granted a special certificate in the subspecialty of pediatric surgery. This certificate must be renewed every 10 years to ensure that every pediatric surgeon is competent and up-to-date with regard to advances in pediatric surgical care.

What differences can a pediatric surgeon make?

Pediatric surgeons specialize in the surgical care of children. They are surgeons who, by training, are oriented toward working with children and understanding their special needs. In addition, they work with various specialists who are also oriented toward children and toward providing high-quality, safe, and emotionally supportive care for their patients. When a pediatric surgeon performs an operation, it is the culmination of an orderly and detailed process involving pediatricians, family physicians, and other medical specialists who work together to treat the whole child.

For pediatric surgeons, one of the most satisfying and fulfilling aspects of their profession is that the majority of their patients will live long into the 21st century.

Pediatric surgeons are able to save whole lifetimes, and have the opportunity to follow their patients through a productive young life into adulthood.

Chapter 5

Surgery in Older Adults

Have you been told by your doctor that you need surgery? If so, you're not alone. Millions of older Americans have surgery each year.

For most surgeries, you will have time to find out about the operation, talk about other treatments with your surgeon (medical doctor who does the operation), and decide what to do. You also have time to get a second opinion.

Questions to Ask

Deciding to have surgery can be hard, but it may be easier once you know why you need surgery. Talk with your surgeon about the operation. It may help to take a member of your family or a friend with you. Don't hesitate to ask the surgeon any questions you might have. For example, do the benefits of surgery outweigh the risks? Risks may include infections, bleeding a lot, or a reaction to the anesthesia (medicine that puts you to sleep).

Your surgeon should be willing to answer your questions. If you don't understand the answers, ask the surgeon to explain more clearly. Answers to the following questions will help you make an informed decision about your treatment:

- What is the surgery? Do I need it now, or can I wait?

- Can another treatment be tried instead of surgery?

"Age Page: Considering Surgery?" by the National Institute on Aging (NIA, www.nia.nih.gov), part of the National Institutes of Health, April 12, 2012.

- How will the surgery affect my health and lifestyle?

- What kind of anesthesia will be used? What are the side effects and risks of having anesthesia?

- Will I be in pain? How long will the pain last?

- When will I be able to go home after the surgery?

- What will the recovery be like? How long will it take to feel better?

- What will happen if I don't have the surgery?

- Is there anything else I should know about this surgery?

Choosing a Surgeon

Your primary care doctor may suggest a surgeon to you. Your state or local medical society can tell you about your surgeon's training. Try to choose a surgeon who operates often on medical problems like yours.

Getting a Second Opinion

Getting a second opinion means asking another doctor about your surgical plan. It is a common medical practice. Most doctors think it's a good idea. With a second opinion, you will get expert advice from another surgeon who knows about treating your medical problem. A second opinion can help you make a good decision.

You can ask your surgeon to send your medical records to the second doctor. This can save time and money since you may not have to repeat tests. When getting a second opinion, be sure to tell the doctor about all your symptoms and the type of surgery that has been suggested.

Medicare may help pay for a second opinion. If you have a private supplemental health insurance plan, find out if it covers a second opinion.

Informed Consent

Before having any surgery, you will be asked to sign a consent form. This form says that the surgeon has told you about the operation, the risks involved, and what results to expect. It's important to talk about all your concerns before signing this form. Your surgeon should be willing to take the time needed to make sure you know what is likely to happen before, during, and after surgery.

Outpatient Surgery

Outpatient surgery, sometimes called same-day surgery, is common for many types of operations. Outpatient surgery can be done in a special part of the hospital or in a surgical center. You will go home within hours after the surgery. Outpatient surgery can cost less than an overnight hospital stay. Your doctor will tell you if outpatient surgery is right for you.

Planning for Surgery

There are many steps you can take to make having surgery a little easier.

Before surgery:

- Make sure you have your preoperation tests and screenings, such as blood tests and X-rays.
- Be sure you have all your insurance questions answered.
- Make plans for any medical equipment or help with health care you will need when you go home.
- Arrange for an adult to drive you home and stay with you for the first 24 hours after surgery.
- Get written instructions about your care, a phone number to call if you have a problem, and prescription medicines you'll need at home.

The day of surgery:

- Leave your jewelry at home.
- Don't wear make-up or contact lenses to surgery.

Following surgery:

- Make sure you follow all your doctor's directions once you're home.
- Go for your scheduled postoperative check-up.
- Ask your doctor when you can return to your normal activities.

Paying for Surgery

The total cost of any surgery includes many different bills. Your surgeon can tell you how much he or she charges. You may also be billed by other doctors, such as the anesthesiologist. There will be hospital charges as well. To find out what the hospital will cost, call the hospital's business office.

If you have Medicare or secondary or supplemental health insurance, check to see what part of the costs it will pay. Talk to your surgeon if you can't afford the surgery.

In Case of Emergency Surgery

An accident or sudden illness may result in emergency surgery. That's why you should always carry the following information with you:

- Your doctor's name and phone number

- Family names and phone numbers

- Ongoing medical problems

- Medicines you take, including prescription and over-the-counter drugs

- Allergies to medicines

- Health insurance information and policy numbers

Make copies of this information to keep in your wallet and glove compartment of your car—just in case you need emergency care.

Chapter 6

Surgery Statistics

Chapter Contents

Section 6.1

Inpatient Surgery Statistics

Excerpted from "National Hospital Discharge Survey: 2006 Annual
Summary," by the National Center for Health Statistics (www.cdc.gov/nchs),
part of the Centers for Disease Control (CDC), December 2010.

Patient and Hospital Characteristics

- There were an estimated 34.9 million discharges from nonfederal short-stay hospitals in 2006. Those discharges used an estimated 166.3 million days of care and were hospitalized for an average of 4.8 days per stay.

- About 77 percent of inpatients discharged from nonmetropolitan hospitals were from facilities with fewer than 100 beds, while hospitals of the same bed size accounted for only 13 percent of all inpatient discharges among metropolitan hospitals. Sixteen percent of all discharges from nonfederal short-stay hospitals in 2006 were from hospitals not in metropolitan areas.

- In 2006, 12 percent of the U.S. population was age 65 and over; however, this age group used approximately 43 percent of the total days of care and comprised 38 percent of all inpatient discharges. This compares to 20 percent of the U.S. population who were under age 15 who accounted for only 7 percent of the total days of care and 7 percent of all inpatient discharges.

- Regionally, the average length of stay in days for nonfederal short-stay hospitals in the United States ranged from 4.2 in the Midwest to 5.3 in the Northeast.

- The status at discharge for 77.2 percent of all inpatients was described as routine or discharged to home.

Procedures

- In 2006, 28.1 million surgical procedures and 17.9 million nonsurgical procedures were performed on hospital inpatients.

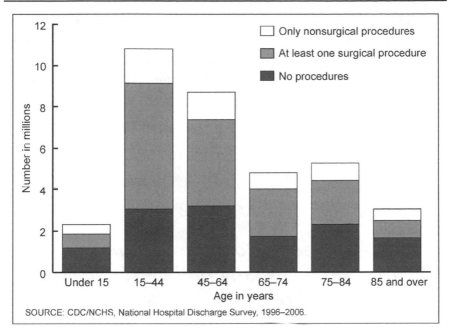

Figure 6.1. *Number and type of procedures for inpatient discharges, by age group: United States, 2006.*

- Of the 8.7 million discharges of inpatients age 45–64, 4.2 million (48%) had at least one surgical procedure (See Figure 6.1.).

- Among the 444,000 coronary artery bypass grafts performed in 2006, only 27.7 percent were performed on women.

- The rate of total hip replacement among inpatients age 65 and over (33.8 per 10,000 population) was over two times that of their counterparts age 45–64 (12.3 per 10,000 population).

Deliveries and Newborn Infants

- In 2006, approximately 4.1 million discharges were for delivery; their average stay was 2.6 days. Over one-half of all deliveries resulted in a length of stay of two or fewer days.

- The rate of episiotomies per 100 vaginal deliveries decreased from 43.2 in 1996 to 16.0 in 2006.

- Fifty-four percent of newborn infants were discharged in 2006 without any illness or risk-related diagnoses. These newborn infants

43

had an average length of stay of 2.1 days compared with 4.9 days among newborns with at least one illness or risk-related diagnosis.

• In 2006, 56.1 percent of all male newborn infants were circumcised during the birth hospitalization compared with 60.2 in 1996.

Section 6.2

Operating Room Procedures Account for Nearly Half of Hospitals' Treatment Costs

By the Agency for Healthcare Research and Quality
(AHRQ, www.ahrq.gov), March 2011.

Although only a quarter of patient stays in U.S. hospitals in 2007 involved procedures that were conducted in operating rooms, such stays accounted for 47 percent of hospitals' costs. This totalled $161 billion for patients receiving procedures, according to a new study by researchers at the Agency for Healthcare Research and Quality (AHRQ) that was published in the December 2010 issue of the *Archives of Surgery*.

The researchers found that one-third of the 15 million operating room procedures that year involved people aged 65 and older and that older patients were two to three times more likely to undergo surgery than younger patients. Surgical patients tended to be less severely ill than non-surgical patients, but their daily cost was double—$2,900 versus $1,400 a day. Fifteen procedures accounted for half of hospitals' costs for surgical patient stays and one-quarter of overall hospital costs. Four of the most expensive procedures—angioplasty, cesarean section delivery, knee replacement, and spinal fusion—increased in volume by between 20 percent and 46 percent between 1997 and 2007, while heart bypass surgery plummeted by 70 percent. More than half of all procedures were elective.

According to the study authors, Anne Elixhauser, PhD, and Roxanne M. Andrews, PhD, the findings highlight the important role that inpatient surgical procedures play in U.S. health care. The study is based on data in AHRQ's Nationwide Inpatient Sample, a database of hospital inpatient stays in short-term, nonfederal hospitals, which includes all patients, regardless of their type of insurance, as well as the uninsured.

Section 6.3

U.S. Outpatient Surgeries on the Rise

By the Centers for Disease Control and Prevention
(CDC, www.cdc.gov), January 28, 2009.

The number of outpatient surgery visits in the United States increased from 20.8 million visits in 1996 to 34.7 million visits in 2006, according to a report from the Centers for Disease Control and Prevention. Outpatient surgery visits accounted for about half of all surgery visits in 1996 but nearly two thirds of all surgery visits in 2006, the report said.

The report, *Ambulatory Surgery in the United States, 2006*, contains the first data on outpatient surgery visits since 1996. The data were collected from 142 hospitals and 295 freestanding centers as part of the National Survey of Ambulatory Surgery (NSAS).

The outpatient surgery visits to freestanding centers increased three-fold from 1996 to 2006, whereas the rate for outpatient surgery visits to hospital centers was relatively unchanged. Visits to hospital centers, at 19.9 million, continued to outnumber those to freestanding centers, at 14.9 million (57 percent compared to nearly 43 percent).

The report also found the following in 2006:

- An estimated 57.1 million surgical and nonsurgical procedures were performed during 34.7 million outpatient surgery visits in 2006.

- Females had significantly more ambulatory surgery visits (20 million) than males (14.7 million).

- The procedures performed most often during outpatient surgery visits included endoscopies of the large intestine (5.8 million)

45

and small intestine (3.5 million) and extraction of lens for cataract surgery (3.1 million).

- The leading diagnosis for outpatient surgery visits was cataract, with three million visits, followed by benign tumor (neoplasm) with two million visits, and malignant tumor with 1.2 million visits.

- The average time spent in the operating room during an outpatient surgery visit varied from 61.7 minutes for hospital centers to 43.2 minutes for freestanding centers. Time spent in surgery and recovery and overall visit time were also higher for hospital centers.

- More than half of outpatient surgery visits (53 percent) were paid by private insurance.

The National Survey of Ambulatory Surgery is a nationally representative survey that covers surgery visits by children and adults and procedures performed in both hospital-based and freestanding surgery centers. It excludes federal, military, and VA hospitals. Data were collected from medical records at the facilities.

Section 6.4

Statistics on Bariatric and Metabolic Surgery

Overview

- Metabolic and bariatric surgery results in significant weight loss and helps prevent, improve, or resolve more than 40 obesity-related diseases or conditions including Type 2 diabetes, heart disease, and certain cancers.[1,2,3]

- Patients may lose as much as 60% of excess weight six months after surgery, and 77% of excess weight as early as 12 months after surgery.[4]

- Clinical studies demonstrate significant improvements in safety,[5,6] showing risk of death from metabolic and bariatric surgery is about 0.1%,[7] which is less than gallbladder (0.7%) and hip replacement (0.93%) surgery.[8,9]

- In the United States, approximately 200,000 adults have metabolic and bariatric surgery each year, which is about 1% of the surgically eligible population.[10]

- Estimates suggest, third-party payers will recover metabolic and bariatric surgery costs within two to four years after surgery, as a result of the reductions in costs associated with treating obesity-related conditions.[11]

Safety and Risks

Federal Agency for Healthcare Research and Quality (AHRQ)[12] and recent clinical studies report significant improvements in metabolic and bariatric surgery safety.

Primary reasons for improved safety include increased use of laparoscopy,[6] advancements in surgical techniques,[13] and establishment of ASMBS and American College of Surgeons (ACS) accreditation programs.

Laparoscopic bariatric operations increased from 20.1% in 2003 to 90.2% in 2008.[7]

Overall likelihood of major complications is about 2.5%. Individual complication rates include:[5,6]

- gastric bypass—3.6%;

- sleeve gastrectomy—2.2%;

- adjustable gastric band—0.9%.

Overall mortality rate is about 0.1%. Individual complication rates include:[7,14]

- gastric bypass—0.1%;

- sleeve gastrectomy—0.19%;

- adjustable gastric band—0.02%.

Clinical evidence shows risks of morbid obesity outweigh risks of metabolic and bariatric surgery.[15,16]

- Individuals with morbid obesity or BMI≥30 have a 50–100% increased risk of premature death compared to individuals of healthy weight.[17]

- Studies show metabolic and bariatric surgery increases life span.[18,19]

- Gastric bypass patients may improve life expectancy by 89%.

- Patients may reduce risk of premature death by 30–40%.

Effectiveness

- Studies show patients typically lose the most weight one to two years after surgery, and maintain substantial weight loss with improvements in obesity-related conditions.[20]

- Patients may lose as much as 60% of excess weight six months after surgery, and 77% of excess weight as early as 12 months after surgery.[4]

- On average, five years after surgery patients maintain 50% of their excess weight loss.[19]

Metabolic and Bariatric Surgery Impact on Mortality

- Metabolic and bariatric surgery help to improve or resolve more than 40 obesity-related diseases and conditions,[3] including Type 2 diabetes, heart disease, certain cancers, sleep apnea, GERD [gastroesophageal reflux disease], high blood pressure, high cholesterol, sleep apnea and joint problems.[21,22,23] See Table 6.1.

- 60% reduction in mortality from cancer, with the largest reductions seen in breast and colon cancers.[19,24]

- 56% reduction in mortality from coronary artery disease.

- 92% reduction in mortality from Type 2 diabetes.

- 40% overall reduction in mortality in gastric bypass patients.[19]

Laparoscopic Gastric Bypass

- Stomach reduced to size of walnut and then attached to middle of small intestine, bypassing a section of the small intestine (duodenum and jejunum) limiting absorption of calories

- Risks include allergic reactions to medicines, blood clots in the legs, blood loss, breathing problems, heart attack or stroke during or after surgery, and infection.[24]

Laparoscopic Adjustable Gastric Band (LAGB)

- Adjustable silicone band filled with saline wrapped around upper part of stomach, creating small pouch that restricts food intake

- Risks include the gastric band eroding through the stomach, the gastric band slipping partly out of place, gastritis, heartburn, stomach ulcers, infection in the port, injury to the stomach, intestines, or other organs during surgery, poor nutrition, and scarring inside the belly.[23]

Table 6.1. Medical Outcomes of Bariatric Surgery

Condition/Disease	% Resolved or Improved	% Resolved[25]
Type 2 Diabetes	86	76.8
Hypertension	78.5	61.7
Obstructive Sleep Apnea	85.7	83.6
Hyperlipidemia	78.5	61.7

Sleeve Gastrectomy

- Stomach divided and stapled vertically, removing more than 85%, creating tube or banana-shaped pouch restricting amount of food that can be consumed and absorbed by the body

- Risks include gastritis, heartburn, stomach ulcers, injury to the stomach, intestines, or other organs during surgery, leaking from the line where parts of the stomach have been stapled together, poor nutrition, scarring inside the belly that could lead to a future blockage in the bowel, and vomiting.[25]

Economics of Bariatric Surgery

- Metabolic and bariatric surgery approximately costs between $11,500 and $26,000.[26]

- On average, health care costs for morbidly obese patients were reduced by 29% within five years following bariatric surgery, due to the reduction or elimination of obesity-related conditions.[27]

- Estimates suggest, third-party payers will recover metabolic and bariatric surgery costs within two to four years following a patient's procedure, as a result of the reduction in costs associated with treating obesity-related conditions.[28]

- According to expert analysis, surgical treatment of morbid obesity results in individual worker productivity gain of $2,765 per year for U.S. employers.[29]

References

1. Chikunguw, S., Patricia, W., Dodson, J. G., et al. (2009). Durable resolution of diabetes after Roux-en-Y gastric bypass associated with maintenance of weight loss. *Surgery for Obesity and Related Diseases.* 5(3) p. S1

2. Torquati, A., Wright, K., Melvin, W., et al. (2007). Effect of gastric bypass operation on Framingham and actual risk of cardiovascular events in class II to III obesity. *Journal of the American College of Surgeons.* 204(5) pp. 776–782. Accessed March 2012 from http://www.ncbi.nlm.nih.gov/pubmed/17481482

3. Kaplan, L. M. (2003). Body weight regulation and obesity. *Journal of Gastrointestinal Surgery.* 7(4) pp. 443–51. Doi:10.1016/

S1091-255X(03)00047-7. Accessed March 2012 from http://edulife.com.br/dados%5CArtigos%5CNutricao%5CObesida de%20e%20Sindrome%20Metabolica%5CBody%20weight%20 regulation%20and%20obesity.pdf

4. Wittgrove, A. C., Clark, G. W., (2000). Laparoscopic gastric bypass, Roux-en-Y: 500 patients: Technique and results, with 3–60 month follow-up. *Obesity Surgery.* 10(3) pp. 233–239. Accessed March 2012 from http://www.lapbypass.com/pdf/ LapGBP_500Patients.pdf

5. Birkmeyer N. J., Dimick J. B., Share D., et al. (2010). Hospital complication rates with bariatric surgery in Michigan. *Journal of the American Medical Association.* 304(4) pp. 435–442. Accessed March 2012 from http://jama.ama-assn.org/content /304/4/435.full.pdf+html

6. Encinosa, W. E., Bernard, D. M., Du D., et al. (2009). Recent improvements in bariatric surgery outcomes. *Medical Care.* 47(5) pp. 531–535. Accessed March 2012 from http://www.ncbi.nlm .nih.gov/pubmed/19318997

7. Nguyen, N. T., Masoomi, H., Magno, C. P., et al. (2011). Trends in use of bariatric surgery, 2003–2008. *Journal of the American College of Surgeons.* 213(2) pp. 261–266. doi:10.10161j. jamcollsurg.2011.04.030

8. Pedersen, A. B., Baron, J. A., Overgaard, S., et al. (2009). Short- and long-term mortality following primary total hip replacement for osteoarthritis. *Journal of Bone and Joint Surgery.* 93-B(2) pp. 172–177 Accessed March 2012 from http://www .ncbi.nlm.nih.gov/pubmed/21282754

9. Dolan, J. P., Diggs, B. S., Sheppard, B. C., et al. (2009). National mortality burden and significant factors associated with open and laparoscopic cholecystectomy: 1997–2006. *Journal of Gastrointestinal Surgery.* 13(12) pp.2292-2301. Accessed March 2012 from http://www.ncbi.nlm.nih.gov/pubmed/19727976

10. American Society for Metabolic & Bariatric Surgery. (2009). All estimates are based on surveys with ASMBS membership and bariatric surgery industry reports.

11. Crémieux, P. Y., Buchwald, H., Shikora, S. A., et al (2008). A study of economic impact of bariatric surgery. *The American Journal of Managed Care.* 14(9) pp. 589–596 Accessed March

2012 from http://www.ajmc.com/publications/issue/2008/
2008-09-vol14-n9/Sep08-3582p589-596

12. Encinosa, W. E., Bernard, D. M., Du D., et al. (2009). Recent improvements in bariatric surgery outcomes. *Medical Care.* 47(5) pp. 531–535

13. Poirier, P., Cornier, M. A., Mazzone, T., et al. (2011). Bariatric surgery and cardiovascular risk factors. *Circulation: Journal of the American Heart Association.* 123 pp. 1–19. Accessed March 2012 from http://circ.ahajournals.org/content/123/15/1683.full.pdf

14. Brethauer, S. A., Hammel, J. P., Schauer, P. R., (2005). Systematic review of sleeve gastrectomy as staging and primary bariatric procedure. SOARD. (5) pp. 469–475 Accessed March 2012 from https://my.clevelandclinic.org/Documents/Bariatric_Surgery/Systematic_Review_of_Sleeve_2009.pdf

15. Christou, N. V., Sampalis F., Moishe Lieberman, M., et al. (2004). Surgery decreases long-term mortality, morbidity, and health care use in morbidly obese patients. *Annals of Surgery.* 240(3) pp. 416–424 Accessed March 2012 from http://www.ncbi.nlm.nih.gov/pmc/articles/PMC1356432/pdf/20040900s00003p416.pdf

16. Schauer, D. P., Arterburn, D.E., Livingston, E.H., et al. (2010). Decision modeling to estimate the impact of gastric bypass surgery on life expectancy for the treatment of morbid obesity. *Archives of Surgery.* 145(1) pp.57–62 Accessed March 2012 from http://www.ncbi.nlm.nih.gov/pubmed/20083755

17. U.S. Department of Health and Human Services Office of the Surgeon General. (2007). Overweight and obesity: health consequences. Accessed May 2011 from http://www.surgeongeneral.gov/topics/obesity/calltoaction/fact_consequences.htm

18. Sjöström. L., Narbro, K., Sjöström, D., et al. (2007). Effects of bariatric surgery on mortality in Swedish obese subjects. *New England Journal of Medicine.* 357 pp. 741–752 Accessed March 2012 from http://www.nejm.org/doi/pdf/10.1056/NEJMoa066254

19. Adams, T. D., Gress, R. E., Smith, S. C., et al. (2007). Long-term mortality after gastric bypass surgery. *New England Journal of Medicine.* 357 pp. 753–761 Accessed March 2012 from http://www.nejm.org/doi/full/10.1056/NEJMoa066603

20. Buchwald, H., Estok, R., Fahrbach, K., et al. (2009). Weight and type 2 diabetes after bariatric surgery: Systematic review and meta-analysis. *American Journal of Medicine.* 122(3) pp. 205–206 Accessed March 2012 from http://www.ncbi.nlm.nih.gov/pubmed/19272486

21. U.S. National Library of Medicine—National Institutes of Health. (2011). Laparoscopic gastric banding surgery. Accessed March 2012 from http://www.nlm.nih.gov/medlineplus/ency/article/007199.htm

22. U.S. National Library of Medicine—National Institutes of Health. (2011). Gastric bypass surgery. Accessed March 2012 from http://www.nlm.nih.gov/medlineplus/ency/article/007199.htm

23. U.S. National Library of Medicine—National Institutes of Health. (2011). Vertical sleeve gastrectomy. Accessed March 2012 from http://www.nlm.nih.gov/medlineplus/ency/article/007435.htm

24. Christou, N. V., Lieberman, M., Sampalis, F., et al. (2008). Bariatric surgery reduces cancer risk in morbidly obese patients. *Surgery for Obesity and Related Diseases.* 4(6) pp. 691–695 Accessed March 2012 from http://www.ncbi.nlm.nih.gov/pubmed/19026373

25. Buchwald, H., Avidor, Y., Braunwald, E., et al. (2004). Bariatric surgery: a systematic review and meta-analysis. *Journal of the American Medical Association.* 292(12) pp. 1724–1737. Accessed March 2012 from http://jama.ama-assn.org/content/292/14/1724.full

26. Salem, L., Jensen, C. C., Flum, R. D. (2005). Are bariatric surgical outcomes worth their cost? A systematic review. *American College of Surgeons.* pp. 270–278

27. Sampalis J. S., Liberman M., Auger S., et al. (2004). Impact of weight reduction surgery on health care costs in morbidly obese patients. *Obesity Surgery.* 14(7) pp. 939–47

28. Crémieux, P. Y., Buchwald, H., Shikora, S. A., et al (2008). A study of economic impact of bariatric surgery. *The American Journal of Managed Care.* 14(9) pp. 589–596

29. Van Gemert, W. G., Adang, E. M., Kop, M., et al. (1999). A prospective cost-effectiveness analysis of vertical banded gastroplasty for treatment of morbid obesity. *Obesity Surgery.* 9(5) pp. 484–91

Section 6.5

Baby Boomers Trigger Major Increase in Knee Replacement Surgeries

By Carolyn M. Clancy, MD, from the Agency for Healthcare Research and Quality (AHRQ, www.ahrq.gov), January 3, 2012.

Whether it's music, lifestyles, or a refuse-to-age outlook, Baby Boomers think of themselves as trailblazers. Now, that generation born between 1946 and 1964 can claim credit for another first—a dramatic increase in knee replacement surgeries.

Women and men between the ages of 45 and 64 were more than twice as likely to have had knee replacement surgery in 2009 than in 1997, recent data from the Agency for Healthcare Research and Quality (AHRQ) show. The rates among women were even higher.

Knee replacement surgery is most common in people whose knees have been damaged by osteoarthritis (OA), rheumatoid arthritis, or injury. Due to their age and fondness for sports, Baby Boomers fit neatly into each category.

The percentage of people who have osteoarthritis, the most common type of arthritis, grows with age. About 27 million Americans have this condition, and, after age 45, it is more common in women. Osteoarthritis occurs when the cartilage that coats the end of each bone breaks down. This can cause the bones to rub against each other, causing pain and stiffness.

Knee pain may also be caused by rheumatoid arthritis, a less common form of arthritis that occurs when the membrane surrounding the joint becomes inflamed. Over time, inflammation damages cartilage, resulting in pain and stiffness. Rheumatoid arthritis affects about 1.3 million people—more women than men. It often begins in middle age, but can occur in children and young adults.

Arthritis after a serious knee injury or repeated stress is another reason for knee replacement surgery. Pain caused by ligament tears or bone fractures caused by sports injuries, for example, may be managed non-surgically for years. Over time, however, pain and limited knee function causes some patients to consider knee replacement surgery.

If you have knee pain from one of these causes, you've probably heard about treatments that are intended to relieve pain and even postpone the need for surgery. Some, but not all, of these options work, a review of 86 research reports funded by AHRQ has found.

What Has Been Shown to Work?

- **Exercise:** Becoming more active—whether through walking, swimming, or water aerobics—can reduce pain and make movement easier. Physical therapy may also help, so ask your doctor if you would benefit.

- **Maintaining a healthy weight:** A 10 percent weight loss combined with a moderate exercise program reduced knee pain in patients with knee osteoarthritis by 50 percent, a recent study by Wake Forest University researchers has found.

- **Pain medicines:** Medicines can relieve osteoarthritis pain, AHRQ's research review concluded. Your doctor or nurse may prescribe an over-the-counter or prescription medicine.

What Usually Does Not Help?

- **Glucosamine and chondroitin:** Some people take nutritional supplements to help build new cartilage. Studies have found that people who take these supplements report less pain, but people who don't take the supplements report the same result.

- **Joint lubrication shots:** This treatment is a gel-like substance given by a shot into the knee. Studies have found that most people who get the shots do not improve very much.

- **Arthroscopic knee surgery:** In this procedure, a flexible tool is inserted into the knee, which is used to rinse the joint. It can be helpful for other types of knee problems, but not for knee osteoarthritis.

If conservative treatments don't provide relief from pain, it may be time to consider knee replacement surgery. The good news is that this procedure has been shown to give a better quality of life that makes it worth the cost, a government-funded study has found. The benefits of this procedure are even better if the surgery is done at a hospital that does a large number of knee replacement procedures.

Before you have surgery, prepare yourself for the best possible outcome by asking questions of your surgeon. You will feel more in control of your health if you have a good idea of what to expect before, during, and after surgery.

Chapter 7

Recent Research and Trends in Surgery and Patient Outcomes

Chapter Contents

Section 7.1

Certain Hospital Characteristics Influence Mortality after Complications Following High-Risk Surgery

By the Agency for Healthcare Research and Quality
(AHRQ, www.ahrq.gov), April 2011.

Managing complications after surgery is an important part of hospital care, particularly for patients who undergo high-risk surgeries. Such patients may die after a major complication; hospitals call this "failure to rescue." Although hospitals with low and high mortality rates may have similar complication rates, there can be marked differences in failure-to-rescue rates. A September 2010 study has found that failure-to-rescue rates vary widely depending on the hospital. In addition, hospitals with the lowest rates have certain characteristics that can be attributed to better outcomes.

Researchers used 7-year data from the American Hospital Association's annual survey as well as from the Nationwide Inpatient Sample, an Agency for Healthcare Research and Quality (AHRQ) database on hospital admissions. A total of 8,862 patients at 672 hospitals were identified who had undergone removal of their pancreas (pancreatectomy), considered a high-risk surgery. The researchers examined the association between five hospital characteristics and failure-to-rescue rates: nurse-to-patient ratios, the teaching status of the hospital, the level of technology available, hospital size, and average daily census.

In general, patients undergoing this surgery at very high-mortality hospitals had a 16-fold increase in the odds of death compared with patients receiving the surgery at very low-mortality hospitals, as well as higher complication rates (33 percent vs. 18 percent). Close to a 10-fold difference was observed in failure-to-rescue rates between very low and very high mortality hospitals. Characteristics associated with favorable failure-to-rescue rates included being admitted to a teaching hospital with more than 200 beds and an average daily census of greater than 50 percent capacity. Increased nurse-to-patient ratios and strong use of hospital technology also had a positive influence. The study was supported in part by AHRQ.

Source: "Hospital characteristics associated with failure to rescue from complications after pancreatectomy," by Amir A. Ghaferi, MD, MS, Nicholas H. Osborne, MD, MS, John D. Birkmeyer, MD, and Justin B. Dimick, MD, MPH, in the September 2010 *Journal of the American College of Surgeons* 211(3), pp. 325–330.

Section 7.2

Trauma Patients with Hospital-Acquired Infections Have Poor Outcomes, Including Increased Mortality Risk

By the Agency for Healthcare Research and Quality
(AHRQ, www.ahrq.gov), March 2012.

Among all hospital admissions, trauma patients are at especially high risk when it comes to developing hospital-acquired infections (HAIs). When these infections occur, they are a leading cause of death in these individuals. A July 2011 study found that trauma patients with HAIs have longer hospital stays, increased risk of dying, and higher inpatient costs.

The researchers examined the relationship between four different HAIs—sepsis, pneumonia, *Staphylococcus* infections, and *Clostridium difficile*-associated disease—and three outcome measures including in-hospital mortality, length of hospital stay, and inpatient costs. They analyzed the records on 155,891 trauma patients obtained from the 2005 and 2006 Nationwide Inpatient Sample.

All three outcome measures were significantly higher in patients with HAIs than in trauma patients without these infections. Patients with sepsis had the highest risk of dying in the hospital, with close to a sixfold higher odds of mortality compared to patients without HAIs. Among the other infections, there was a 1.5- to 1.9-fold higher odds of dying in the hospital. When costs were analyzed, patients with HAIs had health care expenditures 2- to 2.5-fold higher compared with non-infected patients. Those with HAIs also stayed in the hospital twice as long as patients without HAIs. The researchers call for more patient safety initiatives to reduce HAIs and related poor outcomes in this patient population. The study was supported in part by the Agency for Healthcare Research and Quality.

Source: "Increases in mortality, length of stay, and cost associated with hospital-acquired infections in trauma patients," by Laurent G. Glance, MD, Pat W. Stone, PhD, Dana B. Mukamel, PhD. and Andrew W. Dick, PhD, in the July 2011 *Archives of Surgery* 146(7), pp. 794–801.

Section 7.3

Presurgical Medical Consultants May Not Result in Better Care for Patients

"Consultations on Major Surgeries Bring Higher Costs and Longer Stays But Not Care Improvements," by the Agency for Healthcare Research and Quality (AHRQ, www.ahrq.gov), April 2008.

Just 1 in 10 major surgeries involves the services of a medical consultant in the days before and after an operation. Further, these discussions do not result in higher quality care for the patient, a study published in the November 26, 2007 *Archives of Internal Medicine*, found. Andrew D. Auerbach, MD, MPH, undertook the study to understand the effect of consultations the day before, the day of, or the day after a major surgery in terms of costs and length of hospital stay.

Dr. Auerbach, from the Department of Medicine at the University of California, San Francisco, and his colleagues examined records for patients seen at the University's medical center from May 1, 2004, to May 31, 2006. Of the 1,282 patients studied, less than 10 percent underwent a surgical consultation. Those who received consultations had diabetes (29 percent), vascular disease (35 percent), or kidney failure (24 percent), and tended to have severe systemic, life-threatening diseases.

Costs almost doubled for patients who received consultations ($155,020) compared with those who did not ($74,237), and their median hospital stay was longer (10 days vs. 6 days). The authors suggest costs may be higher when consultants are brought in because they may request additional lab tests or procedures. Patients seen by generalists stayed in the hospital as long as those seen by consulting specialists but were more likely to pay less and receive therapies to prevent venous thromboembolism (a blocked blood vessel that can develop after an operation).

Care quality may not have improved when consultants were included for a couple of reasons. One, medical consultants may have been respecting their colleague's turf and opted to answer just the question they were asked. Two, the consultant's advice may not have been heeded. This scenario presents an opportunity to improve the consultation process, the authors suggest. This study was funded in part by the Agency for Healthcare Research and Quality.

Source: "Opportunity missed: Medical consultation, resource use, and quality of care of patients undergoing major surgery," by Dr. Auerbach, Mladen A. Rasic, M.D., Neil Sehgal, M.P.H., and others in the November 26, 2007 *Archives of Internal Medicine* 167(21), pp. 2338–44.

Section 7.4

Medical Tourism:
Going Overseas for Surgical Procedures

What is medical tourism?

Medical tourism is the practice of traveling internationally for elective or non-elective medical procedures. The Deloitte Center for Health Solutions estimates approximately 540,000 Americans traveled abroad for medical care in 2008, and this number could reach more than 1.6 million by 2012.

Why do patients seek treatment outside the United States?

Patients cite increased affordability and greater access to medical care as the primary reasons for traveling abroad for care.

What are the most common procedures sought by medical tourists?

The top non-cosmetic procedures sought by medical tourists include heart bypass, heart valve replacement, hip replacement, knee replacement, and hysterectomy and other gynecological procedures. Common cosmetic and plastic surgery procedures include abdominoplasty, eyelid surgery, breast augmentation/reduction, cosmetic skin refinishing and body contouring, facelifts and implant surgery, liposuction, and rhinoplasty.

Does medical tourism carry risks?

Yes, and some of those risks can be life-threatening. They include:

- exposure to infectious diseases in the host country;
- substandard quality of care;
- travel-related health complications.

How can patients ensure high quality of care and safety?

Patients should research and choose facilities accredited by organizations such as the Joint Commission International (JCI). Most hospitals feature this information on their websites, and patients can find those accredited by JCI at www.jointcommissioninternational.org. While accredited facilities very often have qualified physicians, patients should research licensing and outcomes data for both surgeons and anesthesiologists, as well.

What are medical tourism companies?

Medical tourism companies equip patients with valuable information to help facilitate the process. They often do everything from transferring medical records to coordinating travel logistics.

What are the benefits and risks of using medical tourism companies?

Medical tourism companies offer a variety of convenient services and are therefore worth considering. But patients should research these companies carefully because they vary in quality of service. Other drawbacks can be additional fees, favoritism toward certain facilities or countries, and increased risk of miscommunication as a result of third-party involvement.

Should patients involve their local medical providers in the process?

Yes. Local medical providers will likely play a key role throughout the process, ideally from administering preoperative exams to providing aftercare, especially if complications occur.

What role do insurance companies play?

Patients should be informed of coverage and reimbursement policies from their providers. Never assume any procedure is covered.

What other factors should patients consider?

- Patients should prepare for an extended hospital stay, as some people develop postoperative complications or simply need more time to recover.

- Know your medications and how to access them, and expect your physician to prescribe additional ones before, during or after their procedure, which may cost extra.

- Be sure to coordinate local postoperative care and financing ahead of time.

Part Two

Preparing for Surgery

Chapter 8

How to Find a Qualified Surgeon

Most of us have some criteria for making important decisions in life. But suppose that your doctor recommends that you consider having an operation. How do you go about finding a qualified surgeon? If you or someone you know is considering elective surgery, you should be aware that there are some ways to objectively evaluate your surgeon. The American College of Surgeons—the largest international organization of surgeons in the world—recommends that you look for the following criteria: 1) board certification; 2) hospital or ambulatory center accreditation; and 3) Fellowship in the American College of Surgeons.

Check for Board Certification

In order for a physician to become board certified in a surgical specialty, he or she must complete the required years of residency training in that specialty, and then demonstrate his or her knowledge by successfully completing a rigorous comprehensive examination. Specialty boards certify physicians that meet certain published standards. There are 24 specialty boards that are recognized by the American Board of Medical Specialties (ABMS) and the American Medical Association (AMA).

"Looking for a Qualified Surgeon? Here's How," reprinted with permission from www.facs.org. © 2012 American College of Surgeons. All rights reserved.

A specialist has graduated medical school and received a MD (Medical Doctorate) or DO (Doctor of Osteopathy). The physician then completes three to eight years of additional training in an accredited residency program. Each specialist must pass a written examination given by a specialty board. Fifteen of the specialty boards also require an oral examination. All of the ABMS Boards issue a time-limited certificate, which are valid for 6 to 10 years. In order to retain certification, physicians must become recertified and must show continuing education in the specialty. You can review a brief description of the surgical specialty areas on the American College of Surgeons website (www.facs.org).

You can check on specialty certification of specific physicians through the ABMS website (www.abms.org), through the link: "Is Your Doctor Certified?" Click on "Is Your Doctor Certified?" and enter your search information. In addition, verbal verification of a physician's board certification is available through the ABMS toll-free telephone service. Call: 866-ASK-ABMS (275-2267). You can also check verification in *The Official ABMS Directory of Board Certified Medical Specialists,* published annually. The *Directory* can be found in many medical schools and public libraries. Written verification is available by contacting the individual specialty board in the physician's field of practice.

In most cases, a surgeon who is board certified and/or a Fellow of the American College of Surgeons will have certificates verifying these credentials on display in their office. If not, another way is to simply ask the surgeon for his or her credentials. Or you can phone your state or county medical association for assistance.

Check for Facility Accreditation

Your operation should be performed in an accredited hospital, outpatient surgery center, or cancer treatment center. Accreditation means that the hospital or surgical center is committed to providing high quality health care and that it has demonstrated commitment to meeting high patient safety standards.

Hospitals are accredited and evaluated by The Joint Commission (TJC). A hospital accredited by TJC means that the hospital has met The Joint Commission's quality and safety standards. You can check to see if a hospital has been TJC-accredited by visiting www.qualitycheck .org and entering your search information.

Surgical centers are accredited and evaluated by the Accreditation Association for Ambulatory Health Care (AAAH) and TJC. Accreditation by AAAH is a voluntary process that involves a self-assessment by the organization and a thorough review by expert surveyors. Visit the AAAH site (www.aaahc.org) to see if your surgical center is accredited. Once you enter the AAAH website, click the heading "Search For Accredited Organizations" [near the bottom of the page] to access a list of facilities in your area.

Cancer Treatment Center

Cancer treatment facilities are accredited by the Commission on Cancer (CoC). Accreditation as a cancer center is granted only to those facilities that have voluntarily committed to provide the best in cancer diagnosis and treatment and are able to comply with established CoC standards. Each cancer program must undergo a rigorous evaluation and review of its performance and compliance with the CoC standards every three years. Participating programs are concerned with the continuum of care from prevention and early detection, pretreatment evaluation, and staging, to optimal treatment, rehabilitation, surveillance for recurrent disease, support services, and end-of-life care. Approximately 80 percent of all newly diagnosed cancer patients in the United States are treated in the more than 1,500 facilities that are accredited by the CoC. You can find an accredited cancer center by going to www.facs.org/cancerprogram/index.html and then go to the bottom of the page to "Find a CoC Cancer Program Near You."

Check for Membership in the American College of Surgeons

The letters FACS after a surgeon's name indicates that he or she is a Fellow of the American College of Surgeons (ACS). Fellows of the College are board-certified surgeons whose education, training, professional qualifications, surgical competence, and ethical conduct have been reviewed and evaluated prior to admittance and have been found to be consistent with the high standards of the American College of Surgeons. Not all surgeons are accepted into Fellowship in the College and there are some surgeons who may choose not to become Fellows. The letters FACS after a surgeon's name indicates that the surgeon has submitted to a process to obtain voluntary credential and performance evaluation by their peers.

You can find a member of the American College of Surgeons in the Fellowship Database at web2.facs.org/acsdir/default_public.cfm or call 312-202-5263 for a list of Fellows in your area.

Chapter 9

How to Get a Second Opinion

Getting a Second Opinion before Surgery

What Is a Second Opinion?

A second opinion is when a doctor other than your regular doctor gives his or her view about your health problem and how it should be treated. Getting a second opinion can help you make a more informed decision about your care. Medicare Part B (Medical Insurance) helps pay for a second opinion before surgery. When your doctor says you have a health problem that needs surgery, you have the right to the following:

- Know and understand your treatment choices.

- Have another doctor look at those choices with you (second opinion).

- Participate in treatment decisions by making your wishes known.

When to Get a Second Opinion

If your doctor says you need surgery to diagnose or treat a health problem that isn't an emergency, you should consider getting a second

This chapter contains text excerpted from "Getting a Second Opinion before Surgery," by the Centers for Medicare and Medicaid Services (CMS, www.medi care.gov), June 2010, and from "How to Get a Second Opinion," by the Office on Women's Health (www.womenshealth.gov), part of the U.S. Department of Health and Human Services, September 10, 2008.

opinion. It's up to you to decide when and if you will have surgery. You might also want a second opinion if your doctor tells you that you should have certain kinds of major non-surgical procedures. Medicare doesn't pay for surgeries or procedures that aren't medically necessary, such as cosmetic surgery. This means that Medicare won't pay for second opinions for surgeries or procedures that aren't medically necessary. Don't wait for a second opinion if you need emergency surgery. Some types of emergencies may require surgery right away, such as the following:

- Acute appendicitis
- Blood clot or aneurysm
- Accidental injuries

Finding a Doctor for a Second Opinion

Make sure the doctor giving the second opinion accepts Medicare. To find a doctor for a second opinion, you can do the following:

- Visit www.medicare.gov and select Resource Locator to find doctors who accept Medicare.
- Call 800-MEDICARE (800-633-4227). TTY users should call 877-486-2048. Ask for information about doctors who accept Medicare.
- Ask your doctor for the name of another doctor to see for a second opinion. Don't hesitate to ask; most doctors want you to get a second opinion. You can also ask another doctor you trust to recommend a doctor.
- Ask your local medical society for the names of doctors who treat your illness or injury. Your local library can help you find your local medical society.

What to Do When You Get a Second Opinion

Before you visit the second doctor, you should do the following:

- Ask your doctor to send your medical records to the doctor giving the second opinion. That way, you may not have to repeat the tests you already had.
- Call the second doctor's office and make sure they have your records.
- Write down a list of questions to take with you to the appointment.
- Ask a friend or loved one to go to the appointment with you.

During the visit with the second doctor, you should do the following:

- Tell the doctor what surgery you are considering.

- Tell the doctor what tests you already had.

- Ask the questions you have on your list and encourage your friend or loved one to ask any questions that he or she may have.

Note: The second doctor may ask you to have additional tests performed as a result of the visit. Medicare will help pay for these tests just as it helps pay for other services that are medically necessary.

What If the First and Second Opinions Are Different?

If the second doctor doesn't agree with the first, you may feel confused about what to do. In that case, you may want to do the following:

- Talk more about your condition with your first doctor.

- Talk to a third doctor. Medicare helps pay for a third opinion. Getting a second opinion doesn't mean you have to change doctors. You decide which doctor you want to do your surgery.

Does Medicare Pay for a Second Opinion before Surgery?

Medicare Part B helps pay for a second opinion and related tests just as it helps pay for other services that are medically necessary. If you have Medicare Part B and are in Original Medicare, here is what you and Medicare pay:

- Medicare pays 80% of the Medicare-approved amount for a second opinion.

- Your share is usually 20% of the Medicare-approved amount after you pay your yearly Part B deductible.

- The Part B deductible may increase each year.

If the second opinion doesn't agree with the first opinion, Medicare pays80% of the Medicare-approved amount for a third opinion.

How to Get a Second Opinion

Even though doctors may get similar medical training, they can have their own opinions and thoughts about how to practice medicine. They can have different ideas about how to diagnose and treat conditions or diseases. Some doctors take a more conservative, or traditional, approach to treating their patients. Other doctors are more aggressive and use the newest tests and therapies. It seems like we learn about new advances in medicine almost every day.

Many doctors specialize in one area of medicine, such as cardiology or obstetrics or psychiatry. Not every doctor can be skilled in using all the latest technology. Getting a second opinion from a different doctor might give you a fresh perspective and new information. It could provide you with new options for treating your condition. Then you can make more informed choices. If you get similar opinions from two doctors, you can also talk with a third doctor.

Ask your doctor for a recommendation: Ask for the name of another doctor or specialist, so you can get a second opinion. Don't worry about hurting your doctor's feelings. Most doctors welcome a second opinion, especially when surgery or long-term treatment is involved.

Ask someone you trust for a recommendation: If you don't feel comfortable asking your doctor for a referral, then call another doctor you trust. You can also call university teaching hospitals and medical societies in your area for the names of doctors. Some of this information is also available on the internet.

Check with your health insurance provider: Call your insurance company before you get a second opinion. Ask if they will pay for this office visit. Many health insurance providers do. Ask if there are any special procedures you or your primary care doctor needs to follow.

Ask to have medical records sent to the second doctor: Ask your primary care doctor to send your medical records to the new doctor. You need to give written permission to your current doctor to send any records or test results to a new doctor. You can also ask for a copy of your own medical records for your files. Your new doctor can then examine these records before your office visit.

Learn as much as you can: Ask your doctor for information you can read. Go to a local library. Search the internet. Find a teaching hospital or university that has medical libraries open to the public. The information you find can be hard to understand, or just confusing. Make a list of your questions, and bring it with you when you see your new doctor.

Do not rely on the internet or a telephone conversation: When you get a second opinion, you need to be seen by a doctor. That doctor will perform a physical examination and perhaps other tests. The doctor will also thoroughly review your medical records, ask you questions, and address your concerns.

Chapter 10

How to Prepare for Surgery

Are you facing surgery? You are not alone. Every year, more than 15 million Americans have surgery.

Most operations are not emergencies and are considered elective surgery. This means that you have time to learn about your operation to be sure it is the best treatment for you. You also have time to work with your surgeon to make the surgery as safe as possible.

Your regular doctor is your primary care doctor. He or she may be the doctor who suggests that you have surgery and may refer you to a surgeon. You may also want to find another surgeon to get a second opinion, to confirm if surgery is the right treatment for you. You might want to ask friends or coworkers for the names of surgeons they have used.

This text gives you some questions to ask your primary care doctor and surgeon before you have surgery. It also gives the reasons for asking these questions. The answers will help you make the best decisions.

Your doctors should welcome questions. If you do not understand the answers, ask the doctor to explain them clearly. Bring a friend or relative along to help you talk with the doctor. Research shows that patients who are well informed about their treatment are more satisfied with their results.

Excerpted from "Having Surgery? What You Need to Know," by the Agency for Healthcare Research and Quality (AHRQ, www.ahrq.gov), October 2005. Reviewed by David A. Cooke, MD, FACP, October 10, 2012.

Why do I need an operation?

There are many reasons to have surgery. Some operations can relieve or prevent pain. Others can reduce a symptom of a problem or improve some body function.

Some surgeries are done to find a problem. Surgery can also save your life. Your doctor will tell you the purpose of the procedure. Make sure you understand how the proposed operation will help fix your medical problem. For example, if something is going to be repaired or removed, find out why it needs to be done.

What operation are you recommending?

Ask your surgeon to explain the surgery and how it is done. Your surgeon can draw a picture or a diagram and explain the steps in the surgery.

Is there more than one way of doing the operation? One way may require more extensive surgery than another. Some operations that once needed large incisions (cuts in the body) can now be done using much smaller incisions (laparoscopic surgery).

Some surgeries require that you stay in the hospital for one or more days. Others let you come in and go home on the same day. Ask why your surgeon wants to do the operation one way over another.

Are there alternatives to surgery?

Sometimes, surgery is not the only answer to a medical problem. Medicines or treatments other than surgery, such as a change in diet or special exercises, might help you just as well—or more. Ask your surgeon or primary care doctor about the benefits and risks of these other choices. You need to know as much as possible about these benefits and risks to make the best decision.

One alternative to surgery may be watchful waiting. During a watchful wait, your doctor and you check to see if your problem gets better or worse over time. If it gets worse, you may need surgery right away. If it gets better, you may be able to wait to have surgery or not have it at all.

How much will the operation cost?

Even if you have health insurance, there may be some costs for you to pay. This may depend on your choice of surgeon or hospital. Ask what your surgeon's fee is and what it covers. Surgical fees often also include some visits after the operation. You also will get a bill from the hospital for your care and from the other doctors who gave you care during your surgery.

Before you have the operation, call your insurance company. They can tell you how much of the costs your insurance will pay and what share you will have to pay. If you are covered by Medicare, call 800-MEDICARE (800-633-4227) to find out your share of surgery costs.

What are the benefits of having the operation?

Ask your surgeon what you will gain by having the operation. For example, a hip replacement may mean that you can walk again with ease.

Ask how long the benefits will last. For some procedures, it is not unusual for the benefits to last for a short time only. You may need a second operation at a later date. For other procedures, the benefits may last a lifetime.

When finding out about the benefits of the operation, be realistic. Sometimes patients expect too much and are disappointed with the outcome or results. Ask your doctor if there is anything you can read to help you understand the procedure and its likely results.

What are the risks of having the operation?

All operations have some risk. This is why you need to weigh the benefits of the operation against the risks of complications or side effects.

Complications are unplanned events linked to the operation. Typical complications are infection, too much bleeding, reaction to anesthesia, or accidental injury. Some people have a greater risk of complications because of other medical conditions. There also may be side effects after the operation.

Often, your surgeon can tell you what side effects to expect. For example, there may be swelling and some soreness around the incision.

There is almost always some pain with surgery. Ask your surgeon how much pain there will be and what the doctors and nurses will do to help stop the pain. Controlling the pain will help you to be more comfortable while you heal. Controlling the pain will also help you get well faster and improve the results of your operation.

What if I don't have this operation?

Based on what you learn about the benefits and risks of the operation, you might decide not to have it. Ask your surgeon what you will gain—or lose—by not having the operation now. Could you be in more pain? Could your condition get worse? Could the problem go away?

What kind of anesthesia will I need?

Anesthesia is used so that surgery can be performed without unnecessary pain. Your surgeon can tell you whether the operation calls for local, regional, or general anesthesia and why this form of anesthesia is best for your procedure.

Local anesthesia numbs only a part of your body and only for a short period of time. For example, when you go to the dentist, you may get a local anesthetic called Novocain. It numbs the gum area around a tooth. Not all procedures done with local anesthesia are painless.

Regional anesthesia numbs a larger portion of your body—for example, the lower part of your body—for a few hours. In most cases, you will be awake during the operation with regional anesthesia. General anesthesia numbs your entire body.

You will be asleep during the whole operation if you have general anesthesia.

Anesthesia is quite safe for most patients. It is usually given by a specialized doctor (anesthesiologist) or nurse (nurse anesthetist).

Both are highly skilled and have been trained to give anesthesia. If you decide to have an operation, ask to meet with the person who will give you anesthesia. It is okay to ask what his or her qualifications are. Ask what the side effects and risks of having anesthesia are in your case. Be sure to tell him or her what medical problems you have—including allergies and what medicines you have been taking. These medicines may affect your response to the anesthesia. Be sure to include both prescription and over-the-counter medicines, like vitamins and supplements.

How long will it take me to recover?

Your surgeon can tell you how you might feel and what you will be able to do—or not do—the first few days, weeks, or months after surgery. Ask how long you will be in the hospital. Find out what kind of supplies, equipment, and help you will need when you go home. Knowing what to expect can help you get better faster.

Ask how long it will be before you can go back to work or start regular exercise again. You do not want to do anything that will slow your recovery. For example, lifting a 10-pound bag of potatoes may not seem to be too much a week after your operation, but it could be. You should follow your surgeon's advice to make sure you recover fully as soon as possible.

Chapter 11

Preparing Your Child for Surgery

Preparing Yourself

Your child needs elective surgery and a date has been scheduled. Unlike emergency surgery, an elective procedure isn't done as an immediate matter of life and death. Having an elective procedure gives you the time to prepare your child psychologically for the hospital and the surgery.

Good preparation can help kids feel less anxious about the anesthesia and surgery and get through the recovery period faster. But, like parents everywhere, you're probably uncertain about the best way to prepare your child.

The key is to provide information at your child's level of understanding, correct misunderstandings, and get rid of fears and feelings of guilt. Help your child understand why the surgery is needed and become familiar with the hospital and some of the procedures he or she will undergo.

Kids of all ages cope much better if they have an idea of what's going to happen and why it's necessary. To do that, prepare yourself first and correct any misconceptions of your own. If a parent is anxious and nervous, a child will often reflect these feelings and behaviors as well. It's a good idea to educate yourself, feel comfortable with the process, and make sure all your questions are answered.

Ask Questions

The horror stories you heard from grandparents and parents about traumatic parent/child separations and very limited hospital visiting hours belong to days gone by. Hospitals have changed enormously and have become more family-friendly and patient-centered. For example, many surgeries are now "same-day" procedures requiring no overnight or prolonged stays; most kids are back home, in their own beds, the same night.

Furthermore, most U.S. hospitals permit at least one parent to stay with the child at all times except during the operation. After the surgery, you may return to your child in the recovery room. As your child awakens, he or she will not even realize you left.

Ask the doctors, nurses, or staff for the information you need about what will take place so that you can prepare your child and deal with your own fears or concerns. To parents, one of the most fearful aspects of surgery is anesthesia. Anesthesia is much safer today than in the past, but still carries some risk. You should discuss any concerns you have in advance with the anesthesiologist.

When hospitalization is required overnight or longer, most hospitals avoid separation anxiety by permitting at least one parent to stay with the child day and night. Check with the hospital about its rules regarding parents staying over and when other close family members can visit.

As soon as your child is able, he or she may be playing with other children, toys, and games in a children's recreation room—even if that involves taking along an intravenous (IV) bag on a rolling support.

Explain the Problem

Now that you're more at ease, start preparing your child. Begin by explaining the reason for the surgery in simple, nonthreatening words. Explain—at your child's level of understanding—about the medical problem and why surgery is necessary. Don't use alarming language like "the doctor will cut you," "open you up," or "sew you with a needle." Say that the doctor will fix the problem, and explain that many kids have this problem and must get it fixed at the hospital.

Although they seldom express it, kids may fear that their parents aren't telling them everything—that their health problem is worse than they've been led to believe. To build trust, don't mislead your child—tell as much of the truth as your child can understand.

Handle Fears

Many kids fear that an operation will be painful. It can help to explain that a special doctor, called an anesthesiologist, gives medicine to make patients sleep very deeply so they won't feel anything during the operation and once it's finished, they'll wake up. (Older kids, in particular, need special assurances that they will wake up.)

Again, avoid frightening language—don't say, "You'll be given gas" or "You'll be put to sleep." Young kids may confuse "gas" with the fuel that can poison or kill and "put to sleep" with what can happen to sick pets.

Explain that you'll be there when your child wakes up—and a favorite toy can come along, too. Tell your child that if anything feels sore right after the operation, a doctor or nurse can give medication that will make it feel better.

Common surgery-related fears of young children are the possibility of separation from (or abandonment by) parents and the possibility of pain. School-age kids also fear needles, knives, and damage to their bodies. Give a child this age clear, rational information as well as assurances that the surgery is to fix an existing problem, not create a new one.

The fears of teens go well beyond those of younger kids. Besides pain, change of appearance, and disfigurement, a teen might be afraid of losing control, missing out on events, being embarrassed or humiliated in public, and sounding childish by expressing fear, anxiety, or pain. A teen may also be afraid of waking up during the operation—or not waking up afterward.

Anticipate these fears, then emphasize that expressing fear, anxiety, and response to pain is quite normal (and OK) at any age, even adulthood. Correct any misconceptions about disfigurement or injury. And explain that anesthesia is very safe today and that patients do not wake up during operations but will certainly wake up afterward.

Encourage your teen to read up on the medical condition and share the information with the family. Reading and sharing information is an excellent coping mechanism.

One further fear that affects kids of all ages is being seen naked and having their "private parts" touched. If the operation involves the genital or anal area, your child will cope better if you explain in advance that although it might be embarrassing, doctors and nurses will need to examine these private areas, especially to check if they're healing after the operation. Explain that doctors, nurses, and parents are the only exceptions to the rules about privacy.

Encourage your child's questions about the health problem and hospital experience, so that other fears and anxieties can be expressed. Take all questions seriously and answer them to the best of your ability. If you don't know an answer, tell your child that you'll find it out, and explain that the doctors and nurses are happy to answer questions, too.

Relieve Guilt

Children often believe that their medical problem and operation are really punishments for "being bad." They may not say so, but they may feel guilty and believe that they've brought events on themselves.

Explain that the medical problem is not the result of anything your child may have done or failed to do, and that the operation is not a punishment, but simply the way to "fix" the problem.

On the other hand, if the medical problem was caused by an accident that could have been avoided by obeying safety rules, make sure your child understands the reason for the rules and will follow them in the future.

Explaining What Will Happen

Find books, appropriate to your child's level of understanding, about what to expect at the hospital. Reading together and discussing the surgery will make the hospital seem less threatening. Discuss each idea and encourage your child's questions.

Young kids also will benefit from practicing on a doll or stuffed teddy bear with toy doctor-kit "instruments." Your child can take the toy's "temperature" and "pulse" and listen to its "heartbeat" and "breathing."

Ask your doctor for suggested videos or multimedia tools for parents or kids that can help explain the procedure.

As you discuss the hospital and surgery, remember that in addition to your words, your nonverbal cues convey assurance: Your tone of voice, facial expressions, gestures, and body language send powerful messages. If you appear fearful, your child is likely to feel fearful regardless of the words you use.

Pre-Operative Orientation and Tour

Many hospitals offer special pre-operative children's programs, family orientations, and hospital tours, conducted by specially trained nurses or licensed child-life specialists. Child-life specialists are a valuable resource for parents and children. They are professionals trained to talk to kids and teens about medical procedures, comfort them if they're upset or need extra support, and organize "play time" for hospitalized kids and teens to get together and hang out.

Call the hospital to schedule a pre-operative tour, program, or orientation as soon as possible, even from the doctor's office when the appointment for the surgery is made. It's best to schedule the appointment for a few days before the surgery.

An orientation program can remove the mystery of the surgery for kids and their families by making the hospital familiar and friendly and the experience predictable.

On the Day of Surgery

When you arrive on the day of surgery, your young child can play with toys and books you bring from home or sit on your lap and be cuddled during the waiting time.

You won't be allowed to stay in the operating room during the surgery, but afterward, you'll be escorted to the recovery room to be with your child as he or she awakens. Upon discharge, you'll receive instructions for further recuperation at home and for a follow-up visit to the surgeon.

During recovery, there may be times of discomfort for your child. It can help to explain that your child may be sore or uncomfortable, but will get better.

Distracting your child, whether with a new book or a visit from a relative or friend, also can make recovery more pleasant. Just make sure your child gets plenty of time to rest and recuperate.

Chapter 12

Choosing a Hospital

When you're sick, you may go to the closest hospital or the hospital where your doctor practices. But which hospital is the best for your individual needs? Research now shows that some hospitals do a better job taking care of patients with certain conditions than other hospitals.

When you have a life-threatening emergency, always go to the nearest hospital. However, if you're planning to have surgery, or if you have a condition like heart disease and know you may need hospital care in the future, this information may help you learn about your hospital choices. Understanding your choices will help you have a more informed discussion with your doctor or other health care provider.

Before You Get Started

Make the most of your appointments with your doctor or other health care provider to learn about your condition and health care needs:

- Before your appointment, make a list of things you want to talk about (such as recent symptoms, drug side effects, or other general health questions). Bring this list to your appointment.

Excerpted from "Guide to Choosing a Hospital," by the Centers for Medicare and Medicaid Services (CMS, www.medicare.gov), May 2010.

- Bring any prescription drugs, over-the-counter drugs, vitamins, and supplements to your appointment and review them with your doctor or provider.

- During your appointment, take notes. Then, take a moment to repeat back to the doctor or provider what you were told. Ask any questions you may have.

- Consider bringing along a trusted family member or friend.

- Ask if there's any written information about your condition that you can take with you.

- Call the office if you have questions when you get home.

Learn about the Care You Need and Your Hospital Choices

Talk to your doctor/health care provider about the following:

- Find out which hospitals they work with.

- Ask which hospitals they think give the best care for your condition (for example, have enough staffing, coordinate care, promote medication safety, and prevent infection).

- Ask how well these hospitals check and improve their quality of care.

- Ask if the hospitals participate in Medicare.

- Based on your condition, ask your doctor/health care provider questions such as the following:

  - Which hospitals have the best experience with your condition?

  - Should you consider a specialty hospital, teaching hospital (usually part of a university), community hospital, or one that does research or has clinical trials related to your condition?

  - If you need a surgeon or other type of specialist, what is his or her experience and success treating your condition?

  - Who will be responsible for your overall care while you're in the hospital?

  - Will you need care after leaving the hospital and, if so, what kind of care? Who will arrange this care?

- Are there any alternatives to hospital care?

Think about Your Personal and Financial Needs

Check your hospital insurance coverage:

- Do you need permission from your health plan (like a pre-authorization or a referral) before you're admitted for hospital care?

- If you need care that's not emergency care, do you have to use certain hospitals? Do you have to see certain surgeons or specialists?

- Do you have to pay more to use a hospital (surgeon or specialist) that doesn't participate in your plan?

- Do you need to meet certain requirements to get care after you leave the hospital?

- If you don't have insurance, call the hospital before you're admitted, and ask to speak to someone about setting up a payment plan or other resources to help with payment.

Think about your preferences:

- Do you want a hospital near family members or friends?

- Does the hospital have convenient visiting hours and other rules that are important to you? For example, can a relative or someone helping with your care stay overnight in the room with you?

Find and Compare Hospitals Based on Your Condition and Needs

Use the Hospital Compare web tool at www.hospitalcompare.hhs.gov to do the following and more:

- Find hospitals by name, city, county, state, or ZIP code.

- Check the results of patient surveys (what patients said about their hospital experiences).

- Compare the results of certain measures of quality that show how well these hospitals treat certain conditions.

Search online for other sources to compare the quality of the hospitals you're considering. Some states have laws that require hospitals to report data about the quality and cost of their care and post the data online.

Discuss Your Hospital Options, and Choose a Hospital

- Talk with family members or friends about the hospitals you're comparing.

- Talk to your doctor or health care provider how the hospital information you gathered applies to you.

- Choose the hospital that's best for you.

Hospital Quality Quick Check

Here's a quick summary of what to look for when comparing hospitals. Look for a hospital that:

- has the best experience with your condition;

- checks and improves the quality of its care;

- performs well on measures of quality, including a national patient survey, that are published on the Hospital Compare web tool;

- participates in Medicare;

- meets your needs in terms of location and other factors, like visiting hours;

- is covered by your health plan.

Chapter 13

Choosing Ambulatory Care

Choosing quality health care services for yourself, a family member, or a close friend is one of the most important decisions you will ever make. Knowing what to look for and what to ask will help you choose an ambulatory care organization that provides quality care and best meets your needs—or those of a loved one.

Ambulatory care services include those provided by community health centers, medical practices, outpatient clinics, student health services, urgent/emergency care centers, and specialty services such as cardiac catheterization centers, imaging centers, and surgery centers.

Begin by asking your doctor or insurance case manager to recommend several conveniently located ambulatory care organizations. Visit or call each one and talk with the manager or other staff members about the organization's services, policies, history, and staff credentials. Then use the following questions to determine whether the organization meets your needs.

General Questions

- Does the organization explain your rights and responsibilities as a patient? Ask to see a copy of the organization's patient rights and responsibilities.

"Helping You Choose Quality Ambulatory Care," © The Joint Commission, 2012. Reprinted with permission.

- Do you know the organization's policy regarding visitors? Are family members allowed in the recovery area?

- Does the organization maintain the confidentiality of patient files? How is confidentiality maintained and under what circumstances is specific patient information released?

- Does the organization have a written description of its services and fees? Is the organization able to help you find financial assistance if you need it? Will your insurance company reimburse you for the procedure?

- Is the organization licensed or certified by an appropriate state agency? Is the organization certified by Medicare?

- Is the organization accredited by a nationally recognized accrediting body such as The Joint Commission? Joint Commission accreditation means the organization voluntarily seeks accreditation and meets national health and safety standards.

Questions about Staff Qualifications

- Are the professionals qualified to offer the services and procedures you need? Are the doctors certified by appropriate medical specialty boards? Do the doctors practice at nearby hospitals? Are staff nurses and other personnel trained in emergency services such as cardiopulmonary resuscitation?

- If anesthesia or sedation is necessary for your procedure, are those who will administer it trained or certified?

- If high-tech equipment such as a laser is used in procedures, is staff properly trained to use and care for the equipment?

Questions about Emergency Care

- Does the organization have a 24-hour telephone number you can call if a complication arises after the procedure? Who will answer the phone and what is the procedure for dealing with such emergencies after hours?

- Does the organization have an emergency patient care plan in case of a power failure or a natural disaster? In case of an emergency, will the organization still provide its services?

- Is the organization affiliated with any area hospitals? What is its transfer plan in case of an emergency?

Questions about Your Specific Care

- What is the organization's success record for the specific medical procedure you need? What is the specific training of the doctor who will be performing the procedure? How often is the procedure performed?

- Does the doctor provide you with information about the procedure and its risks?

- Are the doctor and staff receptive to your questions?

To find out if the ambulatory care organization you are considering is accredited by the Joint Commission, see Quality Check at www .qualitycheck.org. Quality Check is a guide to all Joint Commission accredited health care organizations and programs.

Quality Check also provides Quality Reports that include information on the organization's performance and how it compares to other organizations nationwide and statewide. If a report is not available on Quality Check or you would like a printed copy, call the Customer Service Center at 630-792-5800.

Chapter 14

Anesthesia

Chapter Contents

Section 14.1

Anesthesia Basics

Are there different kinds of anesthesia?

There are three main types of anesthesia: Local, regional and general.

Local anesthesia: The anesthetic drug is usually injected into the tissue to numb just the specific location of your body requiring minor surgery, for example, on the hand or foot.

Regional anesthesia: Your anesthesiologist makes an injection near a cluster of nerves to numb the area of your body that requires surgery. You might be awake, or you may be given something to help you relax, sometimes called a sedative. There are several kinds of regional anesthesia. Two of the most frequently used are spinal and epidural anesthesia, which are produced by injections made with great exactness in the appropriate areas of the back. They are frequently preferred for childbirth and prostate surgery.

General anesthesia: You are unconscious and have no awareness or other sensations. There are a number of general anesthetic drugs. Some are gases or vapors inhaled through a breathing mask or tube and others are medications introduced through a vein. During anesthesia, you are carefully monitored, controlled, and treated by your anesthesiologist. A breathing tube may be inserted through your mouth and frequently into the windpipe to maintain proper breathing during this period. The length and level of anesthesia is calculated and constantly adjusted with great precision. At the conclusion of surgery, your anesthesiologist will reverse the process and you will regain awareness in the recovery room.

Is anesthesia safe?

Due to advances in patient safety, the risks of anesthesia are very low. Over the past 25 years, anesthesia-related deaths have decreased from two deaths per 10,000 anesthetics administered to one death per 200,000 to 300,000 anesthetics administered.

Certain types of illnesses, such as heart disease, high blood pressure, and obesity, can increase your anesthesia risks. Even so, anesthesiologists routinely bring even very sick patients through major operations safely.

What are the risks of anesthesia?

All operations and all anesthesia have some risks, and they are dependent upon many factors including the type of surgery and the medical condition of the patient. Fortunately, adverse events are very rare. Your anesthesiologist takes precautions to prevent an accident from occurring.

The specific risks of anesthesia vary with the particular procedure and the condition of the patient. You should ask your anesthesiologist about any risks that may be associated with your anesthesia.

What type of education and training does an anesthesiologist have?

Anesthesiologists have four years of medical school and an additional four of advanced training as in anesthesiology. In addition, some anesthesiologists elect to complete a fellowship and spend an additional year of specialty training in a specific area like pain management, cardiac anesthesia, pediatric anesthesia, neuroanesthesia, obstetric anesthesia, or critical care medicine.

What is the difference between an anesthesiologist and nurse anesthetist?

An anesthesiologist is a physician who specializes in anesthesia care and a nurse anesthetist is a nurse with extra training in administering anesthetics. Both work together on anesthesia care teams, led by anesthesiologists who make critical, medical decisions for patient care.

As physicians, anesthesiologists go through years and years of rigorous training. Anesthesiologists have at least eight years of postgraduate education and training, while nurse anesthetists have two to three years.

Nurse anesthetists are able to perform the technical aspects of the administration of anesthesia, but anesthesiologists have the education, skills, and training to fully manage patients and respond to medical complications.

Should I continue to take my medications prior to surgery?

It is important to tell the doctors providing your care what medications you are taking prior to surgery so that they can be involved in making the decision about stopping or continuing these medications. Some examples of common medications are [the following]:

- Aspirin and Plavix are drugs that are used to prevent blood from clotting. They are used to treat patients with certain disorders of the heart and blood vessels. Because of the way aspirin and Plavix work, they can cause increased bleeding when you get a cut or undergo surgery. If you are taking either of these drugs, you should talk to your primary care physician about stopping them before surgery. The decision to stop aspirin or Plavix is based on the reason why you need to be on the drugs (your medical condition) and on the risk of bleeding from the surgery.

- Diuretics (water pills) are commonly prescribed for treating high blood pressure. This class of drugs can cause changes to electrolyte levels, such as potassium. If you take diuretics, your anesthesiologist may perform certain laboratory testing before surgery.

- Diabetic patients are commonly treated with insulin or oral agents. Your anesthesiologist may decrease your usual morning insulin dose or discontinue your oral agents before surgery. Always speak with an anesthesiologist or your regular doctor to discuss your particular medications, before any surgical procedure.

Could herbal medicines, vitamins, and other dietary supplements affect my anesthesia if I need surgery?

Anesthesiologists are conducting research to determine exactly how certain herbs and dietary supplements interact with certain anesthetics. They are finding that certain herbal medicines may prolong the effects of anesthesia. Others may increase the risks of bleeding or raise blood pressure. Some effects may be subtle and less critical, but for anesthesiologists anticipating a possible reaction is better than reacting to an unexpected condition. So it is very important to tell your doctor about everything you take before surgery.

What happens during a preanesthesia visit with my anesthesiologist?

The preanesthesia visit is an important visit when you will have a chance to learn about your options for anesthesia and to ask questions.

It is also a time when the anesthesia care team can review your medical records, do a focused physical exam, and make decisions about ordering additional tests and consultations.

The interview with the anesthesiologist is a key part of this review. During this interview, the anesthesiologist may ask questions that cover the following:

- Your general health, including any recent changes

- Allergies to medications or other items

- Chronic (long-term) medical problems, such as high blood pressure, heart disease, diabetes, asthma, acid reflux and sleep apnea

- Recent hospital admissions, including surgery or procedures

- Previous experiences with anesthesia, especially any problems

Some people keep their own health records on paper or in an electronic format. To help you answer these questions it is a good idea to bring any documents that describe your health history, as well as a list of all your medications.

When there are different anesthesia alternatives, such as general or regional (nerve block) anesthesia, your anesthesiologist may give you information about these options and then ask about your preferences.

At the conclusion of your visit, you should:

- have clear instructions on when to stop eating and drinking before surgery;

- know what medications you should or should not take on the day of surgery (and sometimes even a few days leading up to surgery);

- know what type of anesthesia will be given to you (keep in mind that things may change between the day of your pre-operative visit and your procedure that result in modifying the anesthesia plan).

How will my anesthesiologist know how much anesthesia to give me?

There is no single or right amount of anesthesia for all patients. Every anesthetic must be tailored to the individual, and to the operation or procedure that the person is having. Individuals have different responses to anesthesia. Some of these differences are genetic, or inborn, and some differences are due to changes in health or illness.

The amount of anesthesia needed can differ according to such things as age, weight, gender, medications being taken, or specific illnesses (such as heart or brain conditions).

Among the things the anesthesiologist measures or observes, and uses to guide the type and amount of anesthetic given are heart rate and rhythm, blood pressure, breathing rate or pattern, oxygen and carbon dioxide levels, and exhaled anesthetic concentration. Because every patient is unique, the anesthesiologist must carefully adjust anesthetic levels for each individual patient.

Why do I need to have an empty stomach prior to surgery?

It is very important that patients have an empty stomach before any surgery or procedure that needs anesthesia. When anesthesia is given, it is common for all the normal reflexes to relax. This condition makes it easy for stomach contents to go backwards into the esophagus (food tube) and mouth or even the windpipe and lungs. Because the stomach contains acid, if any stomach contents do get into the lungs, they can cause a serious pneumonia, called aspiration pneumonitis.

Can I smoke cigarettes before I have surgery?

You should stay off cigarettes for as long as you can before and after surgery. This will help you have the best possible results from your surgery. For example, quitting will reduce the chances you will have problems like a wound infection after the operation. It is especially important that you not smoke the morning of surgery—just like you don't eat the morning of surgery, don't smoke.

Many people find that surgery is also an excellent opportunity to quit smoking for good because most people do not have cravings for cigarettes while in the hospital, and your chances of successfully quitting are almost doubled if you try it around the time of surgery.

What are the different types of sedation?

Sedation allows patients to be comfortable during certain surgical or medical procedures. Sedation can provide pain relief as well as relief of anxiety that may accompany some treatments or diagnostic tests.

During light or moderate sedation, patients are awake and able to respond appropriately to instructions. However, during deep sedation, patients are likely to sleep through a procedure with little or no memory. Breathing can slow and supplemental oxygen is often given during deep sedation.

What is a blood transfusion?

Blood transfusion is an important medical treatment that can save lives. When blood is lost during surgery or from other kinds of trauma, fluids are given to replace the blood. These fluids are essential for the heart and circulation. However, they do not contain essential platelets and proteins that are needed to carry oxygen to tissues, clot when tissues are injured, and fight infection. Only a blood transfusion provides these things.

Who might need a blood transfusion?

Individuals who lose blood during surgery or from other kinds of trauma may need a blood transfusion. In particular, individuals who start off with lower blood counts and those with heart disease, circulation problems, or other major illnesses are more likely to receive a blood transfusion.

Do anesthesiologists administer blood transfusions?

Anesthesiologists administer approximately half the blood transfusions in the United States and are experts in making the risk and benefit assessments needed during a transfusion. Anesthesiologists are committed to the responsible use of the blood supply and to make the best decisions for patients.

How can I help prevent wrong site surgery?

While wrong site surgery is very uncommon, anesthesiologists feel that even one case is too many. The most important things you can do as a patient to prevent wrong site surgery is to make sure your consent form is accurate and to be involved in the process of clearly marking the intended site.

Also, before surgery, there will be a "time out" precaution. While you may be sedated or under anesthesia at this time, all health care providers in the room will stop, pause, and listen while the entire team confirms the correct site.

Should my IV [intravenous] site continue to be sore and swollen weeks after surgery?

Phlebitis is a term that means inflammation of a blood vessel. Phlebitis occurs quite commonly after the insertion of an IV. There is a wide variation because it depends on how phlebitis is defined, such as the place the IV is inserted, the duration that the IV has been in place, the type of material that the IV is made of, the length of the IV catheter, and on the existence of other disorders such as diabetes. If you continue to feel pain and have swelling for more than three weeks you should connect with your physician.

Section 14.2

What Is Anesthesia Awareness?

"Q&A: Anesthesia Awareness During Surgery," © 2012, reprinted with permission from the American Society of Anesthesiologists, 520 N. Northwest Highway, Park Ridge, Illinois, 60068-2573. All rights reserved. For additional information, visit www.lifelinetomodernmedicine.com.

Why does awareness during surgery happen and why are some patients at risk?

Anesthesiologists are committed first and foremost to protecting the life of the patient and making the patient as comfortable as possible. In some high-risk surgeries, such as trauma, cardiac surgery, emergency cesarean delivery, or in situations involving a patient whose condition is unstable, using the usual dose of anesthetic drugs could harm the patient. In these and other critical or emergency situations, there can be a greater risk of awareness during surgery because the patient cannot be put safely into a deeper anesthetic state.

In addition, some patients may react differently to the same level or type of anesthesia. Different medications can mask important signs that anesthesia professionals monitor to help determine the depth of anesthesia. In other rare instances, technical failure or human error may contribute to unexpected episodes of awareness.

What should the patient do before surgery to minimize the risk of intraoperative awareness?

There are several steps the patient should take before surgery to ensure the safest and most comfortable outcome:

- Meet with your anesthesiologist before surgery to discuss all anesthesia options.

- Tell your anesthesiologist about any problems with previous anesthetics, including any history of intraoperative awareness.

- Discuss all medications you are taking, both prescription and over-the-counter. This information is vital to creating an anesthetic plan specifically for your needs.

- If you are concerned about awareness during surgery, tell your anesthesiologist and ask questions about what precautions are taken to avoid it. Don't be afraid to voice your concerns.

What will the anesthesiologist do during surgery to keep the patient safely under general anesthesia?

During surgery, your anesthesiologist will carefully monitor your vital signs, such as your heart rate, breathing rate, and blood pressure to help gauge the depth of anesthesia. In addition, sophisticated technology is available to gauge the presence of anesthetic in the administered gas mixture. Your anesthesiologist may also use brain function monitors intended to measure the depth of anesthesia. The impact of these technologies on the risk of awareness is unclear, so the decision to use them is often made on a case-by-case basis by the anesthesiologist.

No monitor can completely guarantee a patient will not experience awareness during surgery. But you should feel confident relying on your anesthesiologist to guide you safely through your surgery by relying on his or her clinical experience, training, and judgment combined with appropriate technology.

What should I do if I think I have experienced intraoperative awareness?

If you believe you experienced an episode of awareness during surgery, tell your anesthesiologist or another health care professional as soon as you are able. Your anesthesiologist will tell you the events in the operating room and whether any of them would have contributed to awareness. If necessary, you will be referred to a counselor right away to help deal with the feelings associated with awareness. It is important to note that a variety of anesthetic agents are often used, some of which may create false memories or no memory at all of the various events surrounding surgery.

Section 14.3

Anesthesia's Effectiveness Affected by Obesity

Surgery for obese patients presents special challenges for the anesthesiologist. Even simple monitoring tasks, which are essential and life-preserving for all patients, can be a challenge when the patient is significantly overweight. Veins may be harder to locate, finding an appropriate blood pressure cuff to fit the patient's arm may be a challenge, and medication dosing can vary with heavier individuals.

A patient is considered obese if his or her body mass index is greater than 30. Illnesses associated with obesity, such as type 2 diabetes, obstructive sleep apnea, hypertension, and cardiovascular disease, can have serious implications for patients requiring surgery and anesthesia.

In the operating room, obesity-related changes in anatomy make airway management challenging. Airway obstruction due to obstructive sleep apnea can result in decreased airflow and oxygen in patients receiving even minimal amounts of sedation. Placement of a breathing tube (intubation) may require special equipment and techniques. Anesthesiologists have to anticipate these difficulties, prepare for them, and counsel patients regarding potential complications.

Obese patients who are scheduled for surgery should discuss their condition and their options with their physician. In addition, the patient's anesthesiologist can explain the specific risks associated with anesthesia and obesity. Please note, patients who are considering a weight-loss program prior to surgery should discuss it with their physician first to ensure it will not interfere with the course of procedure.

Section 14.4

Medication Use, Anesthesia Response, and Surgery

"Medication and Surgery Before Your Operation,"
reprinted with permission from www.facs.org. © 2012 American
College of Surgeons. All rights reserved.

Your medications may have to be adjusted before your operation. Some medication can affect your recovery and response to anesthesia. Write down all of the mediations you are taking. Make a list.

Your list should include [the following]:

- Any prescription medications

- Over-the-counter (OTC) medications (such as aspirin or Tylenol)

- Herbs, vitamins, and supplements

Tell your doctor if you smoke and how often you drink alcohol or use other recreational drugs.

Check with your doctor about [the following]:

- When to stop taking all vitamins, herbs, and diet supplements: This could be 10 to 14 days before and up to 7 days after your test or operation.

- How to take your medication on the morning of your operation: You may be instructed to take some of your medications even though you won't be able to eat that morning. Take your medications with a sip of water only.

- How to adjust your insulin the morning of your operation since you will not be eating: The doctor who normally manages your insulin often develops the plan for your operation.

- If you need to adjust your medication that affects blood clotting: These drugs may be adjusted up to 7 days before your operation. Your doctor will let you know when to restart taking these drugs.

List of Medications That Affect Blood Clotting

- Antiplatelet medication: Anagrelide (Agrylin), aspirin (any brand, all doses), cilostazol (Pletal), clopidogrel (Plavix), dipyridamole (Persantine), dipyridamole/aspirin (Aggrenox), enteric-coated aspirin (Ecotrin), ticlopidine (Ticlid).

- Anticoagulant medication: Anisindione (Miradon), Arixtra, enoxaparin (Lovenox) injection, Fragmin, heparin injection, Pradaxa, pentosan polysulfate (Elmiron), warfarin (Coumadin), Xarelto.

- Nonsteroidal anti-inflammatory drugs: Celebrex, diclofenac (Voltaren, Cataflam), diflunisal (Dolobid), etodolac (Lodine), fenoprofen (Nalfon), flurbiprofen (Ansaid), ibuprofen (Motrin, Advil, Nuprin, Rufen), indomethacin (Indocin), ketoprofen (Orudis, Actron), ketorolac (Toradol), meclofenamate (Meclomen), meloxicam (Mobic), nabumetone (Relafen), naproxen (Naprosyn, Naprelan, Aleve), oxaprozin (Daypro), piroxicam (Feldene), salsalate (Salflex, Disalcid), sulindac (Clinoril), sulfinpyrazone tolmetin (Tolectin), Trilisate (salicylate combination).

- Herbs/vitamins: Ajoene birch bark, cayenne, Chinese black tree fungus, cumin, evening primrose oil, feverfew, garlic, ginger, ginkgo biloba, ginseng, grape seed extract, milk thistle, omega-3 fatty acids, onion extract, St. John's wort, turmeric, and vitamins C and E.

The above list includes common medications but is not a complete list.

Chapter 15

Substance Use and Surgery

Chapter Contents

Section 15.1

Alcohol
Use and Heart
Surgery

If you are scheduled for surgery, it is important to be honest with your healthcare providers about your alcohol use. Your recovery from surgery may not go as planned if your healthcare providers don't know your history of alcohol use. Please tell your doctor how many drinks you have per day (or per week).

Excessive alcohol use, defined as drinking more than three drinks per day, can affect the outcome of your surgery. Binge drinking (consuming large amounts of alcohol infrequently, such as on weekends) can also affect the outcome of your surgery.

How Does Alcohol Affect My Surgery?

If you drink more than three drinks a day, you could have a complication, called alcohol withdrawal, after surgery. Alcohol withdrawal is a set of symptoms that people have when they suddenly stop drinking after using alcohol for a long period of time. During withdrawal, a person's central nervous system "overreacts" and causes symptoms such as mild shakiness, sweating, hallucinations, and other, more serious, side effects.

Untreated alcohol withdrawal can cause potentially life-threatening complications after surgery, including tremors, seizures, hallucinations, delirium tremens, and even death. Untreated alcohol withdrawal often leads to a longer stay in the intensive care unit (ICU) and a longer hospital stay. Chronic heavy drinking can also interfere with several organ systems and biochemical controls in the body, causing serious, even life-threatening complications.

ne study, more than half of patients who continued smoking after
urgery developed complications, compared with less than 20 percent
f those who quit. Fewer complications means less time in the hospital
nd a quicker recovery.

What risks will I face during surgery if I do not quit smoking?

Smokers require special consideration and treatment when undergo-
ng surgery. The effects of smoking-related diseases increase both anes-
hetic risks, as well as risks of complications during surgery and recovery.
Conversely, anesthesia is safer and more predictable in nonsmok-
rs due to better functioning of the heart, blood vessels, lungs, and
ervous systems.

Why is it so important to anesthesiologists that I quit smoking before my surgery?

Anesthesiologists are the heart and lung specialists in the operat-
ng room who are responsible for the total-body health of patients.
herefore, they directly witness the immense toll smoking takes on a
erson's body and must manage smoking-related complications.
They also witness the tremendous benefits patients experience as a
esult of not smoking before surgery, and are committed to helping all
atients realize these advantages. It is important that your anesthe-
iologist knows about your smoking so that they can take precautions
reduce your risk of having problems.

What is the best way to quit smoking?

When confronted with surgery, many patients decide to take stock
f their lives and change their behaviors. This defining moment is a
reat opportunity to commit to quitting, as it will have a significant
mpact on your quality of life for years to come.
Whether you are preparing for surgery or just thinking about quit-
ng, free help is always available. By calling 800-QuitNow, you can
nnect with trained specialists who will provide advice along with a
stomized plan to help you quit.

Alcohol Withdrawal Treatment before Surgery

Healthcare providers can offer alcohol withdrawal treatment to
help [the following]:

- Decrease postoperative seizures and delirium tremens

- Decrease the use of restraining devices

- Decrease the incidence of patient falls

- Reduce the use of potent sedative medications

- Decrease the length of stay in the hospital

- Decrease the amount of time a mechanical ventilator is needed

- Lower the incidence of organ failure and biochemical
  complications

How Do I Know If I Am at Risk for Alcohol Withdrawal after Surgery?

To be safe and sure, discuss your drinking pattern and any concerns you may have with your primary care physician or your cardiologist.

Section 15.2

Smoking and Surgery

"Q&A: Stop Smoking," © 2012, reprinted with permission from the American Society of Anesthesiologists, 520 N. Northwest Highway, Park Ridge, Illinois, 60068-2573. All rights reserved. For additional information, visit www.lifelinetomodernmedicine.com.

Why should I quit smoking before I have surgery?

By quitting smoking, you will not only reduce the likelihood of experiencing surgery-related complications, but also improve your overall health and even add years to your life. The benefits of quitting smoking include:

- adding six to eight years to your life;
- reducing your risk of lung cancer and heart disease;
- saving an average of $1,400 each year;
- reducing your loved ones' exposure to second-hand smoke.

Why is it especially important to the anesthesiologist that I quit smoking before my surgery?

Anesthesiologists are the heart and lung specialists in the operating room, and they are responsible for the total-body health of patients. Therefore, they directly witness the immense toll smoking takes on a person's body and must manage smoking-related complications.

Anesthesiologists also witness the tremendous benefits patients experience as a result of not smoking before surgery, and are committed to helping all patients realize these advantages. It is important that your anesthesiologist knows about your smoking so he or she can take precautions to reduce your risk of having problems.

How long before my surgery should I quit smoking?

The earlier you quit, the greater your chances are of avoiding surgery-related complications. It is especially important not to smoke on the day of your surgery. Fortunately, the body begins to heal within hours of

quitting. Twelve hours after a person quits, his or her heart a: already begin to function better as nicotine and carbon monoxi drop. It takes less than a day for blood flow to improve, which the likelihood of postoperative complications. We recommend abstain from smoking for as long as possible before and after but even quitting for a brief period is still beneficial.

Is it worth quitting if I decide to do so right before s such as the day before the procedure? Could this ha negative impact on the outcome of my surgery?

There is some misinformation with regard to deciding to q ing right before surgery. There is no data to support the c that quitting too close to surgery may cause additional coug could impact a patient's lung function. There also is no e any other negative effects of quitting too close to surgery. If to quit smoking the morning of surgery, it can still reduce surgical complications.

If my surgery is minimally invasive, do I still need smoking?

Smoking will impact your body before and after surgery re the type of procedure you have. We recommend that all surgi abstain from smoking for as long as possible before and aft

Before surgery, should I also quit smoking additio stances such as marijuana?

It is critical that patients quit smoking all substances before cluding marijuana. They can have the same detrimental effect as nicotine. For example, they can make patients more or less to anesthetics. The carbon monoxide found in any kind of sr blood pressure, making it more difficult for the blood to carry

Please note: Do not be afraid to tell your anesthesiologist been smoking or using other substances before surgery. Th tion will remain confidential and is important to your car

Should I quit smoking permanently, or can I resu ter surgery? How long should I wait after surgery smoking again?

Continuing to smoke after surgery greatly heighten risks of complications, such as infections in the surgical

Chapter 16

Donating Blood for Surgery

Chapter Contents

Section 16.1

Frequently Asked Questions about Blood Donations

How does the blood donation process work?

Donating blood is a simple thing to do, but can make a big difference in the lives of others. The donation process from the time you arrive until the time you leave takes about an hour and 15 minutes. The donation itself is only about 8–10 minutes on average. The steps in the process are:

Registration

1. You will complete donor registration, which includes information such as your name, address, phone number, and donor identification number (if you have one).

2. You will be asked to show a donor card, driver's license, or two other forms of ID.

Health History and Mini Physical

1. You will answer some questions during a private and confidential interview about your health history and the places you have traveled.

2. You will have your temperature, hemoglobin, blood pressure, and pulse checked.

Donation

1. We will cleanse an area on your arm and insert a brand-new, sterile needle for the blood draw. This feels like a quick pinch and is over in seconds.

2. You will have some time to relax while the bag is filling. (For a whole blood donation, it is about 8–10 minutes. If you are donating platelets, red cells, or plasma by apheresis the collection can take up to two hours.)

3. When approximately a pint of blood has been collected, the donation is complete and a staff person will place a bandage on your arm.

Refreshments

1. You will spend a few minutes enjoying refreshments to allow your body time to adjust to the slight decrease in fluid volume.

2. After 10–15 minutes you can then leave the donation site and continue with your normal daily activities.

3. Enjoy the feeling of accomplishment knowing that you have helped to save lives.

Your gift of blood may help up to three people. Donated red blood cells do not last forever. They have a shelf-life of up to 42 days. A healthy donor may donate every 56 days.

What should I do after donating blood?

After you give blood:

- Take the following precautions:

  - Drink an extra four glasses (eight ounces each) of non-alcoholic liquids.

  - Keep your bandage on and dry for the next five hours, and do not do heavy exercising or lifting.

  - If the needle site starts to bleed, raise your arm straight up and press on the site until the bleeding stops.

  - Because you could experience dizziness or loss of strength, use caution if you plan to do anything that could put you or others at risk of harm. For any hazardous occupation or hobby, follow applicable safety recommendations regarding your return to these activities following a blood donation.

  - Eat healthy meals and consider adding iron-rich foods to your regular diet, or discuss taking an iron supplement with your health care provider, to replace the iron lost with blood donation.

113

- If you get a bruise: Apply ice to the area intermittently for 10–15 minutes during the first 24 hours. Thereafter, apply warm, moist heat to the area intermittently for 10–15 minutes. A rainbow of colors may occur for about 10 days.

- If you get dizzy or lightheaded: Stop what you are doing, lie down, and raise your feet until the feeling passes and you feel well enough to safely resume activities.

- And remember to enjoy the feeling of knowing you have helped save lives.

- Schedule your next appointment.

- If this is your first donation, expect your American Red Cross Donor Card in the mail within 6–8 weeks.

Will it hurt when you insert the needle?

Only for a moment. Pinch the fleshy, soft underside of your arm. That pinch is similar to what you will feel when the needle is inserted.

How long does a blood donation take?

The entire process takes about one hour and 15 minutes; the actual donation of a pint of whole blood unit takes 8 to 10 minutes. However, the time varies slightly with each person depending on several factors including the donor's health history and attendance at the blood drive.

How long will it take to replenish the pint of blood I donate?

The plasma from your donation is replaced within about 24 hours. Red cells need about four to six weeks for complete replacement. That's why at least eight weeks are required between whole blood donations.

Why does the Red Cross ask so many personal questions when I give blood?

The highest priorities of the Red Cross are the safety of the blood supply and our blood donors. Some individuals may be at risk of transferring communicable disease through blood donation due to exposure via travel or other activities or may encounter problems with blood donation due to their health. We ask these questions to ensure that it is safe for patients to receive your blood and to ensure that it is safe for you to donate blood that day.

Section 16.2

Autologous and Directed Blood Donations

Autologous Donations

Autologous donations are donations that individuals give for their own use—for example, before a surgery.

Requirements for an Autologous Donation

- Autologous donations require a doctor's prescription.

- You must call 800-RED-CROSS [800-733-2767] to schedule an appointment in advance and request an Autologous Donation form to be signed by your physician.

- You must be in reasonably good health. You will not be allowed to self-donate if you have an active infection and you may not be allowed if you have a heart condition.

- There is no age limitation for autologous donation.

- Unless otherwise directed by a physician, you may safely donate blood every four to seven days and up to three business days before your surgery as long as you meet the donation guidelines.

- You cannot donate within 72 hours of your surgery.

- Acetaminophen (Tylenol), aspirin, and alcohol should be avoided for 48 hours before your donation.

- Your hemoglobin/hematocrit will be checked and must be at a satisfactory level before donating. A physician may prescribe iron supplements to prevent deferral at the donation site, especially if you have been anemic or are making more than one donation.

- If blood loss during your surgery is less than anticipated, transfusing the autologous blood may not be medically necessary. If the donated blood is not used during surgery, it is discarded since current safety standards do not allow its transfusion to other patients.

Directed Donations

A directed donation occurs when a patient's family and friends donate blood for his or her upcoming procedure. A patient must give consent and have his/her physician submit a written request for the Red Cross to collect blood from the selected donors.

Carefully consider the following:

- There is no evidence that patients can select safer donors than the volunteer blood system provides.

- All donated blood products are tested with the same tests for HIV [human immunodeficiency virus] and other infectious diseases, which further enhances the safety of the blood supply.

- Social pressure associated with directed donations may compromise the reliability of the donor's answers to health-history questions

The Red Cross accepts both directed and regular donations and encourages eligible donors to give blood for patients in need.

Chapter 17

Dealing with Preoperative Anxiety

Chapter Contents

Section 17.1

Overview of Relaxation Techniques and How They Alleviate Anxiety

Excerpted from "Relaxation Techniques for Health: An Introduction," by the National Center for Complementary and Alternative Medicine (NCCAM, www.nccam.nih.gov), part of the National Institutes of Health, August 2011.

Relaxation techniques include a number of practices such as progressive relaxation, guided imagery, biofeedback, self-hypnosis, and deep breathing exercises. The goal is similar in all: To consciously produce the body's natural relaxation response, characterized by slower breathing, lower blood pressure, and a feeling of calm and well-being.

Relaxation techniques (also called relaxation response techniques) may be used by some to release tension and to counteract the ill effects of stress. Relaxation techniques are also used to induce sleep, reduce pain, and calm emotions.

About Relaxation Techniques

Relaxation is more than a state of mind; it physically changes the way your body functions. When your body is relaxed breathing slows, blood pressure and oxygen consumption decrease, and some people report an increased sense of well-being. This is called the relaxation response. Being able to produce the relaxation response using relaxation techniques may counteract the effects of long-term stress, which may contribute to or worsen a range of health problems including depression, digestive disorders, headaches, high blood pressure, and insomnia.

Relaxation techniques often combine breathing and focused attention on pleasing thoughts and images to calm the mind and the body. Most methods require only brief instruction from a book or experienced practitioner before they can be done without assistance. These techniques may be most effective when practiced regularly and combined with good nutrition, regular exercise, and a strong social support system.

The relaxation response techniques covered in this text include:

- **Autogenic training:** When using this method, you focus on the physical sensation of your own breathing or heartbeat and picture your body as warm, heavy, and/or relaxed.

- **Biofeedback:** Biofeedback-assisted relaxation uses electronic devices to teach you how to consciously produce the relaxation response. Biofeedback is sometimes used to relieve conditions that are caused or worsened by stress.

- **Deep breathing or breathing exercises:** To relax using this method, you consciously slow your breathing and focus on taking regular and deep breaths.

- **Guided imagery:** For this technique, you focus on pleasant images to replace negative or stressful feelings and relax. Guided imagery may be directed by you or a practitioner through storytelling or descriptions designed to suggest mental images (also called visualization).

- **Progressive relaxation** (also called Jacobson's progressive relaxation or progressive muscle relaxation): For this relaxation method, you focus on tightening and relaxing each muscle group. Progressive relaxation is often combined with guided imagery and breathing exercises.

- **Self-hypnosis:** In self-hypnosis you produce the relaxation response with a phrase or nonverbal cue (called a suggestion). Self-hypnosis may be used to relieve pain (tension headaches, labor, or minor surgery) as well as to treat anxiety and irritable bowel syndrome.

Mind and body practices, such as meditation and yoga are also sometimes considered relaxation techniques.

How Relaxation Techniques May Work

To understand how consciously producing the relaxation response may affect your health, it is helpful to understand how your body responds to the opposite of relaxation—stress.

When you're under stress, your body releases hormones that produce the fight-or-flight response: Heart rate and breathing rate go up and blood vessels narrow (restricting the flow of blood). This response allows energy to flow to parts of your body that need to take action, for example, the muscles and the heart. However useful this response may be in the short term, there is evidence that when your body remains in a stress state for a long time, emotional or physical damage can occur. Long-term or chronic stress (lasting months or years) may reduce your body's ability to fight off illness and lead to or worsen certain health conditions. Chronic stress may lead to high blood pressure, headaches, stomachache, and other symptoms. Stress may worsen certain conditions, such as asthma. Stress also has been linked to depression, anxiety, and other mental illnesses.

In contrast to the stress response, the relaxation response slows the heart rate, lowers blood pressure, and decreases oxygen consumption and levels of stress hormones. Because relaxation is the opposite of stress, the theory is that voluntarily creating the relaxation response through regular use of relaxation techniques could counteract the negative effects of stress.

Section 17.2

Presurgery Program Teaches Anxiety Reduction

"UC Irvine Medical Center Offers 'Mind, Body and Spirit' Program," July 6, 2009. Reprinted with permission from the University of California Medical Center, www.healthcare.uci.edu. © 2009 Regents of the University of California. All rights reserved.

UC Irvine Medical Center now offers patients a one-of-a-kind program called "Preparing for Surgery—Mind, Body, and Spirit" that teaches techniques shown to improve patient outcomes, reduce postoperative pain, and even lower the amount of pain medication needed after surgery.

"Surgery can be a life-altering experience," said Dr. Zeev N. Kain, chair of UC Irvine's Department of Anesthesiology & Perioperative Care and associate dean for clinical research. "Anxiety is connected to and focuses pain, so our goal is to teach patients how to cope with their surgery and reduce anxiety before surgery and pain after surgery."

"This is a unique program. It's not just a lecture about anesthesia and surgery," he said. "It addresses the real mind-body connection and the way a patient experiences pain."

Dr. Abraham Rosenbaum, assistant professor of clinical anesthesiology, and perioperative nurse Karen Bopp lead the twice-monthly sessions at UC Irvine Douglas Hospital. Patients are encouraged to attend a session one to four weeks prior to surgery and to bring a support person, such as a spouse, friend or child. The "Preparing for Surgery—Mind, Body, and Spirit" sessions are free and last about two hours.

Patients scheduled for surgery often experience fear of the unknown and fear of not being in control. "It's natural to feel that way," said Bopp. "Patients need to know what to expect and to understand what things are normal aspects of the surgical process."

The first part of each session addresses events surrounding the surgery, including anesthesia, and provides a general description of events in the operating room. In addition, patients are able to ask questions about their procedures.

In the session's second part, patients are taught such relaxation techniques as yoga breathing, guided imagery, and meditation. The intent is to give them tools to use before and after surgery to reduce their anxiety levels and cope with their stress.

"Research shows that patients have improved outcomes when these approaches—discussing the surgery and learning relaxation techniques—are combined prior to surgery," Kain said.

He has long researched the relationship between anxiety and pain among children undergoing surgery, publishing studies in such journals as *Pediatrics* and *Anesthesiology*. Since leaving Yale University and coming to UCI in 2008, Kain has continued to seek ways to alleviate preoperative anxiety and postoperative pain in all surgical patients.

The results observed in the "Mind, Body, and Spirit" sessions may be used in research designed to further physicians' understanding of how stress and anxiety contribute to pain, said Rosenbaum.

Section 17.3

Hypnosis Helps Reduce Stress Surrounding Surgery

The first task for many psychologists who use hypnosis is telling patients what hypnosis is and what it isn't.

"If you watch hypnosis on TV, the subject always ends up clucking like a chicken, being naked, or assassinating a president," says Eric Willmarth, PhD, founder of Michigan Behavioral Consultants and past president of APA Div. 30 (Society of Psychological Hypnosis).

Even though stage hypnotists and TV shows have damaged the public image of hypnosis, a growing body of scientific research supports its benefits in treating a wide range of conditions, including pain, depression, anxiety, and phobias.

"Hypnosis works and the empirical support is unequivocal in that regard. It really does help people," says Michael Yapko, PhD, a psychologist and fellow of the American Society of Clinical Hypnosis. "But hypnosis isn't a therapy in and of itself. Most people wouldn't regard it that way."

Hypnosis can create a highly relaxed state of inner concentration and focused attention for patients, and the technique can be tailored to different treatment methods, such as cognitive-behavioral therapy. Patients also can become more empowered by learning to hypnotize themselves at home to reduce chronic pain, improve sleep, or alleviate some symptoms of depression or anxiety.

Hypnosis has been used for centuries for pain control, including during the Civil War when Army surgeons hypnotized injured soldiers before amputations. Recent studies have confirmed its effectiveness as a tool to reduce pain. Among the leading researchers in the field is Guy H. Montgomery, PhD, a psychologist who has conducted extensive research on hypnosis and pain management at Mount Sinai School of Medicine, where he is director of the Integrative Behavioral Medicine Program.

In one study, Montgomery and colleagues tested the effectiveness of a 15-minute pre-surgery hypnosis session versus an empathic listening session in a clinical trial with 200 breast cancer patients. In a 2007 article in the *Journal of the National Cancer Institute* (Vol. 99, No. 17), the team reported that patients who received hypnosis reported less post-surgical pain, nausea, fatigue, and discomfort. The study also found that the hospital saved $772 per patient in the hypnosis group, mainly due to reduced surgical time. Patients who were hypnotized required less of the analgesic lidocaine and the sedative propofol during surgery.

"Hypnosis helps patients to reduce their distress and have positive expectations about the outcomes of surgery," Montgomery says. "I don't think there is any magic or mind control."

In a 2009 article in *Health Psychology* (Vol. 28, No. 3), Montgomery and colleagues reported on another study, which found that a combination of hypnosis and cognitive-behavioral therapy could reduce fatigue for breast cancer patients undergoing radiation therapy.

Research has also shown the benefits of hypnosis for burn victims. In a 2007 report in *Rehabilitation Psychology* (Vol. 52, No. 3), Shelley Wiechman Askay, PhD, David R. Patterson, PhD, and colleagues at the University of Washington Medical School found that hypnosis before wound debridements significantly reduced pain reported by patients on one pain rating questionnaire.

No Cure-All

People vary widely in their ability to respond to hypnotic suggestions, a trait which can be measured by standardized scales. But it isn't well understood what causes the varying levels of "hypnotizability" or their significance.

Yapko says few clinicians use hypnotizability scales because responses to a structured test don't predict how a patient will respond to hypnosis in treatment. He served as guest editor for a recent special issue of the *International Journal of Clinical and Experimental Hypnosis* (Vol. 58, No. 2) that examined research on hypnosis and depression. In an editorial, Yapko urged more research and a rejection of outdated views that hypnosis can precipitate suicide or psychosis in depressed patients. Other articles examined how hypnosis can be integrated with cognitive-behavioral therapy or used with depressed patients and their families.

Willmarth says he doesn't always use hypnotizability scales with his patients, but will try a hypnosis session and measure the patient's response to see if it is effective. "You have to be a little bit willing to fail in order to do it often enough to succeed," he says.

Hypnosis may not succeed in all cases and can actually be detrimental in some instances, especially in the realm of retrieving memories.

Joseph P. Green, PhD, a psychology professor at Ohio State University at Lima, has researched how hypnotic suggestions can produce distorted or false memories. He also found that people may believe hypnotically induced memories are more reliable, mirroring a mistaken cultural belief that hypnosis acts like a truth serum. Hypnosis is "on thin ice" when used to recover memories, as is the case with most other memory retrieval techniques, Green says.

Hypnosis got a bad name in the 1990s when some therapists convinced patients they had been molested or abused as children because of hypnotically induced memories, which often had no evidence to support them. As a result, many innocent people were wrongly accused of abuse in hundreds of court cases, Yapko says.

"People didn't really understand the suggestibility of memory," he says. "That whole issue has pretty much fallen by the wayside now" because of advances in research.

In a 2007 decision, the Supreme Court of Canada established a precedent that post-hypnosis evidence is inadmissible in court because of its unreliability. In *R. v. Trochym,* the court overturned a murder conviction after a witness changed her timeline of events following a hypnosis session that was requested by detectives. The jury wasn't told that the witness had been hypnotized or that she had changed her recollection.

"In sum, while it is not generally accepted that hypnosis always produces unreliable memories, neither is it clear when hypnosis results in pseudo-memories or how a witness, scientist, or trier of fact might distinguish between fabricated and accurate memories," the decision stated.

Up in Smoke

Smokers also should be wary of the plethora of hypnosis programs and tapes peddled online with guarantees of instant success. "Despite the widespread use, the science warranting that popularity is suspect," Green says.

Green began studying hypnosis and smoking cessation more than 25 years ago after seeing overblown claims from itinerant hypnotists who held weekend sessions in hotels before moving on to the next town. In an article in the *American Journal of Clinical Hypnosis* (Vol. 52, No. 3), Green and Binghamton University psychology professor

Steven Jay Lynn, PhD, wrote about the body of research on hypnosis and smoking cessation and found mixed results.

In a literature review published in 2000 (*International Journal of Clinical and Experimental Hypnosis,* Vol. 48, No. 2), Green and Lynn analyzed 59 studies on hypnosis and smoking cessation. While hypnosis was more successful than no treatment, it was generally equivalent to other smoking-cessation methods. However, many studies had combined hypnosis with cognitive-behavioral therapy or other treatment methods, so it was impossible to determine the effectiveness of hypnosis alone. Green says hypnosis may help smokers quit, but more research needs to be done. In a 2008 report published by the Cochrane Library, Neil C. Abbot, operations director for ME Research UK, and colleagues examined nine randomized trials and also found insufficient evidence to recommend hypnosis as a specific treatment for smoking cessation.

Learning the Ropes

While more research is being conducted on the benefits of hypnosis, graduate schools are lagging behind in incorporating hypnosis training into psychology programs, say Yapko, Willmarth, and Montgomery. "The universities have really dropped the ball by thinking hypnosis is a side-show rather than being relevant to effective psychotherapy," Yapko says.

Some graduate schools may not be convinced of the effectiveness of hypnosis or the research supporting its use, but other schools have developed clinical hypnosis classes, including Saybrook University's Graduate College of Mind-Body Medicine in San Francisco, where Willmarth teaches a hypnosis course. At Washington State University, psychology professor Arreed Barabasz, PhD, directs the hypnosis laboratory and teaches graduate-level hypnosis courses and research seminars. He also is editor-in-chief of the *International Journal of Clinical and Experimental Hypnosis*.

Since many psychologists have never taken a hypnosis class as part of their education, they often seek training later in their careers. It can be bewildering to find a class, though, since a search for "hypnosis training" generates more than 600,000 hits on Google.

"You can go anyplace on the weekend and get a hypnosis certification," Willmarth says. "You have thousands of lay hypnosis schools that are willing to train anyone who will pay the tuition."

To make sure psychologists don't end up with charlatan teachers, Willmarth recommends courses approved by the American Society of Clinical Hypnosis. ASCH also offers a certification in clinical hypnosis for licensed health-care professionals with at least a master's degree. Certification requires at least 40 hours of ASCH-approved workshop training, 20 hours of individualized training, and two years of independent practice using clinical hypnosis.

Willmarth says interest in clinical hypnosis is growing and more psychologists are learning how hypnosis can help their patients.

"It goes in waves," he says. "Right now, we're on an upswing."

Chapter 18

Understanding Informed Consent

Informed consent involves much more than just reading and signing a piece of paper. Rather, it involves two essential parts: A document and a process.

The informed consent document provides a summary of the clinical trial (including its purpose, the treatment procedures and schedule, potential risks and benefits, alternatives to participation, etc.) and explains your rights as a participant. It is designed to begin the informed consent process, which consists of conversations between you and the research team. If you then decide to enter the trial, you give your official consent by signing the document. You can keep a copy and use it as an information resource throughout the course of the trial.

The informed consent process provides you with ongoing explanations that will help you make educated decisions about whether to begin or continue participating in a trial. Researchers and health professionals know that a written document alone may not ensure that you fully understand what participation means. Therefore, before you make your decision, the research team will discuss with you the trial's purpose, procedures, risks and potential benefits, and your rights as a participant. If you decide to participate, the team will continue to update you on any new information that may affect your situation. Before, during, and even after the trial, you will have the opportunity

Excerpted from "A Guide to Understanding Informed Consent," by the National Cancer Institute (NCI, www.cancer.gov), part of the National Institutes of Health, March 2006. Reviewed by David A. Cooke, MD, FACP, October 10, 2012.

to ask questions and raise concerns. Thus, informed consent is an ongoing, interactive process, rather than a one-time information session.

Myth and Reality

You may find it helpful to confront some of the most common misperceptions about informed consent and clinical trials. Even if these do not represent your thinking about informed consent, they can serve as a helpful reminder of what the process is really about before you go through it.

Myth: Informed consent is designed primarily to protect the legal interests of the research team.

Reality: The purpose of the process is to protect you and other participants by providing access to information that can help you make an informed choice. It also is designed to make you aware of your rights as a participant.

Myth: The most important part of this process is signing the informed consent document.

Reality: Actually, the heart of this process is your ongoing interaction and discussions with the research team and other medical personnel—before, during, and after the trial. The document is designed to get this conversation started.

Myth: My doctor knows best; he or she can tell me whether or not I should consent to participate.

Reality: Your doctor is likely to be a valuable source of advice and information, but only you can make this decision. No one—not even medical experts—can predict whether a treatment, screening, prevention, or supportive care method under evaluation in a trial will prove successful. The informed consent process is designed to help you weigh all of the information and make the right choice for you or your child.

Myth: Once I sign the consent form, I have to enroll and stay enrolled in the trial.

Reality: That's not true. Even after you sign the form, you are free to change your mind and decide not to participate. You also have the right to leave a clinical trial at any time for any reason, without forfeiting access to other treatment.

Myth: Medical personnel are busy, so I can't really expect them to keep me informed as the trial progresses or listen to my questions.

Reality: The research team has a duty to keep you informed, make sure that you understand the information they provide, and answer your questions. If you ever feel that you are not getting what you need, do not hesitate to speak up. You will be given the name and phone number of a key contact person who can answer your questions throughout the course of the trial. Keep in mind that people like you are making this research possible through their willingness to participate.

A Checklist of Questions to Ask the Research Team

The following questions deal with many of the areas that should be covered in the informed consent document. To double-check that you have all the information you need, consider bringing this checklist to a meeting with the research team. You also may wish to fill it out as you read the informed consent document, both to ensure your own understanding of the trial and to create a ready reference written in your own words. Many of these questions are specific to treatment trials, but the checklist still should prove useful if you are considering a prevention, screening, or supportive care trial.

The Study

1. What is the purpose of the study?

2. Why do researchers think the approach may be effective?

3. Who will sponsor the study?

4. Who has reviewed and approved the study?

5. How are study results and safety of participants being checked?

6. How long will the study last?

7. What will my responsibilities be if I participate?

8. Whom can I speak with about questions I have during and after the trial? To find out the study results?

9. What steps will be taken to protect my privacy and the confidentiality of my medical records?

Possible Risks and Benefits

1. What are my possible short-term benefits?

2. What are my possible long-term benefits?

3. What are my short-term risks, such as side effects?

4. What are my possible long-term risks?

5. What other options do people with my risk of cancer or type of cancer have?

6. How do the possible risks and benefits of this trial compare with those options?

Participation and Care

1. What kinds of therapies, procedures, and /or tests will I have during the trial?

2. Will they hurt, and if so, how long?

3. How do the tests in the study compare with those I would have outside of the trial?

4. Will I be able to take my regular medications while in the clinical trial?

5. Where will I have my medical care?

6. Will I have to be hospitalized? If so, how often and for how long?

7. Who will be in charge of my care?

8. What type of follow-up care is part of the study?

Personal Issues

1. How could being in the study affect my daily life?

2. Can I talk to other people in the study?

Cost Issues

1. Will I have to pay for any part of the trial such as tests or the study drug?

2. If so, what will the charges likely be?

3. What is my health insurance likely to cover?

4. Who can help answer any questions from my insurance company or health plan?

5. Will there be many travel or child care costs that I need to consider while I am in the trial?

Chapter 19

Ensuring Patient Safety

Chapter Contents

Section 19.1

Twenty Tips to Prevent Medical Errors

"20 Tips to Help Prevent Medical Errors," by the Agency for Healthcare Research and Quality (AHRQ, www.ahrq.gov), September 2011.

One in seven Medicare patients in hospitals experience a medical error. But medical errors can occur anywhere in the health care system: In hospitals, clinics, surgery centers, doctors' offices, nursing homes, pharmacies, and patients' homes. Errors can involve medicines, surgery, diagnosis, equipment, or lab reports. They can happen during even the most routine tasks, such as when a hospital patient on a salt-free diet is given a high-salt meal.

Most errors result from problems created by today's complex health care system. But errors also happen when doctors and patients have problems communicating. These tips tell what you can do to get safer care.

The best way you can help to prevent errors is to be an active member of your health care team. That means taking part in every decision about your health care. Research shows that patients who are more involved with their care tend to get better results.

Medicines

1. Make sure that all of your doctors know about every medicine you are taking. This includes prescription and over-the-counter medicines and dietary supplements, such as vitamins and herbs.

2. Bring all of your medicines and supplements to your doctor visits. "Brown bagging" your medicines can help you and your doctor talk about them and find out if there are any problems. It can also help your doctor keep your records up-to-date and help you get better quality care.

3. Make sure your doctor knows about any allergies and adverse reactions you have had to medicines. This can help you to avoid getting a medicine that could harm you.

4. When your doctor writes a prescription for you, make sure you can read it. If you cannot read your doctor's handwriting, your pharmacist might not be able to either.

5. Ask for information about your medicines in terms you can understand—both when your medicines are prescribed and when you get them:

    • What is the medicine for?

    • How am I supposed to take it and for how long?

    • What side effects are likely? What do I do if they occur?

    • Is this medicine safe to take with other medicines or dietary supplements I am taking?

    • What food, drink, or activities should I avoid while taking this medicine?

6. When you pick up your medicine from the pharmacy, ask: Is this the medicine that my doctor prescribed?

7. If you have any questions about the directions on your medicine labels, ask. Medicine labels can be hard to understand. For example, ask if "four times daily" means taking a dose every 6 hours around the clock or just during regular waking hours.

8. Ask your pharmacist for the best device to measure your liquid medicine. For example, many people use household teaspoons, which often do not hold a true teaspoon of liquid. Special devices, like marked syringes, help people measure the right dose.

9. Ask for written information about the side effects your medicine could cause. If you know what might happen, you will be better prepared if it does or if something unexpected happens.

Hospital Stays

10. If you are in a hospital, consider asking all health care workers who will touch you whether they have washed their hands. Handwashing can prevent the spread of infections in hospitals.

11. When you are being discharged from the hospital, ask your doctor to explain the treatment plan you will follow at home. This includes learning about your new medicines, making

sure you know when to schedule follow-up appointments, and finding out when you can get back to your regular activities. It is important to know whether you should keep taking the medicines you were taking before your hospital stay. Getting clear instructions may help prevent an unexpected return trip to the hospital.

Surgery

12. If you are having surgery, make sure that you, your doctor, and your surgeon all agree on exactly what will be done. Having surgery at the wrong site (for example, operating on the left knee instead of the right) is rare. But even once is too often. The good news is that wrong-site surgery is 100 percent preventable. Surgeons are expected to sign their initials directly on the site to be operated on before the surgery.

13. If you have a choice, choose a hospital where many patients have had the procedure or surgery you need. Research shows that patients tend to have better results when they are treated in hospitals that have a great deal of experience with their condition.

Other Steps

14. Speak up if you have questions or concerns. You have a right to question anyone who is involved with your care.

15. Make sure that someone, such as your primary care doctor, coordinates your care. This is especially important if you have many health problems or are in the hospital.

16. Make sure that all your doctors have your important health information. Do not assume that everyone has all the information they need.

17. Ask a family member or friend to go to appointments with you. Even if you do not need help now, you might need it later.

18. Know that "more" is not always better. It is a good idea to find out why a test or treatment is needed and how it can help you. You could be better off without it.

19. If you have a test, do not assume that no news is good news. Ask how and when you will get the results.

20. Learn about your condition and treatments by asking your doctor and nurse and by using other reliable sources. For example, treatment options based on the latest scientific evidence are available from the Effective Health Care website (www.effectivehealthcare.ahrq.gov/options). Ask your doctor if your treatment is based on the latest evidence.

Section 19.2

Ten Things You Can Do to Be a Safe Patient

"Patient Safety: Ten Things You Can Do to Be a Safe Patient,"
by the Centers for Disease Control and Prevention (CDC, www.cdc.gov),
February 3, 2011.

You go to the hospital to get well, right? Of course, but did you know that patients can get infections in the hospital while they are being treated for something else? Here are 10 things you can do to be a safe patient.

Do you plan to go to the hospital today for an emergency? No one does. Imagine a scenario like the following:

- Your mother starts having chest pain.

- Your son breaks his ankle during football practice.

- Your spouse is in a car accident.

You rush to the hospital.

Thankfully, you are told that your loved one is going to recover, but will spend some time in the hospital. However, extra time in the hospital can also put patients at risk for a healthcare-associated infection (HAI), such as a blood, surgical site, or urinary tract infection.

Every day, patients get infections in healthcare facilities while they are being treated for something else. These infections can have devastating emotional, financial, and medical effects. Worst of all, they can be deadly.

Healthcare procedures can leave you vulnerable to germs that cause HAIs. These germs can be spread in healthcare settings from patient to patient on unclean hands of healthcare personnel or through the improper use or reuse equipment.

These infections are not limited to hospitals. For example, in the past 10 years alone, there have been more than 30 outbreaks of hepatitis B and hepatitis C in non-hospital healthcare settings such as outpatient clinics, dialysis centers, and long-term care facilities.

Fortunately, the solution is clear. To prevent HAIs, everyone—you, your healthcare providers, and your visitors—should follow infection prevention procedures as described below.

What can you do as a patient or loved one of a patient? Here are 10 ways to be a safe patient:

1. Speak up. Talk to your doctors about any worries you have about your safety and ask them what they are doing to protect you.

2. Keep hands clean. If you do not see your providers clean their hands, please ask them to do so. Also remind your loved ones and visitors. Washing hands can prevent the spread of germs.

3. Ask if you still need a central line catheter or urinary catheter. Leaving a catheter in place too long increases the chances of getting an infection.

4. Ask your healthcare provider, "Will there be a new needle, new syringe, and a new vial for this procedure or injection?" Healthcare providers should never reuse a needle or syringe on more than one patient.

5. Be careful with medications. Avoid taking too much medicine by following package directions. Also, to avoid harmful drug interactions, tell your doctor about all the medicines you are taking.

6. Get smart about antibiotics. Help prevent antibiotic resistance by taking all your antibiotics as prescribed, and not sharing your antibiotics with other people. Remember that antibiotics don't work against viruses like the ones that cause the common cold.

7. Prepare for surgery. There are things you can do to reduce your risk of getting a surgical site infection. Talk to your doctor to learn what you should do to prepare for surgery. Let your doctor know about other medical problems you have.

8. Watch out for *C. diff* (aka *Clostridium difficile*). Tell your doctor if you have severe diarrhea, especially if you are also taking an antibiotic.

9. Know the signs and symptoms of infection. Some skin infections, like MRSA, appear as redness, pain, or drainage at an IV catheter site or surgical incision site, and a fever. Tell your doctor if you have these symptoms.

10. Get your flu shot. Protect yourself against the flu and other complications by getting vaccinated.

By following these 10 steps you can help make healthcare safer and help prevent healthcare-associated infections.

Section 19.3

Wrong-Site Surgery: Help Avoid Mistakes in Your Surgery

"Speak Up: Help Avoid Mistakes in Your Surgery," © The Joint Commission, 2009. Reprinted with permission.

Mistakes can happen during surgery. Surgeons can do the wrong surgery. They can operate on the wrong part of your body. Or they can operate on the wrong person. Hospitals and other medical facilities that are accredited by The Joint Commission must follow a procedure that helps surgeons avoid these mistakes. (Facilities that are accredited by The Joint Commission are listed on The Joint Commission's Quality Check website: www.qualitycheck.org.)

Mistakes can also happen before or after surgery. A patient can take the wrong medicine. Or they don't understand the instructions about how to take care of themselves. As a patient, you can make your care safer by being an active, involved, and informed member of your health care team.

Preparing for Your Surgery

Ask your doctor:

- Are there any prescription or over-the-counter medicines that you should not take before your surgery?

- Can you eat or drink before your surgery?

- Should you trim your nails and remove any nail polish?

- If you have other questions, write them down.

Take your list of questions with you when you see your doctor. Ask someone you trust to:

- take you to and from the surgery facility;

- be with you at the hospital or surgery facility.

This person can make sure you get the care you need to feel comfortable and safe.

Before You Leave Home

- Shower and wash your hair. Do not wear make-up. Your caregivers need to see your skin to check your blood circulation.

- Leave your jewelry, money, and other valuables at home.

At the Surgery Facility

The staff will ask you to sign an Informed Consent form. Read it carefully. It lists:

- your name;

- the kind of surgery you will have;

- the risks of your surgery;

- that you talked to your doctor about the surgery and asked questions;

- your agreement to have the surgery.

Make sure everything on the form is correct. Make sure all of your questions have been answered. If you do not understand something on the form—speak up.

For your safety, the staff may ask you the same question many times. They will ask:

- who you are;

- what kind of surgery you are having;

- the part of your body to be operated on.

They will also double-check the records from your doctor's office.

Before Your Surgery

- A health care professional will mark the spot on your body to be operated on. Make sure they mark only the correct part and no-where else. This helps avoid mistakes.

- Marking usually happens when you are awake. Sometimes you cannot be awake for the marking. If this happens, a family member or friend or another health care worker can watch the marking. They can make sure that your correct body part is marked.

- Your neck, upper back, or lower back will be marked if you are having spine surgery. The surgeon will check the exact place on your spine in the operating room after you are asleep.

- Ask your surgeon if they will take a time out just before your surgery. This is done to make sure they are doing the right surgery on the right body part on the right person.

After Your Surgery

- Tell your doctor or nurse about your pain. Hospitals and other surgical facilities that are accredited by The Joint Commission must help relieve your pain.

- Ask questions about medicines that are given to you, especially new medicines. What is it? What is it for? Are there any side effects? Tell your caregivers about any allergies you have to medicines. If you have more questions about a medicine, talk to your doctor or nurse before taking it.

- Find out about any IV (intravenous) fluids that you are given. These are liquids that drip from a bag into your vein. Ask how long the liquid should take to run out. Tell the nurse if it seems to be dripping too fast or too slow.

- Ask your doctor if you will need therapy or medicines after you leave the hospital.

- Ask when you can resume activities like work, exercise, and travel.

Chapter 20

What Medicare Covers If You Are Having Surgery

If you're enrolled in Original Medicare, finding out if Medicare will cover a service or supply that you need isn't always easy. Generally, Medicare covers services (such as lab tests, surgeries, and doctor visits) and supplies (like wheelchairs and walkers) that Medicare considers medically necessary to treat a disease or condition. What Medicare covers may be based on several factors, such as the following:

- Federal laws describing Medicare benefits, or state laws that tell what services a particular type of practitioner is licensed to provide

- National coverage decisions made by Medicare about whether a particular item or service is covered nationally under Medicare's rules

- Local coverage decisions made by local companies in each state that process claims for Medicare

These companies decide whether an item or service is medically necessary and should be covered in that area under Medicare's rules.

There may be other coverage rules and policies that also apply. Some services may only be covered when provided in certain settings or covered for patients with certain conditions. For example, some surgeries, such as organ transplants, can only be done in certain approved

Excerpted from "Learning What Medicare Covers and How Much You Pay," by the Centers for Medicare and Medicaid Services (CMS, www.medicare.gov), October 2010.

hospitals. If you're in a Medicare Advantage Plan or Other Medicare Plan, you may have different rules, but your plan must give you at least the same coverage as Original Medicare.

Where can I learn more about what Medicare covers?

1. Talk to your doctor or other health care provider about why you need the service or supply and ask whether he or she thinks Medicare will cover it. Your doctor or provider knows more than anyone about your individual medical needs.

2. Check your *Medicare & You* handbook mailed to you each fall.

3. Call 800-MEDICARE to see if they have information on any related local or national coverage policies.

If there is a service or supply that Medicare usually covers that your doctor, health care provider, or supplier thinks Medicare won't cover in your specific case, he or she must give you a Medicare notice, such as an Advance Beneficiary Notice of Non coverage, and ask you to sign it. Read this notice carefully to understand your options and payment responsibilities. You'll be asked if you want to get the items or services listed on the notice and you will have to pay for them if Medicare doesn't.

I'm having surgery. How do I find out how much I'll have to pay?

For surgeries or procedures, it may be difficult to know the exact costs in advance because no one can tell you with certainty the amount or type of services you will need. For example, if you experience complications during surgery, your costs could be higher. If you're having surgery or a procedure, there are some things you can do in advance to determine approximately what your share of the cost may be:

*   Ask the doctor or health care provider if they can tell you how much the surgery or procedure will cost and how much you'll have to pay. Learn how Medicare covers inpatient versus outpatient hospital services. Visit http://go.usa.gov/im9 to view or print the publication, Are You a Hospital Inpatient or Outpatient? If you have Medicare—Ask! You can also call 800-MEDICARE (800-633-4227) for a free copy. TTY users should call (877-486-2048).

- Look at your last Medicare Summary Notice to see if you met the deductible for Part A (Hospital Insurance) if you expect to be admitted to the hospital, or the deductible for Part B (Medical Insurance) for a doctor's visit and other outpatient care. You will need to pay the deductible amounts before Medicare will start to pay. After Medicare starts to pay, you may have copayments for the care you get.

- Check with any other insurance you may have such as Medigap (Medicare Supplement Insurance), Medicaid, or an employer retiree insurance plan, to see what they will pay. If you belong to a Medicare Health Plan, contact the plan for more information.

- Call the hospital or facility and ask them to tell you the copayment for the specific surgery or procedure the doctor is planning. It's important to remember that if you need other unexpected services, your costs may be higher.

- Ask your doctor, surgeon, or other health care provider, or their staff what kind of care or services you may need after your surgery or procedure and how much you'll have to pay.

Chapter 21

Advanced Care Planning

What is an advance directive?

Advance directive is a general term that describes two types of legal documents:

- Living will
- Healthcare power of attorney

These documents allow you to instruct others about your future healthcare wishes and appoint a person to make healthcare decisions if you are not able to speak for yourself. Each state regulates the use of advance directives differently.

What is a living will?

A living will allows you to put in writing your wishes about medical treatments for the end of your life in the event that you cannot communicate these wishes directly. Different states name this document differently. For example, it may be called a directive to physicians, healthcare declaration, or medical directive. Regardless of what it is called, its purpose is to guide your family and doctors in deciding about the use of medical treatments for you at the end of life.

Excerpted from "End of Life Decisions," © 2008 National Hospice and Palliative Care Organization. © 2011 Revised. All rights reserved. Reprinted with permission. For the complete text of this booklet, and additional information, visit www .caringinfo.org.

Your legal right to accept or refuse treatment is protected by the Constitutions and case law.

However, your state law may define when the living will goes into effect, and may limit the treatments to which the living will applies. You should read your state's document carefully to ensure that it reflects your wishes. You can add further instructions or write your own living will to cover situations that the state suggested document might not address. Even if your state does not have a living will law, it is wise to put your wishes about the use of life-sustaining medical treatments in writing as a guide to healthcare providers and loved ones.

What is the difference between a will, a living trust, and a living will?

A will (last will and testament) and living trusts are both financial documents; they allow you to plan who receives your financial assets and property. A living will deals with medical issues while you are alive. It allows you to express your preferences about your medical care at the end of life.

Wills and living trusts are complex legal instruments, for which you will need and want legal advice to complete them. Although a living will is a legal document, you do not need a lawyer to complete it.

What is a healthcare power of attorney?

This can also be called a healthcare proxy, appointment of a healthcare agent, or durable power of attorney for healthcare. The person you appoint may be called your healthcare agent, surrogate, attorney-in-fact, or healthcare proxy. The person you appoint usually is authorized to deal with all medical situations when you cannot speak for yourself. Thus, he or she can speak for you if you become temporarily incapacitated—after an accident, for example—as well as if you become permanently incapacitated because of illness or injury.

What is the difference between financial power of attorney, a financial durable power of attorney, and a healthcare power of attorney?

A financial power of attorney and a financial durable power of attorney are both legal documents that let you appoint someone to make financial decisions for you. A power of attorney is effective only while you still handle your own finances, whereas a durable power of attorney remains valid even after you have lost the ability to make financial decisions due to illness and injury.

A healthcare power of attorney (which in some states is called a durable power of attorney for medical or healthcare) only permits the appointed person to make medical decisions for you if you cannot make those decisions yourself. It does not authorize the person to handle your financial affairs, and normally does not empower him or her to make decisions while you can still make them.

Generally, the law requires your agent to make the same medical decisions that you would have made, if possible. To help your agent do this, it is essential that you discuss your values about the quality of life that is important to you and the kinds of decisions you would make in various situations. These discussions along with a living will will help your agent to form a picture of your views regarding the use of medical treatments.

Why bother with an advance directive if I want my family to make the necessary decisions for me?

Depending on your state's laws, your family might not be allowed to make decisions about life sustaining treatment for you without a living will stating your wishes. Some states' laws do permit family members to make all medical decisions for their incapacitated loved ones.

However, other states require clear evidence of the person's own wishes or a legally designated decision maker.

Even in states that do permit family decision-making, you should still prepare advance directives for three reasons:

- You can name the person with whom you are most comfortable (this person does not need to be a family member) to make sure your wishes are honored.

- Your living will makes your specific wishes known.

- It is a gift to loved ones faced with making decisions about your care.

Should I prepare a living will and also use a medical power of attorney to appoint an agent?

Yes, each document offers something the other does not. Together they provide the best insurance that your wishes will be honored.

Benefits of appointing a healthcare agent: The person who you appoint as your agent can respond as your care needs and conditions changes in a way that no document can. In addition, you are legally authorizing that person to make decisions based not only on what you expressed in writing or verbally, but also on the knowledge of you as a person.

Benefits of having a living will: If your agent must decide whether or not to begin, continue or discontinue medical treatment, your living will can reassure your agent that he or she is following your wishes. Further, if the person you appointed as an agent is unavailable or unwilling to speak for you, or if other people challenge a decision about medical treatments, your living will can guide your caregivers.

What if I do not have anyone to appoint as my agent?

If you do not have anyone to appoint as your agent, it is especially important that you complete a clear living will and that you talk about it with anyone who might be involved with your healthcare. This might include family members, even if you do not want them to be your agent.

It also could include social workers, spiritual caregivers, visiting nurses, or aids who are helping you in some way. You should discuss it with any physicians that you see regularly and give them a copy to put in your medical record. If you are admitted to a hospital or long-term care facility, you should have a copy of your living will made a part of your medical record.

When will my advance directive go into effect?

Your advance directive becomes legally valid as soon as you sign them in front of the required witnesses. However, they normally do not go into effect unless you are unable to make your own decisions. Each state establishes its own guidelines for when an advance directive becomes active. The rules may differ for living wills and healthcare power of attorney, as described below.

Living will: In most states, before your living will can guide medical decision making, two physicians must certify that you are unable to make medical decisions and that you are in the medical conditions specified in the state's living will law (such as terminal illness or permanent unconsciousness). Other requirements may also apply, depending upon the state.

Healthcare power of attorney: Most healthcare power of attorneys go into effect when your physician concludes that you are unable to make your own decisions. If you regain the ability to make decisions, your agent cannot continue to act for you. Many states have additional requirements that apply only to decisions about life-sustaining medical treatments.

Will my advance directive be honored if I am in an accident or experience a medical crisis at home and emergency technicians are called?

In these emergency situations, unless you are able to speak for yourself emergency personnel are obligated to do what is necessary to stabilize a person for transfer to a hospital, both from accident sites and from a home or other facility. After a physician fully evaluates the person's condition and determines the underlying conditions, an advance directive can be implemented.

Emergency medical technicians cannot honor living wills or healthcare power of attorneys. However, in many localities, the specific crisis of cardiac arrest/respiratory arrest is addressed by a document called a non-hospital Do-Not-Resuscitate Order. These non-hospital DNR orders instruct emergency personnel not to perform cardiopulmonary resuscitation (CPR).

These are physician orders that apply to situations in which the person's heart has stopped beating or breathing has stopped. For all other conditions, emergency medical technicians are still required to treat and transport the person to the nearest hospital for evaluation by a physician. If you wish to find out whether non-hospital DNR orders are available in your locality, contact your local emergency medical services or department of health.

Will my advance directive be honored in another state?

The answer to this question varies from state to state. Some states do honor an advance directive from another state; others will honor out-of-state documents to the extent they match the state's own law; and some states do not address the issue.

If you spend a significant amount of time in more than one state, it is recommended that you complete an advance directive for all the states involved. It will be easier to have your advance directive honored if they are the ones with which the medical facility is familiar.

How can I change what is in my advance directive?

If you want to change anything in an advance directive once you have completed it, you should complete a new document. For this reason you should review your advance directive periodically to endure that the forms still reflect you wishes.

Must my advance directive be witnessed?

Yes, every state has some type of witnessing requirement. Most require two adult witnesses; some also require a notary. Some states give you the option of having two witnesses or a notary alone as a witness. The purpose of witnessing is to confirm that you really are the person who signed the document, you were not forced to sign it, and you appeared to understand what you were doing. The witnesses do not need to know the content of the document.

Generally, a person you appoint as your agent or alternative agent cannot be a witness. In some states your witnesses cannot be any relatives by blood or marriage, or anyone who would benefit from your estate. Some states prohibit your doctor and employees of a healthcare institution in which you are a resident from acting as a witness. To ensure it is done correctly read the instructions carefully to see who can and cannot be a witness on your state-specific form.

What should I do with my completed advance directive?

Make several photocopies of the completed documents. Keep the original documents in a safe but easily accessible place, and tell others where you put them; you can note on the photocopies the locations where the originals are kept. Do not keep your advance directive in a safe deposit box. Other people may need access to them.

Give photocopies to your agent and alternate agent. Be sure your doctors have copies of your advance directives and give copies to everyone who might be involved with your healthcare, such as your family, clergy, or friends. Your local hospital might also be willing to file your advance directive in case you are admitted in the future. If you have surgery or are being admitted to a hospital, bring a copy with you and ask for it to be placed in your medical record.

Do healthcare providers run any legal risk by honoring advance directives?

No. Most advance directives statutes state explicitly that providers run no legal risk for honoring valid advance directives.

What if my healthcare provider will not honor my advance directive?

In many states, healthcare providers can refuse to honor an advance directive for ethical, moral, or religious reasons. For this reason, it is important to ask in advance if a healthcare provider has personal views or if an institution has any policy that would prevent them from honoring a person's treatment choices. If you know that your personal doctor is unable or unwilling to carry out your wishes, it would be wise to change to a physician who will respect them.

Who would make decisions about my medical care if I did not complete an advance directive?

There is not a simple answer to this question. In general, physicians consult with families when the person cannot make decisions. A number of states have passed surrogate decision making statutes. These laws create a decision-making process by identifying the individuals who may make decisions for a person who has no advance directive.

Is there a federal law about advance directives?

Yes, the Patient Self-Determination Act (PSDA) is a federal law regarding advance directives. It requires medical facilities that receive Medicaid and Medicare funds to have procedures for handling a person's advance directive, and to tell individuals upon admission about their rights under state law to use advance directives. The PSDA does not set standards for what an advance directive must say; it does not require facilities to provide advance directive forms; and it does not require people to have an advance directive. Rather PSDA's purpose is to make people aware of their rights.

Can I state my wishes about organ donation, cremation, or burial in my advance directive?

Several states permit you to indicate your wishes regarding organ donation. In those states that do not specifically address the issues of organ donation you may state your wishes in your advance directive. However, you should consider expressing your wishes through a form designed for that purpose. You should also make your family aware of your wishes. Since your advance directive and the authority of your agent technically ceases upon your death, you should tell your wishes about cremation or burial to your family or the executor of your estate.

Part Three

Common Types
of Surgery and Surgical
Procedures

Chapter 22

Head and Neck Surgery

Chapter Contents

Section 22.1

Treating Head and Neck Cancer

Excerpted from "Head and Neck Cancers,"
by the National Cancer Institute (NCI, www.cancer.gov),
part of the National Institutes of Health, April 17, 2012.

Cancers that are known collectively as head and neck cancers usually begin in the squamous cells that line the moist, mucosal surfaces inside the head and neck (for example, inside the mouth, the nose, and the throat). These squamous cell cancers are often referred to as squamous cell carcinomas of the head and neck. Head and neck cancers can also begin in the salivary glands, but salivary gland cancers are relatively uncommon. Salivary glands contain many different types of cells that can become cancerous, so there are many different types of salivary gland cancer.

Cancers of the head and neck are further categorized by the area of the head or neck in which they begin.

Cancers of the brain, the eye, the esophagus, and the thyroid gland, as well as those of the scalp, skin, muscles, and bones of the head and neck, are not usually classified as head and neck cancers.

How are head and neck cancers treated?

The treatment plan for an individual patient depends on a number of factors, including the exact location of the tumor, the stage of the cancer, and the person's age and general health. Treatment for head and neck cancer can include surgery, radiation therapy, chemotherapy, targeted therapy, or a combination of treatments.

The patient and the doctor should consider treatment options carefully. They should discuss each type of treatment and how it might change the way the patient looks, talks, eats, or breathes.

What are the side effects of treatment?

Surgery for head and neck cancers often changes the patient's ability to chew, swallow, or talk. The patient may look different after surgery, and the face and neck may be swollen. The swelling usually goes away within a few weeks. However, if lymph nodes are removed, the flow of lymph in the area where they were removed may be slower and lymph could collect in the tissues, causing additional swelling; this swelling may last for a long time.

After a laryngectomy (surgery to remove the larynx) or other surgery in the neck, parts of the neck and throat may feel numb because nerves have been cut. If lymph nodes in the neck were removed, the shoulder and neck may become weak and stiff.

Patients who receive radiation to the head and neck may experience redness, irritation, and sores in the mouth; a dry mouth or thickened saliva; difficulty in swallowing; changes in taste; or nausea. Other problems that may occur during treatment are loss of taste, which may decrease appetite and affect nutrition, and earaches (caused by the hardening of ear wax). Patients may also notice some swelling or drooping of the skin under the chin and changes in the texture of the skin. The jaw may feel stiff, and patients may not be able to open their mouth as wide as before treatment.

Patients should report any side effects to their doctor or nurse, and discuss how to deal with them.

Section 22.2

Brain Surgery

Brain surgery is a procedure to treat problems in the brain and the surrounding structures.

Description

Before surgery, the hair on part of the scalp is shaved, and the area is cleaned. The doctor makes a surgical cut through the scalp. The location of this cut depends on where the problem in the brain is located.

The surgeon creates a hole in the skull and removes a piece, called a bone flap.

If possible, the surgeon will make a smaller hole and insert a tube with a light and camera on the end. This is called an endoscope. The surgery will be done with tools placed through the endoscope. MRI [magnetic resonance imaging] or CT [computed tomography] can help guide the doctor to the proper place in the brain.

During surgery, your surgeon may:

- clip off an aneurysm to prevent blood flow;
- remove a tumor or a piece of tumor for a biopsy;
- remove abnormal brain tissue;
- drain blood or an infection.

The bone flap is usually replaced after surgery, using small metal plates, sutures, or wires. The bone flap may not be put back if your surgery involved a tumor or an infection, or if the brain was swollen. (This is called a craniectomy.)

The time it takes for the surgery depends on the problem being treated.

Why the Procedure Is Performed

Brain surgery may be done if you have:

- a brain tumor;

- bleeding (hemorrhage) in the brain;

- blood clots (hematomas) in the brain;

- weaknesses in blood vessels;

- abnormal blood vessels in the brain (arteriovenous malformations [AVMs]);

- damage to tissues covering the brain (dura);

- infections in the brain (brain abscesses);

- severe nerve or face pain (such as trigeminal neuralgia or tic douloureux);

- skull fracture;

- pressure in the brain after an injury or stroke;

- epilepsy;

- certain brain diseases (such as Parkinson disease) that may be helped with an implanted electronic device.

Risks

Risks for any anesthesia are:

- reactions to medications;

- problems breathing.

Possible risks of brain surgery are:

- Surgery on any one area may cause problems with speech, memory, muscle weakness, balance, vision, coordination, and other functions. These problems may last a short while or they may not go away.

- Blood clot or bleeding in the brain

- Seizures

- Stroke

- Coma

- Infection in the brain, in the wound, or in the skull

- Brain swelling

Before the Procedure

Your doctor will examine you, and may order laboratory and X-ray tests.

Always tell your doctor or nurse:

- if you could be pregnant;
- what drugs you are taking, even drugs, supplements, vitamins, or herbs you bought without a prescription;
- if you have been drinking a lot of alcohol;
- if you take aspirin or anti-inflammatory drugs such as ibuprofen;
- if you have allergies or reactions to medications or iodine.

During the days before the surgery:

- You may be asked to stop taking aspirin, ibuprofen, warfarin (Coumadin), and any other drugs that make it hard for your blood to clot.
- Ask your doctor which drugs you should still take on the day of the surgery.
- Always try to stop smoking. Ask your doctor for help.
- Your doctor or nurse may ask you to wash your hair with a special shampoo the night before surgery.

On the day of the surgery:

- You will usually be asked not to drink or eat anything for 8 to 12 hours before the surgery.
- Take the drugs your doctor told you to take with a small sip of water.
- Your doctor or nurse will tell you when to arrive at the hospital.

After the Procedure

After surgery, you'll be closely monitored by your health care team to make sure your brain is working properly. The doctor or nurse may ask you questions, shine a light in your eyes, and ask you to do simple tasks. You may need oxygen for a few days.

The head of your bed will be kept raised to help reduce swelling of your face or head, which is normal.

Medicines will be given to relieve pain.

You will usually stay in the hospital for three to seven days. You may need physical therapy (rehabilitation).

Outlook (Prognosis)

How well you do after brain surgery depends on the condition being treated, your general health, which part of the brain is involved, and the specific type of surgery.

Section 22.3

Ear Tube Surgery for Ear Infections

"Middle Ear Infections and Ear Tube Surgery," October 2011, reprinted with permission from www.kidshealth.org. This information was provided by KidsHealth®, one of the largest resources online for medically reviewed health information written for parents, kids, and teens. For more articles like this, visit www.KidsHealth.org, or www.TeensHealth.org. Copyright © 1995–2012 The Nemours Foundation. All rights reserved.

Why Surgery?

Many kids get middle ear infections (otitis media, or OM), usually between the ages of 6 months and 2 years.

Some kids are particularly susceptible because of environmental and lifestyle factors (like attendance at a group childcare, secondhand tobacco smoke exposure, and taking a bottle to bed).

Although these infections are relatively easy to treat, a child who has multiple ear infections that do not get better easily or has evidence of hearing loss or speech delay may be a candidate for ear tube surgery.

During this surgery, small tubes are placed in the eardrums to ventilate the area behind the eardrum and keep the pressure equalized to atmospheric pressure in the middle ear.

About Otitis Media

The middle ear is an air-filled cavity located behind the eardrum. When sound enters the ear, it makes the eardrum vibrate, which in turn makes tiny bones in the middle ear vibrate. This transmits sound signals to the inner ear, where nerves relay the signals to the brain.

A small passage leading from the middle ear to the back of the nose—called the eustachian tube—equalizes the air pressure between the middle ear and the outside world. (When your ears pop while yawning or swallowing, the eustachian tubes are adjusting the air pressure in the middle ears.)

Infection

Bacteria or viruses can enter the middle ear through the eustachian tube and cause an infection—this often occurs when a child has had a cold or other respiratory infection. When the middle ear becomes infected, it may fill with fluid or pus, particularly if the infection is bacterial.

Pressure from this buildup pushes on the eardrum and causes pain, and because the eardrum cannot vibrate, the child may experience a temporary decrease in hearing.

With treatment, a bacterial infection can be quickly cleared up. In most kids the fluid will resolve over time and hearing will be restored. Some research suggests that long periods of hearing loss in young children can lead to delays in speech development and learning.

Symptoms and Diagnosis

Symptoms of otitis media include:

- pulling or rubbing the ears because of ear pain;
- fever;
- fussiness or irritability;
- fluid leaking from the ear;
- changes in appetite or sleeping patterns;
- trouble hearing.

Call your doctor if you think your child has an ear infection. He or she will perform a physical examination and look at your child's eardrums. If the doctor suspects a bacterial infection (often based on the presence of pus behind the eardrum), he or she may elect to wait and see if the immune system will clear the infection without the use of antibiotics.

If symptoms persist (fever and pain) for more than 48 hours, then antibiotics may be prescribed. This is important to know since unnecessary use of antibiotics can lead to resistant bacteria.

In some instances, the doctor will insert a needle through the eardrum to remove a sample of the pus from the middle ear for a laboratory culture. Called a tympanocentesis, this procedure can help the doctor decide which antibiotic to use.

Treatment

Although ear tube surgery is a relatively common procedure, surgery is not the first choice of treatment for otitis media. Antibiotics are often used to treat bacterial ear infections but many ear infections are viral and cannot be treated with antibiotics. These infections need to get better on their own, and only time can help them heal.

But if your child has frequent ear infections that don't clear up easily or a hearing loss or speech delay, the doctor may suggest surgery to drain fluid from the middle ear and insert a ventilation tube.

Because most kids have had infections in both ears, surgery is often done in both; this is called a bilateral myringotomy, or BMT. A tiny tube, called a pressure equalization (PE) or tympanostomy tube, is inserted into the eardrum to ventilate and equalize pressure in the middle ear. This will help to prevent future infections and the accumulation of fluid, and will help normalize hearing.

The presence of the tiny hole in the eardrum from the tube doesn't impair hearing (in fact, kids with a speech or language delay from hearing loss often will see a normalization of their hearing). Depending on the type used, the tube remains in place for about 6 months to 18 months or more.

Tympanostomy Tube Surgery

If your child is old enough to understand what surgery is, talk about what happens during ear tube surgery:

- Because your child will receive general anesthesia, the surgery will be performed in a hospital so that an anesthesiologist can monitor your child. The procedure takes about 10 to 15 minutes.

- The surgeon will make a small hole in the eardrum and remove fluid from the middle ear using suction. Because the surgeon can reach the eardrum through the ear canal, there is no visible incision or stitches.

- The surgeon will finish by inserting a small metal or plastic tube into the hole in the eardrum.

Afterward, your child will wake up in the recovery area. In most cases, the total time spent in the hospital is a few hours. Very young children or those with significant medical problems may stay longer.

After Surgery

A tympanostomy tube helps prevent recurring ear infections by allowing air into the middle ear. Other substances, including water, may sometimes enter through the tube, but this is rarely a problem. Your surgeon might recommend earplugs for regular bathing or swimming.

In most cases, surgery to remove a tympanostomy tube isn't necessary. The tube usually falls out on its own, pushed out as the eardrum heals. A tube generally stays in the ear anywhere from 6 months to 18 months, depending on the type of tube used.

If the tube remains in the eardrum beyond two to three years, however, it probably will be removed surgically to prevent a perforation in the eardrum or accumulation of debris around the tube.

Although effective in reducing chronic ear infections, ear tubes are not always a permanent cure for otitis media. Up to 25% of kids who need ear tubes before the age of 2 may need them again.

Section 22.4

Cochlear Implant Surgery

"Cochlear Implants," by the National Institute on Deafness
and Other Communication Disorders (NIDCD, www.nidcd.nih.gov),
part of the National Institutes of Health, March 2011.

What is a cochlear implant?

A cochlear implant is a small, complex electronic device that can help to provide a sense of sound to a person who is profoundly deaf or severely hard-of-hearing. The implant consists of an external portion that sits behind the ear and a second portion that is surgically placed under the skin. An implant has the following parts:

- A microphone, which picks up sound from the environment

- A speech processor, which selects and arranges sounds picked up by the microphone

- A transmitter and receiver/stimulator, which receive signals from the speech processor and convert them into electric impulses

- An electrode array, which is a group of electrodes that collects the impulses from the stimulator and sends them to different regions of the auditory nerve

An implant does not restore normal hearing. Instead, it can give a deaf person a useful representation of sounds in the environment and help him or her to understand speech.

How does a cochlear implant work?

A cochlear implant is very different from a hearing aid. Hearing aids amplify sounds so they may be detected by damaged ears. Cochlear implants bypass damaged portions of the ear and directly stimulate the auditory nerve. Signals generated by the implant are sent by way of the auditory nerve to the brain, which recognizes the signals as sound. Hearing through a cochlear implant is different from normal hearing and takes time to learn or relearn. However, it allows many people to recognize warning signals, understand other sounds in the environment, and enjoy a conversation in person or by telephone.

How does someone receive a cochlear implant?

Use of a cochlear implant requires both a surgical procedure and significant therapy to learn or relearn the sense of hearing. Not everyone performs at the same level with this device. The decision to receive an implant should involve discussions with medical specialists, including an experienced cochlear-implant surgeon. The process can be expensive. For example, a person's health insurance may cover the expense, but not always. Some individuals may choose not to have a cochlear implant for a variety of personal reasons. Surgical implantations are almost always safe, although complications are a risk factor, just as with any kind of surgery. An additional consideration is learning to interpret the sounds created by an implant. This process takes time and practice. Speech-language pathologists and audiologists are frequently involved in this learning process. Prior to implantation, all of these factors need to be considered.

Section 22.5

Sinus Surgery

"Endoscopic Sinus Surgery," by Marc Dubin, MD, Jivianne Lee, MD, Troy D. Woodard, MD, and Sarah K. Wise, MD, revised April 2012. © American Rhinologic Society (www.american-rhinologic.org). Reprinted with permission.

Sinus surgery has truly evolved in the last several years. This procedure was once performed through external incisions (incisions on the face and in the mouth), required extensive nasal packing, caused significant patient discomfort, and was often followed by a lengthy recovery. With recent advances in technology, including the nasal endoscope, this procedure is now commonly performed without incisions and entirely through the nose. The nasal endoscope is a small lighted metal telescope placed into the nostril, which allows the surgeon to visualize the nose and sinuses. In current practice, endoscopic sinus surgery usually requires minimal nasal packing and is associated with relatively mild pain and short recovery times.

What are the indications for sinus surgery?

The most common indication for endoscopic sinus surgery is chronic rhinosinusitis. Chronic rhinosinusitis is a term applied to various nasal processes which involve inflammation of the nose and sinuses that do not adequately improve with medical management.

Less common indications include (but are not limited to): Recurrent infections (rather than chronic inflammation), complications of sinus infections, nasal polyps, mucoceles, chronic sinus headaches, impaired sense of smell, tumors of the nasal and sinus cavities, cerebrospinal fluid leaks, nasolacrimal duct obstruction, choanal atresia, and the need to decompress the orbit. Additionally, recent advances in endoscopic techniques allow your sinus surgeon to provide access to areas of the brain and pituitary gland for neurosurgeons, or to the orbits (eye sockets) for certain ophthalmology procedures.

169

What therapies should be attempted prior to sinus surgery?

Prior to undergoing endoscopic sinus surgery, patients should talk with their physicians to make sure that all reasonable medical options have been exhausted.

This list of medications that have been recommended for the treatment of sinusitis is quite long. They include both prescription and hundreds of over-the-counter treatments located at your local pharmacy. For acute sinusitis (an infection that typically occurs after a cold and lasts less than four weeks), antibiotics are the main treatment. In addition, nasal saline irrigations or spray are another treatment with little risk and may be added to an antibiotic regimen. While nasal decongestant sprays (pseudoephedrine or oxymetazoline) can be used to improve nasal stuffiness, they should not be used longer than three days, as there is a risk of developing dependence and experiencing rebound stuffiness. In addition, people that have high blood pressure, glaucoma, urinary retention, heart disease, and heartbeat irregularities should consult their doctor before using medicines because they can exacerbate these illnesses.

As an infection progresses beyond four weeks to become a more chronic illness, treatments may change. Antibiotics that cover more types of bacteria may be utilized for longer than the typical 10–14 days. Steroid sprays to decrease inflammation and oral steroids (i.e., prednisone) may also be used. If sinus infections progress longer than four weeks, your physician may order a CT (CAT, or computed tomography) scan of your sinuses and obtain a culture of nasal mucus to help choose the appropriate antibiotic.

Allergy medications (antihistamines, nasal steroids, nasal antihistamine sprays, allergy shots) have a role in treating allergy, which is one of the major causes of nasal swelling. If someone does not have allergies, these treatments are of little benefit (with the possible exception of nasal steroids).

What are the benefits of endoscopic sinus surgery?

If medical options have been unsuccessful in managing your symptoms, endoscopic sinus surgery may have tangible benefits. The overall goal of sinus surgery is to improve the drainage pathway of the sinuses. By opening the natural drainage pathway of the diseased sinus, the frequency, duration, and severity of infections should be reduced.

Although there are patients who have mechanical obstruction due to their particular anatomy, many patients have an intrinsic problem with the lining (mucous membrane) of their nose and sinuses. While the patients with mechanical obstruction, will receive the maximal benefit from surgery (i.e., fixing the plumbing problem), the benefit for patients with mucous membrane disease is also tangible because the larger opening created during surgery will allow better drainage and more medication and rinses to get into the sinuses and help treat the diseased lining.

One of the most important benefits of surgery is the ability to deliver medications (e.g., sprays, rinses, nebulized drugs) to the lining of your sinuses after they have been opened. Therefore, surgery is an adjunct to, not a replacement for, proper medical management.

It is important to note, however, that if you are one of the patients who have diseased mucous membranes or form nasal polyps, no amount of surgery can change this fact. So although surgery plays a role in managing the disease, it may not cure sinus disease with polyps or other types of chronic inflammation. Therefore, it should be emphasized that surgery is not a cure for sinusitis but is one of the multiple steps in managing your disease.

Does anything need to be done in preparation for my sinus surgery?

It is generally recommended that patients avoid any medications that may exacerbate bleeding, such as aspirin and ibuprofen products. In addition, certain vitamins, herbal remedies, and spices including vitamin E, garlic, ginger, gingko, and ginseng may increase your bleeding risk. Some patients may be asked to take antibiotics and/or steroids (i.e., prednisone) to decrease some of the swelling. This will vary greatly from patient to patient and surgeon to surgeon, so if you have any questions about which medications you should or should not take, you must ask your surgeon.

How is endoscopic sinus surgery performed?

Endoscopic sinus surgery may be performed under local or general anesthesia. The procedure involves the use of a small telescope (nasal endoscope) that is inserted into the nasal cavity through the nostril to visualize your nose and sinuses. The goal of the surgery is to identify the narrow channels that connect the paranasal sinuses to the nasal cavity, enlarge these areas, and improve the drainage from the sinuses into the nose.

Most people have four sinuses on each side of their face, for a total of eight sinuses. These are the maxillary, ethmoid, sphenoid, and frontal sinuses. The maxillary sinuses are in your cheek, the ethmoids are between your eyes, the sphenoid sinuses are almost exactly in the center of your head, and the frontal sinuses are in your forehead. It is possible that you may not have all of these sinuses due to developmental differences from person to person, or they may have already been opened by previous procedures.

Sinusitis may affect some or all of your sinuses. Your symptoms, endoscopic exam, and CT scan will determine which sinuses need to be opened.

Sometimes sinus surgery may require simultaneous repair of the nasal septum, which divides the two sides of the nose, or the turbinates, which filter and humidify air inside of the nose.

What is the recovery after endoscopic sinus surgery?

The use of nasal packing will depend on the extent of surgery and the preference of your surgeon. The recovery period will also vary depending on the extent of surgery but postoperative discomfort, congestion, and drainage should significantly improve after the first few postoperative days, with mild symptoms sometimes lingering several weeks after the surgery.

How are the results of endoscopic sinus surgery?

Endoscopic sinus surgery generally yields excellent results, and significant symptomatic improvement is achieved in the vast majority of patients.

What is sinuplasty (or balloon sinuplasty)?

Sinuplasty refers to a procedure, or specifically a surgical device that was developed by a specific device manufacturer. This device is similar to balloon angioplasty, the technology that expands the vessels in someone's heart. These balloons are advanced into the opening of a patient's sinuses and are expanded to open the narrowed channels. Sinuplasty may also be used in conjunction with more traditional endoscopic sinus surgery techniques.

Like all medical advances, the information in the popular press may not reflect reality. Although useful, this new technology is not for everyone, and in many cases is not a substitute for standard techniques. However, in some people it is a technique that may decrease recovery time. Only with a thorough examination, in conjunction with a CT scan, can this be determined by your surgeon.

What are the potential complications of sinus surgery?

Adverse events are rare but may include postoperative bleeding, orbital (visual or eye) complications, complications from the general anesthetic, cerebrospinal fluid leaks, and intracranial complications such as meningitis. However, it is important to realize that chronic sinus infections are located directly beneath the skull base and adjacent to the eye and the failure to treat this problem without surgery may lead to dire consequences, such as involvement of the eye or brain.

What are the alternatives?

Continuing medical therapy alone and avoiding surgery is always an alternative. Medical therapy is chiefly antibiotics and/or steroids along with other medications. As with any surgery, you should feel more than comfortable seeking a second opinion from another surgeon.

What is endoscopic skull base surgery?

Over the course of the last 5 to 10 years, lesions that involve the areas of the skull base and brain that are adjacent to the nose and sinuses have been removed via the nostril, without facial incisions. Using cameras and video equipment similar to that utilized for sinus surgery, these tumors can be removed without facial incisions. Because this technique may be significantly less painful, requires less traction on the brain, and necessitates a shorter hospital stay it is an attractive option for some patients and tumors. It must be emphasized that this technique is not for all patients or tumors, however.

Section 22.6

Adenoidectomy

Often, tonsils and adenoids are surgically removed at the same time. Although you can see the tonsils at the back of the throat, adenoids aren't directly visible. A doctor has to use a telescope to get a peek at them. As an alternative, an X-ray of the head can give the doctor an idea of the size of someone's adenoids.

So, what are adenoids anyway? They're a mass of tissue in the passage that connects the back of the nasal cavity to the throat. By producing antibodies to help the body fight infections, adenoids help to control bacteria and viruses that enter through the nose.

In kids, adenoids usually shrink after about five years of age and often practically disappear by the teen years.

Symptoms of Enlarged Adenoids

Because adenoids trap germs that enter the body, adenoid tissue can temporarily swell as it tries to fight off an infection. These symptoms are often associated with enlarged adenoids:

- Difficulty breathing through the nose

- Breathing through the mouth

- Talking as if the nostrils are pinched

- Noisy breathing

- Snoring

- Stopped breathing for a few seconds during sleep (sleep apnea)

- Frequent "sinus" symptoms

- Ongoing ear middle ear infections or middle ear fluid in a school-aged child

If enlarged adenoids are suspected, the doctor may ask about and then check your child's ears, nose, and throat, and feel the neck along the jaw. To get a really close look, the doctor might order one or more X-rays. For a suspected infection, the doctor may prescribe oral antibiotics.

When Is Surgery Necessary?

If enlarged or infected adenoids keep bothering your child and are not controlled by medication, the doctor may recommend surgically removing them with an adenoidectomy. This may be recommended if your child has one or more of the following:

- Difficulty breathing

- Sleep apnea

- Recurrent infections

- Ear infections, middle ear fluid, and hearing loss requiring a second or third set of ear tubes

Having your child's adenoids removed is especially important when repeated infections lead to sinus and ear infections. Badly swollen adenoids can interfere with the ability of the middle ear space to stay ventilated. This can sometimes lead to infections or middle ear fluid causing a temporary hearing loss. So kids whose infected adenoids cause frequent earaches and fluid buildup might also need an adenoid-ectomy at the time of their ear tube surgery.

And although adenoids can be taken out without the tonsils, if your child is having tonsil problems, they may be removed at the same time. A tonsillectomy with an adenoidectomy is the most common pediatric operation.

What Happens during Surgery?

Surgery, no matter how common or simple the procedure, can be frightening for both kids and parents. You can help prepare your child for surgery by talking about what to expect. During the adenoidectomy:

- Your child will receive general anesthesia. This means the surgery will be performed in an operating room so that an anesthesiologist can monitor your child.

- Your child will be asleep for about 20 minutes.

- The surgeon can get to the tonsils and/or the adenoids through your child's open mouth—there's no need to cut through skin.

- The surgeon removes the adenoids and then cauterizes (or seals) the blood vessels.

Your child will wake up in the recovery area. In most cases, the total time in the hospital is less than five hours. Very young children and those who are significantly overweight, or have a chronic disease such as seizure disorders or cerebral palsy, may need to stay overnight for observation.

The typical recuperation after an adenoidectomy often involves several days of moderate pain and discomfort.

In less than a week after surgery, everything should return to normal. The adenoid area will heal naturally, which means there are no stitches to worry about. There's a small chance any tissue that's left behind can swell, but it rarely causes new problems.

After surgery, a child's symptoms usually disappear immediately, unless there's a lot of swelling that could lead to some temporary symptoms.

Even though some kids need surgery, remember that enlarged adenoids are normal in others. If your child's adenoids aren't infected, the doctor may choose to wait to operate because the adenoids may eventually shrink on their own as adolescence approaches.

Section 22.7

Tonsillectomy

Everybody's heard of tonsils. But not everyone knows what tonsils do or why they may need to be removed. Knowing the facts can help alleviate the fears of both parents and kids facing a tonsillectomy.

Tonsils and Tonsillitis

Tonsils are clumps of tissue on both sides of the throat that help fight infections.

Tonsils may swell when they become infected (tonsillitis). If you look down your child's throat with a flashlight, the tonsils may be red and swollen or have a white or yellow coating on them. Other symptoms of tonsillitis can include:

- sore throat;
- pain or discomfort when swallowing;
- fever;
- swollen glands (lymph nodes) in the neck.

Enlarged tonsils without any symptoms are common among kids. Left alone, enlarged tonsils may eventually shrink on their own over the course of several years.

Don't rely on your own guesses, though—it can be hard to judge whether tonsils are infected. If you suspect tonsillitis, contact your doctor. Recurrent sore throats and infections should also be evaluated by the doctor, who may order a throat culture to check for strep throat.

About Tonsillectomies

Doctors might recommend surgical removal of the tonsils, called a tonsillectomy, for a child who has one or more of the following:

- Persistent or recurrent tonsillitis or strep infections
- Swollen tonsils that make it hard to breathe, particularly during sleep
- Difficulty eating meat or chewy foods
- Sleep difficulty that might be affecting the child's daily activities
- Snoring and obstructive sleep apnea (when someone stops breathing for a few seconds at a time during sleep because enlarged tonsils are partially blocking the airway)

Surgery, no matter how common or simple the procedure, is often frightening for kids and parents. You can help prepare your child for surgery by talking about what to expect. During the tonsillectomy:

- Your child will receive general anesthesia. This means the surgery will be performed in an operating room so that an anesthesiologist can monitor your child.
- The operation will take about 20 to 30 minutes.
- The surgeon can get to the tonsils through your child's open mouth—there's no need to cut through skin.

Your child will wake up in the recovery area. Expect to spend about five hours or a bit longer at the hospital. Most kids go home on the same day, though some may require observation overnight. In general, kids under three years old and those with chronic disease will usually stay overnight for observation.

Rarely, children may show signs of bleeding, which would require a return to the operating room.

Depending on the surgical technique, the typical recuperation after a tonsillectomy may take several days to a week or more. Expect some pain and discomfort due to the exposure of the throat muscles after the tonsils are removed. This can affect your child's ability to eat and drink and return to normal activities.

Intracapsular tonsillectomy, a variation on traditional tonsillectomy techniques, is surgery in which all involved tonsil tissue is removed but a small layer of tonsil tissue is left in place to protect the underlying throat muscles. As a result, the recovery is much faster because most kids experience less pain, don't need as much strong pain medication, and are more willing to eat and drink. Additionally, the risk of bleeding after surgery is significantly less than with a traditional tonsillectomy. Since residual tonsil tissue remains, there is a very slight chance that it can re-enlarge or become infected and require more tonsil surgery, but this occurs in less than 1% of children undergoing intracapsular tonsillectomy.

Section 22.8

Thyroid Surgery

What Is the Thyroid Gland?

The thyroid gland is a butterfly-shaped endocrine gland that is normally located in the lower front of the neck. The thyroid's job is to make thyroid hormones, which are secreted into the blood and then carried to every tissue in the body. Thyroid hormone helps the body use energy, stay warm, and keep the brain, heart, muscles, and other organs working as they should.

General Information

Thyroid operations are advised for patients who have a variety of thyroid conditions, including both cancerous and benign (non-cancerous) thyroid nodules, large thyroid glands (goiters), and over-active thyroid glands.

There are several thyroid operations that a surgeon may perform, including:

- excisional biopsy—removing a small part of the thyroid gland (rarely in use today);
- lobectomy—removing half of the thyroid gland;
- removing nearly all of the thyroid gland (subtotal thyroidec-tomy—leaving a small amount of thyroid tissue bilaterally or

near-total thyroidectomy—leaving about one gm or cm of thyroid tissue on one side); or

- total thyroidectomy, which removes all identifiable thyroid tissue.

There are specific indications for each of these operations. The main risks of a thyroid operation involve possible damage to important structures near the thyroid, primarily the parathyroid glands (which regulate calcium levels) and the recurrent and external laryngeal nerves (which control the vocal cords).

Questions and Considerations

When thyroid surgery is recommended, patients should ask several questions regarding the surgery including:

1. Why do I need an operation?
2. Are there other means of treatment?
3. How should I be evaluated prior to the operation?
4. How do I select a surgeon?
5. What are the risks of the operation?
6. How much of my thyroid gland needs to be removed?
7. What can I expect once I decide to proceed with surgery?
8. Will I lead a normal life after surgery?

Why do I need an operation?

The most common reason for thyroid surgery is to remove a thyroid nodule, which has been found to be suspicious through a fine needle aspiration biopsy. Surgery may be recommended for the following biopsy results:

- Cancer (papillary cancer)
- Possible cancer (follicular neoplasm)
- Inconclusive biopsy

Surgery may be also recommended for nodules with benign biopsy results if the nodule is large, if it continues to increase in size, or if it is causing symptoms (pain, difficulty swallowing, etc.).

Surgery is also an option for the treatment of hyperthyroidism, for large and multinodular goiters, and for any goiter that may be causing symptoms.

Are there other means of treatment?

Surgery is definitely indicated to remove nodules suspicious for thyroid cancer. In the absence of a possibility of thyroid cancer, there may be nonsurgical options of therapy depending on the diagnosis. You should discuss other options for therapy with your physician.

How should I be evaluated prior to the operation?

As for other operations, all patients considering thyroid surgery should be evaluated preoperatively with a thorough and comprehensive medical history and physical exam, including cardiopulmonary (heart) evaluation. An electrocardiogram and a chest X-ray prior to surgery are often recommended for patients who are over 45 years of age or who are symptomatic from cardiac disease. Blood tests may be performed to determine if a bleeding disorder is present. Any patients who have had a change in voice or who have had a previous neck operation should have their vocal cord function evaluated preoperatively. This is necessary to determine whether the recurrent laryngeal nerve that controls the vocal cord muscles is functioning normally. Finally, if medullary thyroid cancer is suspected, patients should be evaluated for coexisting adrenal tumors (pheochromocytomas) and for hypercalcemia and hyperparathyroidism.

How do I select a surgeon?

In general, thyroid surgery is best performed by a surgeon who has received special training and who performs thyroid surgery on a regular basis. The complication rate of thyroid operations is lower when the operation is done by a surgeon who does a considerable number of thyroid operations each year. Patients should ask their referring physician where he or she would go to have a thyroid operation or where he or she would send a family member.

What are the risks of the operation?

The most serious possible risks of thyroid surgery include:

- bleeding that can cause acute respiratory distress;
- injury to the recurrent laryngeal nerve that can cause permanent hoarseness; and

- damage to the parathyroid glands that control calcium levels in the body, causing hypoparathyroidism and hypocalcemia.

These complications occur more frequently in patients with invasive tumors or extensive lymph node involvement, in patients requiring a second thyroid surgery, and in patients with large goiters that go below the collarbone.

Overall the risk of any serious complication should be less than 2%. However, the risk of complications discussed with the patient should be the particular surgeon's risks rather than that quoted in the literature. Prior to surgery, patients should understand the reasons for the operation, the alternative methods of treatment, and the potential risks and benefits of the operation (informed consent).

How much of my thyroid gland needs to be removed?

Your surgeon should explain the planned thyroid operation, such as lobectomy or total thyroidectomy, and the reasons why such a procedure is recommended. For patients with papillary or follicular thyroid cancer many, but not all, surgeons recommend total or near total thyroidectomy when they believe that subsequent treatment with radioactive iodine might be beneficial. For patients with large (>1.5 cm) or more aggressive cancers and for patients with medullary thyroid cancer, more extensive lymph node dissection is necessary to remove possibly involved lymph node metastases.

Thyroid lobectomy may be recommended for overactive one-sided nodules or for benign one-sided nodules that are causing symptoms such as compression, hoarseness, shortness of breath, or difficulty swallowing. A total or near-total thyroidectomy may be recommended for patients with Graves' disease or for patients with enlarged multinodular goiters.

What can I expect once I decide to proceed with surgery?

Once you have met with the surgeon and decided to proceed with surgery, you will be scheduled for your pre-op evaluation and will meet with the anesthesiologist (the person who will put you to sleep during the surgery). You should have nothing to eat or drink after midnight on the day before surgery and should leave valuables and jewelry at home. The surgery usually takes two to two and a half hours, after which time you will slowly wake up in the recovery room. Surgery may be performed through a standard incision in the neck or may be done through a smaller incision with the aid of a video camera (minimally invasive video assisted thyroidectomy). Under special circumstances, thyroid surgery can be performed with the assistance of a robot through a distant incision in either the axilla or the back of the neck. There may be a surgical drain in the incision in your neck (which will be removed the morning after the surgery) and your throat may be sore because of the breathing tube placed during the operation.

Once you are fully awake, you will be moved to a bed in a hospital room where you will be able to eat and drink as you wish. Most patients having thyroid operations are hospitalized for about 24 hours and can be discharged on the morning following the operation. Normal activity can begin on the first postoperative day. Vigorous sports, such as swimming, and activities that include heavy lifting should be delayed for at least 10 days.

Will I be able to lead a normal life after surgery?

Yes. Once you have recovered from the effects of thyroid surgery, you will usually be able to do anything that you could do prior to surgery. Many patients become hypothyroid following thyroid surgery, requiring treatment with thyroid hormone. This is especially true if you had surgery for thyroid cancer. Thyroid hormone replacement therapy may be delayed for several weeks if you are to receive radioactive iodine therapy.

Chapter 23

Eye Surgery

Chapter Contents

Section 23.1

Cataract Surgery

Excerpted from "Facts about Cataract," by the National
Eye Institute (NEI, www.nei.nih.gov), part of the National
Institutes of Health, September 9, 2009.

What is a cataract?

A cataract is a clouding of the lens in the eye that affects vision.
Most cataracts are related to aging. Cataracts are very common in
older people. By age 80, more than half of all Americans either have a
cataract or have had cataract surgery.

A cataract can occur in either or both eyes. It cannot spread from
one eye to the other.

How is a cataract treated?

The symptoms of early cataract may be improved with new eyeglasses, brighter lighting, anti-glare sunglasses, or magnifying lenses.
If these measures do not help, surgery is the only effective treatment.
Surgery involves removing the cloudy lens and replacing it with an
artificial lens.

A cataract needs to be removed only when vision loss interferes with
your everyday activities, such as driving, reading, or watching TV. You
and your eye care professional can make this decision together. Once you
understand the benefits and risks of surgery, you can make an informed
decision about whether cataract surgery is right for you. In most cases,
delaying cataract surgery will not cause long-term damage to your eye
or make the surgery more difficult. You do not have to rush into surgery.

Sometimes a cataract should be removed even if it does not cause
problems with your vision. For example, a cataract should be removed
if it prevents examination or treatment of another eye problem, such as
age-related macular degeneration or diabetic retinopathy. If your eye
care professional finds a cataract, you may not need cataract surgery
for several years. In fact, you might never need cataract surgery. By
having your vision tested regularly, you and your eye care professional
can discuss if and when you might need treatment.

If you choose surgery, your eye care professional may refer you to a specialist to remove the cataract.

If you have cataracts in both eyes that require surgery, the surgery will be performed on each eye at separate times, usually four to eight weeks apart.

Many people who need cataract surgery also have other eye conditions, such as age-related macular degeneration or glaucoma. If you have other eye conditions in addition to cataract, talk with your doctor. Learn about the risks, benefits, alternatives, and expected results of cataract surgery.

What are the different types of cataract surgery?

There are two types of cataract surgery. Your doctor can explain the differences and help determine which is better for you:

- Phacoemulsification, or phaco: A small incision is made on the side of the cornea, the clear, dome-shaped surface that covers the front of the eye. Your doctor inserts a tiny probe into the eye. This device emits ultrasound waves that soften and break up the lens so that it can be removed by suction. Most cataract surgery today is done by phacoemulsification, also called small incision cataract surgery.

- Extracapsular surgery: Your doctor makes a longer incision on the side of the cornea and removes the cloudy core of the lens in one piece. The rest of the lens is removed by suction.

After the natural lens has been removed, it often is replaced by an artificial lens, called an intraocular lens (IOL). An IOL is a clear, plastic lens that requires no care and becomes a permanent part of your eye. Light is focused clearly by the IOL onto the retina, improving your vision. You will not feel or see the new lens.

Some people cannot have an IOL. They may have another eye disease or have problems during surgery. For these patients, a soft contact lens, or glasses that provide high magnification, may be suggested.

What are the risks of cataract surgery?

As with any surgery, cataract surgery poses risks, such as infection and bleeding. Before cataract surgery, your doctor may ask you to temporarily stop taking certain medications that increase the risk of bleeding during surgery. After surgery, you must keep your eye clean, wash your hands before touching your eye, and use the prescribed medications to help minimize the risk of infection. Serious infection can result in loss of vision.

Cataract surgery slightly increases your risk of retinal detachment. Other eye disorders, such as high myopia (nearsightedness), can further increase your risk of retinal detachment after cataract surgery. One sign of a retinal detachment is a sudden increase in flashes or floaters. Floaters are little "cobwebs" or specks that seem to float about in your field of vision. If you notice a sudden increase in floaters or flashes, see an eye care professional immediately. A retinal detachment is a medical emergency. If necessary, go to an emergency service or hospital. Your eye must be examined by an eye surgeon as soon as possible. A retinal detachment causes no pain. Early treatment for retinal detachment often can prevent permanent loss of vision. The sooner you get treatment, the more likely you will regain good vision. Even if you are treated promptly, some vision may be lost.

Talk to your eye care professional about these risks. Make sure cataract surgery is right for you.

Is cataract surgery effective?

Cataract removal is one of the most common operations performed in the United States. It also is one of the safest and most effective types of surgery. In about 90 percent of cases, people who have cataract surgery have better vision afterward.

What happens before surgery?

A week or two before surgery, your doctor will do some tests. These tests may include measuring the curve of the cornea and the size and shape of your eye. This information helps your doctor choose the right type of IOL.

You may be asked not to eat or drink anything 12 hours before your surgery.

What happens during surgery?

At the hospital or eye clinic, drops will be put into your eye to dilate the pupil. The area around your eye will be washed and cleansed.

The operation usually lasts less than one hour and is almost painless. Many people choose to stay awake during surgery. Others may need to be put to sleep for a short time.

If you are awake, you will have an anesthetic to numb the nerves in and around your eye.

After the operation, a patch may be placed over your eye. You will rest for a while. Your medical team will watch for any problems, such as bleeding. Most people who have cataract surgery can go home the same day. You will need someone to drive you home.

What happens after surgery?

Itching and mild discomfort are normal after cataract surgery. Some fluid discharge is also common. Your eye may be sensitive to light and touch. If you have discomfort, your doctor can suggest treatment. After one or two days, moderate discomfort should disappear.

For a few days after surgery, your doctor may ask you to use eyedrops to help healing and decrease the risk of infection. Ask your doctor about how to use your eyedrops, how often to use them, and what effects they can have. You will need to wear an eye shield or eyeglasses to help protect your eye. Avoid rubbing or pressing on your eye.

When you are home, try not to bend from the waist to pick up objects on the floor. Do not lift any heavy objects. You can walk, climb stairs, and do light household chores.

In most cases, healing will be complete within eight weeks. Your doctor will schedule exams to check on your progress.

Can problems develop after surgery?

Problems after surgery are rare, but they can occur. These problems can include infection, bleeding, inflammation (pain, redness, swelling), loss of vision, double vision, and high or low eye pressure. With prompt medical attention, these problems can usually be treated successfully.

Sometimes the eye tissue that encloses the IOL becomes cloudy and may blur your vision. This condition is called an after-cataract. An after-cataract can develop months or years after cataract surgery.

An after-cataract is treated with a laser. Your doctor uses a laser to make a tiny hole in the eye tissue behind the lens to let light pass through. This outpatient procedure is called a YAG [yttrium aluminum garnet] laser capsulotomy. It is painless and rarely results in increased eye pressure or other eye problems. As a precaution, your doctor may give you eyedrops to lower your eye pressure before or after the procedure.

Section 23.2

Glaucoma Surgery

Excerpted from "Glaucoma: What You Should Know,"
by the National Eye Institute (NEI, www.nei.nih.gov), part of
the National Institutes of Health, June 2011.

Glaucoma is a group of diseases that damage the eye's optic nerve
and can result in vision loss and blindness. However, with early detection and treatment, you can often protect your eyes against serious
vision loss.

Glaucoma Surgical Treatments

Immediate treatment for early-stage, open-angle glaucoma can
delay progression of the disease. That's why early diagnosis is very
important.

Glaucoma treatments include medicines, laser trabeculoplasty, conventional surgery, or a combination of any of these.

While these treatments may save remaining vision, they do not
improve sight already lost from glaucoma.

Laser Trabeculoplasty

Laser trabeculoplasty helps fluid drain out of the eye. Your doctor
may suggest this step at any time. In many cases, you will need to keep
taking glaucoma medicines after this procedure.

Laser trabeculoplasty is performed in your doctor's office or eye
clinic. Before the surgery, numbing drops are applied to your eye. As
you sit facing the laser machine, your doctor holds a special lens to
your eye. A high-intensity beam of light is aimed through the lens and
reflected onto the meshwork inside your eye. You may see flashes of
bright green or red light. The laser makes several evenly spaced burns
that stretch the drainage holes in the meshwork. This allows the fluid
to drain better.

Like any surgery, laser surgery can cause side effects, such as inflammation. Your doctor may give you some drops to take home for any
soreness or inflammation inside the eye.

You will need to make several follow-up visits to have your eye pressure and eye monitored.

If you have glaucoma in both eyes, usually only one eye will be treated at a time. Laser treatments for each eye will be scheduled several days to several weeks apart.

Studies show that laser surgery can be very good at reducing the pressure in some patients. However, its effects can wear off over time. Your doctor may suggest further treatment.

Conventional Surgery

Conventional surgery makes a new opening for the fluid to leave the eye. Your doctor may suggest this treatment at any time. Conventional surgery often is done after medicines and laser surgery have failed to control pressure.

Conventional surgery, called trabeculectomy, is performed in an operating room. Before the surgery, you are given medicine to help you relax. Your doctor makes small injections around the eye to numb it. A small piece of tissue is removed to create a new channel for the fluid to drain from the eye. This fluid will drain between the eye tissue layers and create a blister-like filtration bleb.

For several weeks after the surgery, you must put drops in the eye to fight infection and inflammation. These drops will be different from those you may have been using before surgery.

Conventional surgery is performed on one eye at a time. Usually the operations are four to six weeks apart.

Conventional surgery is about 60 to 80 percent effective at lowering eye pressure. If the new drainage opening narrows, a second operation may be needed. Conventional surgery works best if you have not had previous eye surgery, such as a cataract operation.

Sometimes after conventional surgery, your vision may not be as good as it was before conventional surgery. Conventional surgery can cause side effects, including cataract, problems with the cornea, inflammation, infection inside the eye, or low eye pressure problems. If you have any of these problems, tell your doctor so a treatment plan can be developed.

Section 23.3

Macular Degeneration Surgery

Excerpted from "Facts about Age-Related Macular Degeneration,"
by the National Eye Institute (NEI, www.nei.nih.gov), part of the
National Institutes of Health, September 2009.

Perhaps you have just learned that you or a loved one has age-related macular degeneration, also known as AMD. If you are like many people, you probably do not know a lot about the condition or understand what is going on inside your eyes.

What Is AMD?

AMD is a common eye condition among people age 50 and older. It is a leading cause of vision loss in older adults. It gradually destroys the macula, the part of the eye that provides sharp, central vision needed for seeing objects clearly.

In some people, AMD advances so slowly that vision loss does not occur for a long time. In others, the disorder progresses faster and may lead to a loss of vision in one or both eyes. The vision loss makes it difficult to recognize faces, drive a car, read, print, or do close work, such as sewing or fixing things around the house.

Despite the limited vision, AMD does not cause complete blindness. You will be able to see using your side (peripheral) vision.

Treatment Options for AMD

With early diagnosis and proper treatment, you can delay the progression of AMD. The earlier it is detected, the better your chances of keeping your vision. Wet AMD typically results in severe vision loss. However, eye care professionals can try different therapies to stop further vision loss. You should remember that the therapies described in the following are not a cure. The condition may progress even with treatment.

Injections

One option to slow the progression of wet AMD is to inject drugs into your eye. With wet AMD, abnormally high levels of vascular endothelial growth factor (VEGF) are secreted in your eyes. This substance promotes the growth of new abnormal blood vessels. The anti-VEGF injection therapy blocks its effects. If you get this treatment, you may need multiple injections. Your eye care professional may give them monthly. Before each injection, your eye care professional will numb your eye and clean it with antiseptics. To prevent the risk of infection, a doctor may prescribe antibiotic drops.

Photodynamic Therapy

This technique involves laser treatment of select areas of the retina. First, a drug called verteporfin will be injected into a vein in your arm. The drug travels through the blood vessels in your body, including any new, abnormal blood vessels in your eye. Your eye care professional then shines a laser beam into your eye to activate the drug in the blood vessels. Once activated, the drug destroys the new blood vessels and slows the rate of vision loss. This procedure takes about 20 minutes.

Laser Surgery

Eye care professionals sometimes treat certain cases of wet AMD with laser surgery, though this is less common than other treatments. This treatment is performed in a doctor's office or eye clinic. It involves aiming an intense beam of light at the new blood vessels in your eyes to destroy them. However, laser treatment also may destroy some surrounding healthy tissue and cause more blurred vision.

Section 23.4

Laser Eye Surgery (LASIK) for Refractive Disorders

This section includes text from the following documents: "LASIK," "What Is LASIK?", "When Is LASIK Not for Me?", "What Are the Risks and How Can I Find the Right Doctor for Me?", and "What Should I Expect before, during, and after Surgery?" by the U.S. Food and Drug Administration (FDA, www.fda.gov), December 9, 2011.

LASIK

LASIK is a surgical procedure intended to reduce a person's dependency on glasses or contact lenses. LASIK stands for Laser-Assisted In Situ Keratomileusis and is a procedure that permanently changes the shape of the cornea, the clear covering of the front of the eye, using an excimer laser. A mechanical microkeratome (a blade device) or a laser keratome (a laser device) is used to cut a flap in the cornea. A hinge is left at one end of this flap. The flap is folded back revealing the stroma, the middle section of the cornea. Pulses from a computer-controlled laser vaporize a portion of the stroma and the flap is replaced. There are other techniques and many new terms related to LASIK that you may hear about.

What Is LASIK?

The Eye and Vision Errors

The cornea is a part of the eye that helps focus light to create an image on the retina. It works in much the same way that the lens of a camera focuses light to create an image on film. The bending and focusing of light is also known as refraction. Usually the shape of the cornea and the eye are not perfect and the image on the retina is out-of-focus (blurred) or distorted. These imperfections in the focusing power of the eye are called refractive errors. There are three primary types of refractive errors—myopia, hyperopia, and astigmatism. Persons with myopia, or nearsightedness, have more difficulty seeing distant objects as clearly as near objects. Persons with hyperopia, or farsightedness, have more difficulty seeing near objects as clearly as distant objects. Astigmatism is a distortion of the image on the retina caused by irregularities in the cornea or lens of the eye. Combinations of myopia and astigmatism or hyperopia and astigmatism are common. Glasses or contact lenses are designed to compensate for the eye's imperfections. Surgical procedures aimed at improving the focusing power of the eye are called refractive surgery. In LASIK surgery, precise and controlled removal of corneal tissue by a special laser reshapes the cornea, changing its focusing power.

Other Types of Refractive Surgery

Radial keratotomy or RK and Photorefractive keratectomy or PRK are other refractive surgeries used to reshape the cornea. In RK, a very sharp knife is used to cut slits in the cornea changing its shape. PRK was the first surgical procedure developed to reshape the cornea, by sculpting, using a laser. Later, LASIK was developed. The same type of laser is used for LASIK and PRK. Often the exact same laser is used for the two types of surgery. The major difference between the two surgeries is the way that the stroma, the middle layer of the cornea, is exposed before it is vaporized with the laser. In PRK, the top layer of the cornea, called the epithelium, is scraped away to expose the stromal layer underneath. In LASIK, a flap is cut in the stromal layer and the flap is folded back.

Another type of refractive surgery is thermokeratoplasty in which heat is used to reshape the cornea. The source of the heat can be a laser, but it is a different kind of laser than is used for LASIK and PRK. Other refractive devices include corneal ring segments that are inserted into the stroma and special contact lenses that temporarily reshape the cornea (orthokeratology).

When Is LASIK Not for Me?

You are probably not a good candidate for refractive surgery if the following are true:

- You are not a risk taker. Certain complications are unavoidable in a percentage of patients, and there are no long-term data available for current procedures.

- It will jeopardize your career. Some jobs prohibit certain refractive procedures. Be sure to check with your employer/professional society/military service before undergoing any procedure.

- Cost is an issue. Most medical insurance will not pay for refractive surgery. Although the cost is coming down, it is still significant.

- You required a change in your contact lens or glasses prescription in the past year. This is called refractive instability. Patients who are in their early 20s or younger; whose hormones are fluctuating due to disease such as diabetes; who are pregnant or breastfeeding; or who are taking medications that may cause fluctuations in vision are more likely to have refractive instability and should discuss the possible additional risks with their doctor.

- You have a disease or are on medications that may affect wound healing. Certain conditions, such as autoimmune diseases (e.g., lupus, rheumatoid arthritis), immunodeficiency states (e.g., human immunodeficiency virus [HIV]) and diabetes, and some medications (e.g., retinoic acid and steroids) may prevent proper healing after a refractive procedure.

- You actively participate in contact sports. You participate in boxing, wrestling, martial arts, or other activities in which blows to the face and eyes are a normal occurrence.

- You are not an adult. Currently, no lasers are approved for LASIK on persons under the age of 18.

Precautions

The safety and effectiveness of refractive procedures has not been determined in patients with some diseases. Discuss with your doctor if you have a history of any of the following:

- Herpes simplex or Herpes zoster (shingles) involving the eye area

- Glaucoma, glaucoma suspect, or ocular hypertension

- Eye diseases, such as uveitis/iritis (inflammations of the eye)

- Eye injuries or previous eye surgeries

- Keratoconus

Other Risk Factors

Your doctor should screen you for the following conditions or indicators of risk:

- **Blepharitis:** This is an inflammation of the eyelids with crusting of the eyelashes that may increase the risk of infection or inflammation of the cornea after LASIK.

- **Large pupils:** Make sure this evaluation is done in a dark room. Although anyone may have large pupils, younger patients and patients on certain medications may be particularly prone to having large pupils under dim lighting conditions. This can cause symptoms such as glare, halos, starbursts, and ghost images (double vision) after surgery. In some patients these symptoms may be debilitating. For example, a patient may no longer be able to drive a car at night or in certain weather conditions, such as fog.

- **Thin corneas:** The cornea is the thin clear covering of the eye that is over the iris, the colored part of the eye. Most refractive procedures change the eye's focusing power by reshaping the cornea (for example, by removing tissue). Performing a refractive procedure on a cornea that is too thin may result in blinding complications.

- **Previous refractive surgery (e.g., RK, PRK, LASIK):** Additional refractive surgery may not be recommended. The decision to have additional refractive surgery must be made in consultation with your doctor after careful consideration of your unique situation.

- **Dry eyes:** LASIK surgery tends to aggravate this condition.

What Are the Risks and How Can I Find the Right Doctor for Me?

Most patients are very pleased with the results of their refractive surgery. However, like any other medical procedure, there are risks involved. That's why it is important for you to understand the limitations and possible complications of refractive surgery.

Before undergoing a refractive procedure, you should carefully weigh the risks and benefits based on your own personal value system, and try to avoid being influenced by friends that have had the procedure or doctors encouraging you to do so.

Some patients lose vision. Some patients lose lines of vision on the vision chart that cannot be corrected with glasses, contact lenses, or surgery as a result of treatment.

Some patients develop debilitating visual symptoms. Some patients develop glare, halos, and/or double vision that can seriously affect nighttime vision. Even with good vision on the vision chart, some patients do not see as well in situations of low contrast, such as at night or in fog, after treatment as compared to before treatment.

You may be under treated or over treated. Only a certain percent of patients achieve 20/20 vision without glasses or contacts. You may require additional treatment, but additional treatment may not be possible. You may still need glasses or contact lenses after surgery. This may be true even if you only required a very weak prescription before surgery. If you used reading glasses before surgery, you may still need reading glasses after surgery.

Some patients may develop severe dry eye syndrome. As a result of surgery, your eye may not be able to produce enough tears to keep the eye moist and comfortable. Dry eye not only causes discomfort, but can reduce visual quality due to intermittent blurring and other visual symptoms. This condition may be permanent. Intensive drop therapy and use of plugs or other procedures may be required.

Results are generally not as good in patients with very large refractive errors of any type. You should discuss your expectations with your doctor and realize that you may still require glasses or contacts after the surgery.

For some farsighted patients, results may diminish with age. If you are farsighted, the level of improved vision you experience after surgery may decrease with age. This can occur if your manifest refraction (a vision exam with lenses before dilating drops) is very different from your cycloplegic refraction (a vision exam with lenses after dilating drops).

Long-term data are not available. LASIK is a relatively new technology. The first laser was approved for LASIK eye surgery in 1998. Therefore, the long-term safety and effectiveness of LASIK surgery is not known.

There are additional risks if you are considering the following procedures.

Monovision

Monovision is one clinical technique used to deal with the correction of presbyopia, the gradual loss of the ability of the eye to change focus for close-up tasks that progresses with age. The intent of monovision is for the presbyopic patient to use one eye for distance viewing and one eye for near viewing. This practice was first applied to fit contact lens wearers and more recently to LASIK and other refractive surgeries. With contact lenses, a presbyopic patient has one eye fit with a contact lens to correct distance vision, and the other eye fit with a contact lens to correct near vision. In the same way, with LASIK, a presbyopic patient has one eye operated on to correct the distance vision, and the other operated on to correct the near vision. In other words, the goal of the surgery is for one eye to have vision worse than 20/20, the commonly referred to goal for LASIK surgical correction of distance vision. Since one eye is corrected for distance viewing and the other eye is corrected for near viewing, the two eyes no longer work together. This results in poorer quality vision and a decrease in depth perception. These effects of monovision are most noticeable in low lighting conditions and when performing tasks requiring very sharp vision. Therefore, you may need to wear glasses or contact lenses to fully correct both eyes for distance or near when performing visually demanding tasks, such as driving at night, operating dangerous equipment, or performing occupational tasks requiring very sharp close vision (e.g., reading small print for long periods of time).

Many patients cannot get used to having one eye blurred at all times. Therefore, if you are considering monovision with LASIK, make sure you go through a trial period with contact lenses to see if you can tolerate monovision, before having the surgery performed on your eyes. Find out if you pass your state's driver's license requirements with monovision.

In addition, you should consider how much your presbyopia is expected to increase in the future. Ask your doctor when you should expect the results of your monovision surgery to no longer be enough for you to see nearby objects clearly without the aid of glasses or contacts, or when a second surgery might be required to further correct your near vision.

Bilateral Simultaneous Treatment

You may choose to have LASIK surgery on both eyes at the same time or to have surgery on one eye at a time. Although the convenience of having surgery on both eyes on the same day is attractive, this practice is riskier than having two separate surgeries.

If you decide to have one eye done at a time, you and your doctor will decide how long to wait before having surgery on the other eye. If both eyes are treated at the same time or before one eye has a chance to fully heal, you and your doctor do not have the advantage of being able to see how the first eye responds to surgery before the second eye is treated.

Another disadvantage to having surgery on both eyes at the same time is that the vision in both eyes may be blurred after surgery until the initial healing process is over, rather than being able to rely on clear vision in at least one eye at all times.

During Surgery

Malfunction of a device or other error, such as cutting a flap of cornea through and through instead of making a hinge during LASIK surgery, may lead to discontinuation of the procedure or irreversible damage to the eye.

After Surgery

Some complications, such as migration of the flap, inflammation, or infection, may require another procedure and/or intensive treatment with drops. Even with aggressive therapy, such complications may lead to temporary loss of vision or even irreversible blindness.

Under the care of an experienced doctor, carefully screened candidates with reasonable expectations and a clear understanding of the risks and alternatives are likely to be happy with the results of their refractive procedure.

Advertising

Be cautious about slick advertising and/or deals that sound too good to be true. Remember, they usually are. There is a lot of competition resulting in a great deal of advertising and bidding for your business. Do your homework.

What Should I Expect before, during, and after Surgery?

What to expect before, during, and after surgery will vary from doctor to doctor and patient to patient.

Before Surgery

If you decide to go ahead with LASIK surgery, you will need an initial or baseline evaluation by your eye doctor to determine if you are a good candidate. This is what you need to know to prepare for the exam and what you should expect.

If you wear contact lenses, it is a good idea to stop wearing them before your baseline evaluation and switch to wearing your glasses full-time. Contact lenses change the shape of your cornea for up to several weeks after you have stopped using them depending on the type of contact lenses you wear. Not leaving your contact lenses out long enough for your cornea to assume its natural shape before surgery can have negative consequences. These consequences include inaccurate measurements and a poor surgical plan, resulting in poor vision after surgery. These measurements, which determine how much corneal tissue to remove, may need to be repeated at least a week after your initial evaluation and before surgery to make sure they have not changed, especially if you wear RGP or hard lenses

- If you wear soft contact lenses, you should stop wearing them for two weeks before your initial evaluation.

- If you wear toric soft lenses or rigid gas permeable (RGP) lenses, you should stop wearing them for at least three weeks before your initial evaluation.

- If you wear hard lenses, you should stop wearing them for at least four weeks before your initial evaluation.

You should tell your doctor:

- about your past and present medical and eye conditions;
- about all the medications you are taking, including over-the-counter medications and any medications you may be allergic to.

Your doctor should perform a thorough eye exam and discuss:

- whether you are a good candidate;
- what the risks, benefits, and alternatives of the surgery are;
- what you should expect before, during, and after surgery;
- what your responsibilities will be before, during, and after surgery.

You should have the opportunity to ask your doctor questions during this discussion. Give yourself plenty of time to think about the risk/ benefit discussion, to review any informational literature provided by your doctor, and to have any additional questions answered by your doctor before deciding to go through with surgery and before signing the informed consent form.

You should not feel pressured by your doctor, family, friends, or anyone else to make a decision about having surgery. Carefully consider the pros and cons.

The day before surgery, you should stop using:

- creams;
- lotions;
- makeup;
- perfumes.

These products as well as debris along the eyelashes may increase the risk of infection during and after surgery. Your doctor may ask you to scrub your eyelashes for a period of time before surgery to get rid of residues and debris along the lashes.

Also before surgery, arrange for transportation to and from your surgery and your first follow-up visit. On the day of surgery, your doctor may give you some medicine to make you relax. Because this medicine impairs your ability to drive and because your vision may be blurry, even if you don't drive make sure someone can bring you home after surgery.

During Surgery

The surgery should take less than 30 minutes. You will lie on your back in a reclining chair in an exam room containing the laser system. The laser system includes a large machine with a microscope attached to it and a computer screen.

A numbing drop will be placed in your eye, the area around your eye will be cleaned, and an instrument called a lid speculum will be used to hold your eyelids open.

Your doctor may use a mechanical microkeratome (a blade device) to cut a flap in the cornea.

If a mechanical microkeratome is used, a ring will be placed on your eye and very high pressures will be applied to create suction to the cornea. Your vision will dim while the suction ring is on and you may feel the pressure and experience some discomfort during this part of the procedure. The microkeratome, a cutting instrument, is attached to the suction ring. Your doctor will use the blade of the microkeratome to cut a flap in your cornea. Microkeratome blades are meant to be used only once and then thrown out. The microkeratome and the suction ring are then removed.

Your doctor may use a laser keratome (a laser device), instead of a mechanical microkeratome, to cut a flap on the cornea.

If a laser keratome is used, the cornea is flattened with a clear plastic plate. Your vision will dim and you may feel the pressure and experience some discomfort during this part of the procedure. Laser energy is focused inside the cornea tissue, creating thousands of small bubbles of gas and water that expand and connect to separate the tissue underneath the cornea surface, creating a flap. The plate is then removed.

You will be able to see, but you will experience fluctuating degrees of blurred vision during the rest of the procedure. The doctor will then lift the flap and fold it back on its hinge, and dry the exposed tissue.

The laser will be positioned over your eye and you will be asked to stare at a light. This is not the laser used to remove tissue from the cornea. This light is to help you keep your eye fixed on one spot once the laser comes on. Note: If you cannot stare at a fixed object for at least 60 seconds, you may not be a good candidate for this surgery.

When your eye is in the correct position, your doctor will start the laser. At this point in the surgery, you may become aware of new sounds and smells. The pulse of the laser makes a ticking sound. As the laser removes corneal tissue, some people have reported a smell similar to burning hair. A computer controls the amount of laser energy delivered to your eye. Before the start of surgery, your doctor will have programmed the computer to vaporize a particular amount of tissue based on the measurements taken at your initial evaluation. After the pulses of laser energy vaporize the corneal tissue, the flap is put back into position.

A shield should be placed over your eye at the end of the procedure as protection, since no stitches are used to hold the flap in place. It is important for you to wear this shield to prevent you from rubbing your eye and putting pressure on your eye while you sleep, and to protect your eye from accidentally being hit or poked until the flap has healed.

After Surgery

Immediately after the procedure, your eye may burn, itch, or feel like there is something in it. You may experience some discomfort, or in some cases, mild pain and your doctor may suggest you take a mild pain reliever. Both your eyes may tear or water. Your vision will probably be hazy or blurry. You will instinctively want to rub your eye, but don't. Rubbing your eye could dislodge the flap, requiring further treatment. In addition, you may experience sensitivity to light, glare, starbursts, or haloes around lights, or the whites of your eye may look red or bloodshot. These symptoms should improve considerably within the first few days after surgery. You should plan on taking a few days off from work until these symptoms subside. You should contact your doctor immediately and not wait for your scheduled visit, if you experience severe pain, or if your vision or other symptoms get worse instead of better.

You should see your doctor within the first 24 to 48 hours after surgery and at regular intervals after that for at least the first six months. At the first postoperative visit, your doctor will remove the eye shield, test your vision, and examine your eye. Your doctor may give you one or more types of eye drops to take at home to help prevent infection and/or inflammation. You may also be advised to use artificial tears to help lubricate the eye. Do not resume wearing a contact lens in the operated eye, even if your vision is blurry.

You should wait one to three days following surgery before beginning any non-contact sports, depending on the amount of activity required, how you feel, and your doctor's instructions.

To help prevent infection, you may need to wait for up to two weeks after surgery or until your doctor advises you otherwise before using lotions, creams, or make-up around the eye. Your doctor may advise you to continue scrubbing your eyelashes for a period of time after surgery. You should also avoid swimming and using hot tubs or whirlpools for one to two months.

Strenuous contact sports such as boxing, football, karate, etc. should not be attempted for at least four weeks after surgery. It is important to protect your eyes from anything that might get in them and from being hit or bumped.

During the first few months after surgery, your vision may fluctuate. It may take up to three to six months for your vision to stabilize after surgery.

Glare, haloes, difficulty driving at night, and other visual symptoms may also persist during this stabilization period. If further correction or enhancement is necessary, you should wait until your eye measurements are consistent for two consecutive visits at least three months apart before reoperation.

It is important to realize that although distance vision may improve after reoperation, it is unlikely that other visual symptoms such as glare or haloes will improve.

It is also important to note that no laser company has presented enough evidence for the FDA to make conclusions about the safety or effectiveness of enhancement surgery.

Contact your eye doctor immediately, if you develop any new, unusual, or worsening symptoms at any point after surgery. Such symptoms could signal a problem that, if not treated early enough, may lead to a loss of vision.

Chapter 24

Dental and Endodontic Surgery

Chapter Contents

Section 24.1

Traumatic Dental Injuries May Require Surgery

What is endodontic treatment?

Endo is the Greek word for inside and odont is Greek for tooth. Endodontic treatment (involves) the inside of the tooth.

To understand endodontic treatment, it helps to know something about the anatomy of the tooth. Inside the tooth, under the white enamel and a hard layer called the dentin, is a soft tissue called the pulp. The pulp contains blood vessels, nerves, and connective tissue, and creates the surrounding hard tissues of the tooth during development.

The pulp extends from the crown of the tooth to the tip of the roots where it connects to the tissues surrounding the root. The pulp is important during a tooth's growth and development. However, once a tooth is fully mature it can survive without the pulp, because the tooth continues to be nourished by the tissues surrounding it.

Who performs endodontic treatment?

All dentists, including your general dentist, received training in endodontic treatment in dental school. General dentists can perform endodontic procedures along with other dental procedures, but often they refer patients needing endodontic treatment to endodontists.

Endodontists are dentists with special training in endodontic pro-cedures. They provide only endodontic services in their practices be-cause they are specialists. To become specialists, they complete dental school and an additional two or more years of advanced training in endodontics. They perform routine as well as difficult and very complex endodontic procedures, including endodontic surgery. Endodontists are also experienced at finding the cause of oral and facial pain that has been difficult to diagnose.

How will my injury be treated?

Chipped teeth account for the majority of all dental injuries. Dislodged or knocked-out teeth are examples of less frequent, but more severe injuries. Treatment depends on the type, location, and severity of each injury. Any dental injury, even if apparently mild, requires examination by a dentist or an endodontist immediately. Sometimes, neighboring teeth suffer an additional, unnoticed injury that will only be detected by a thorough dental exam.

Chipped or fractured teeth: Most chipped or fractured tooth crowns can be repaired either by reattaching the broken piece or by placing a tooth-colored filling. If a significant portion of the tooth crown is broken off, an artificial crown or cap may be needed to restore the tooth.

If the pulp is exposed or damaged after a crown fracture, root canal treatment may be needed. These injuries require special attention. If breathing through your mouth or drinking cold fluids is painful, bite on clean, moist gauze or cloth to help relieve symptoms until reaching your dentist's office. Never use topical oral pain medications (such as Anbesol) or ointments, or place aspirin on the affected areas to eliminate pain symptoms.

Injuries in the back teeth often include fractured cusps, cracked teeth, and the more serious split tooth. If cracks extend into the root, root canal treatment and a full coverage crown may be needed to restore function to the tooth. Split teeth may require extraction.

Dislodged (luxated) teeth: During an injury, a tooth may be pushed sideways, out of or into its socket. Your endodontist or general dentist will reposition and stabilize your tooth. Root canal treatment is usually needed for permanent teeth that have been dislodged and should be started a few days following the injury. Medication such as calcium hydroxide may be put inside the tooth as part of the root canal treatment. A permanent root canal filling will be placed at a later date.

Children between 7 and 12 years old may not need root canal treatment since their teeth are still developing. For those patients, an endodontist or dentist will monitor the healing carefully and intervene immediately if any unfavorable changes appear. Therefore, multiple follow-up appointments are likely to be needed. New research indicates that stem cells present in the pulps of young people can be stimulated to complete root growth and heal the pulp following injuries or infection.

Knocked-out (avulsed) teeth: If a tooth is completely knocked out of your mouth, time is of the essence. The tooth should be handled very gently, avoiding touching the root surface itself. If it is dirty, quickly and gently rinse it in water. Do not use soap or any other cleaning agent, and never scrape or brush the tooth. If possible, the tooth should be placed back into its socket as soon as possible. The less time the tooth is out of its socket, the better the chance for saving it. Call a dentist immediately.

If you cannot put the tooth back in its socket, it needs to be kept moist in special solutions that are available at many local drug-stores (such as Save-A-Tooth). If those solutions are unavailable, you should put the tooth in milk. Doing this will keep the root cells in your tooth moist and alive for a few hours. Another option is to simply put the tooth in your mouth between your gum and cheek. Do not place the tooth in regular tap water because the root surface cells do not tolerate it.

Once the tooth has been put back in its socket, your dentist will evaluate it and will check for any other dental and facial injuries. If the tooth has not been placed back into its socket, your dentist will clean it carefully and replace it. A stabilizing splint will be placed for a few weeks. Depending on the stage of root development, your dentist or endodontist may start root canal treatment a week or two later. A medication may be placed inside the tooth followed by a permanent root canal filling at a later date.

The length of time the tooth was out of the mouth and the way the tooth was stored before reaching the dentist influence the chances of saving the tooth. Again, immediate treatment is essential. Taking all these factors into account, your dentist or endodontist may discuss other treatment options with you.

Root fractures: A traumatic injury to the tooth may also result in a horizontal root fracture. The location of the fracture determines the long-term health of the tooth. If the fracture is close to the root tip, the chances for success are much better. However, the closer the fracture is to the gum line, the poorer the long-term success rate. Sometimes, stabilization with a splint is required for a period of time.

Do traumatic dental injuries differ in children?

Chipped primary (or baby) teeth can be esthetically restored. Dislodged primary teeth can, in rare cases, be repositioned. However, primary teeth that have been knocked out typically should not be replanted. This is because the replantation of a knocked-out primary tooth may cause further and permanent damage to the underlying permanent tooth that is growing inside the bone.

Children's permanent teeth that are not fully developed at the time of the injury need special attention and careful follow up, but not all of them will need root canal treatment. In an immature permanent tooth, the blood supply to the tooth and the presence of stem cells in the region may enable your dentist or endodontist to stimulate continued root growth.

Endodontists have the knowledge and skill to treat incompletely formed roots in children so that, in some instances, the roots can continue to develop. Endodontists will do all that is possible to save the natural tooth. These specialists are the logical source of information and expertise for children who are victims of dental trauma.

Will the tooth need any special care or additional treatment?

The nature of the injury, the length of time from injury to treatment, how your tooth was cared for after the injury and your body's response all affect the long-term health of the tooth. Timely treatment is particularly important with dislodged or knocked-out teeth in order to prevent root resorption.

Resorption occurs when your body, through its own defense mechanisms, begins to reject your own tooth in response to the traumatic injury. Following the injury, you should return to your dentist or endodontist to have the tooth examined and/or treated at regular intervals for up to five years to ensure that root resorption is not occurring and that surrounding tissues continue to heal. It has to be noted that some types of resorption are untreatable.

Section 24.2

Endodontic Surgery

Why would I need endodontic surgery?

Surgery can help save your tooth in a variety of situations.

Surgery may be used in diagnosis. If you have persistent symptoms but no problems appear on your X-ray, your tooth may have a tiny fracture or canal that could not be detected during nonsurgical treatment. In such a case, surgery allows your endodontist to examine the entire root of your tooth, find the problem, and provide treatment.

Sometimes calcium deposits make a canal too narrow for the instruments used in nonsurgical root canal treatment to reach the end of the root. If your tooth has this calcification, your endodontist may perform endodontic surgery to clean and seal the remainder of the canal.

Usually, a tooth that has undergone a root canal can last the rest of your life and never need further endodontic treatment. However, in a few cases, a tooth may not heal or become infected. A tooth may become painful or diseased months or even years after successful treatment. If this is true for you, surgery may help save your tooth.

Surgery may also be performed to treat damaged root surfaces or surrounding bone.

Although there are many surgical procedures that can be performed to save a tooth, the most common is called apicoectomy or root-end resection. When inflammation or infection persists in the bony area around the end of your tooth after a root canal procedure, your endodontist may have to perform an apicoectomy.

What is an apicoectomy?

In this procedure, the endodontist opens the gum tissue near the tooth to see the underlying bone and to remove any inflamed or infected tissue. The very end of the root is also removed.

A small filling may be placed in the root to seal the end of the root canal, and a few stitches or sutures are placed in the gingiva to help the tissue heal properly.

Over a period of months, the bone heals around the end of the root.

Are there other types of endodontic surgery?

Other surgeries endodontists might perform include dividing a tooth in half, repairing an injured root, or even removing one or more roots. Your endodontist will be happy to discuss the specific type of surgery your tooth requires.

In certain cases, a procedure called intentional replantation may be performed. In this procedure, a tooth is extracted, treated with an endodontic procedure while it is out of the mouth, and then replaced in its socket.

These procedures are designed to help you save your tooth.

Will the procedure hurt?

Local anesthetics make the procedure comfortable. Of course, you may feel some discomfort or experience slight swelling while the incision heals. This is normal for any surgical procedure. Your endodontist will recommend appropriate pain medication to alleviate your discomfort.

Your endodontist will give you specific postoperative instructions to follow. If you have questions after your procedure, or if you have pain that does not respond to medication, call your endodontist.

Can I drive myself home?

Often you can, but you should ask your endodontist before your appointment so that you can make transportation arrangements if necessary.

When can I return to my normal activities?

Most patients return to work or other routine activities the next day. Your endodontist will be happy to discuss your expected recovery time with you.

Does insurance cover endodontic surgery?

Each insurance plan is different. Check with your employer or insurance company prior to treatment.

How do I know the surgery will be successful?

Your dentist or endodontist is suggesting endodontic surgery because he or she believes it is the best option for saving your own natural tooth. Of course, there are no guarantees with any surgical procedure. Your endodontist will discuss your chances for success so that you can make an informed decision.

What are the alternatives to endodontic surgery?

Often, the only alternative to surgery is extraction of the tooth. The extracted tooth must then be replaced with an implant, bridge, or removable partial denture to restore chewing function and to prevent adjacent teeth from shifting. Because these alternatives require surgery or dental procedures on adjacent healthy teeth, endodontic surgery is usually the most biologic and cost-effective option for maintaining your oral health.

No matter how effective modern artificial tooth replacements are—and they can be very effective—nothing is as good as a natural tooth. You've already made an investment in saving your tooth. The pay-off for choosing endodontic surgery could be a healthy, functioning natural tooth for the rest of your life.

Chapter 25

Breast Surgeries

Chapter Contents

Section 25.1

Breast Augmentation

What Is Breast Augmentation Surgery?

Also known as augmentation mammaplasty, breast augmentation surgery involves using implants to fulfill your desire for fuller breasts or to restore breast volume lost after weight reduction or pregnancy.

Breast Augmentation before and after

If you are dissatisfied with your breast size, breast augmentation surgery (either breast enhancement or breast enlargement) is a choice to consider. Breast augmentation can:

- increase fullness and projection of your breasts;

- improve the balance of your figure;

- enhance your self-image and self-confidence.

Also known as augmentation mammaplasty, the procedure involves using implants to fulfill your desire for fuller breasts or to restore breast volume lost after weight reduction or pregnancy.

Implants also may be used to reconstruct a breast after mastectomy or injury.

Many patients find it helpful to review breast augmentation before and after photos.

What It Won't Do

Breast augmentation does not correct severely drooping breasts. If you want your breasts to look fuller and to be lifted due to sagging, a breast lift may be required in conjunction with breast augmentation.

Breast lifting can often be done at the same time as your augmentation or may require a separate operation. Your plastic surgeon will assist you in making this decision.

Is It Right for Me?

Breast augmentation is a highly individualized procedure and you should do it for yourself, not to fulfill someone else's desires or to try to fit any sort of ideal image. Pictures of breast augmentation procedures performed by ASPS Member Surgeons may help you in the decision-making process.

Breast augmentation may be a good option for you if:

* you are physically healthy;

* you have realistic expectations;

* your breasts are fully developed;

* you are bothered by the feeling that your breasts are too small;

* you are dissatisfied with your breasts losing shape and volume after pregnancy, weight loss, or with aging;

* your breasts vary in size or shape;

* one or both breasts failed to develop normally.

Preparing for Breast Augmentation Surgery

After researching the basics about breast enhancement or breast enlargement, many patients want to know what to expect before breast augmentation surgery.

Prior to breast surgery, your ASPS Member Surgeon may ask you to:

* get lab testing or a medical evaluation;

* take certain medications or adjust your current medications;

* get a baseline mammogram before surgery and another one after surgery to help detect any future changes in your breast tissue;

* stop smoking well in advance of your breast augmentation surgery;

* avoid taking aspirin, anti-inflammatory drugs, and herbal supplements as they can increase bleeding.

215

Special instructions you receive will cover:

- what to do on the day of surgery;

- postoperative care and follow-up;

- breast implant registry documents (when necessary).

Your plastic surgeon will also discuss where your procedure will be performed. Breast augmentation surgery may be performed in an accredited office-based surgical center, outpatient ambulatory surgical center, or a hospital.

You'll Need Help

If your breast augmentation is performed on an outpatient basis, be sure to arrange for someone to drive you to and from surgery and to stay with you for at least the first night following surgery.

Breast Implant Risks and Safety Information

The success and safety of your breast augmentation procedure depends very much on your being completely candid during your consultation. By being actively involved your consultation about breast augmentation, problems, concerns, and questions you may have can be addressed by your ASPS Member Surgeon. You'll be asked a number of questions about your health, desires, and lifestyle.

Be prepared to discuss:

- why you want breast augmentation surgery, your expectations, and desired outcome;

- medical conditions, drug allergies, and medical treatments;

- use of current medications, vitamins, herbal supplements, alcohol, tobacco, and drugs;

- previous surgeries;

- family history of breast cancer and results of any mammograms or previous biopsies.

Your surgeon may also:

- evaluate your general health status and any pre-existing health conditions or risk factors;

- examine your breasts, and may take detailed measurements of their size and shape, skin quality, placement of your nipples;

- take photographs for your medical record;

- discuss your options and recommend a course of treatment;

- discuss likely outcomes of breast augmentation surgery and any risks or potential complications;

- discuss the use of anesthesia during your breast augmentation procedure.

Important Facts about Breast Augmentation Risks and Complications

The decision to have breast augmentation surgery is extremely personal and you'll have to decide if the benefits will achieve your goals and if the risks of breast implant safety and potential complications are acceptable.

Your plastic surgeon and/or staff will explain in detail the risks associated with surgery. You will be asked to sign consent forms to ensure that you fully understand the procedure you will undergo and any risks or potential complications.

The risks of breast implants and complications after breast augmentation include:

- unfavorable scarring;

- bleeding (hematoma);

- infection;

- poor healing of incisions;

- changes in nipple or breast sensation, may be temporary or permanent;

- capsular contracture, which is the formation of firm scar tissue around the implant;

- implant leakage or rupture;

- wrinkling of the skin over the implant;

- anesthesia risks;

- fluid accumulation;

- blood clots;

- pain, which may persist;

- deep vein thrombosis, cardiac and pulmonary complications;

- possibility of revisional surgery.

Although there potentially may be complications with breast implants, they do not impair breast health. Careful review of scientific research conducted by independent groups such as the Institute of Medicine has found no proven link between breast implants and autoimmune or other systemic diseases.

Other important considerations:

- Breast implants are not guaranteed to last a lifetime and future surgery may be required to replace one or both implants.

- Pregnancy, weight loss, and menopause may influence the appearance of augmented breasts over the course of your lifetime.

Section 25.2

Breast Reduction

What Is Breast Reduction Surgery?

Also known as reduction mammaplasty, breast reduction surgery removes excess breast fat, glandular tissue, and skin to achieve a breast size in proportion with your body and to alleviate the discomfort associated with overly large breasts.

Breast Reduction Surgery: Health and Beauty for Life

Overly large breasts can cause some women to have both health and emotional problems. In addition to self-image issues, you may also experience physical pain and discomfort.

The weight of excess breast tissue can impair your ability to lead an active life. The emotional discomfort and self-consciousness often associated with having large pendulous breasts is as important an issue to many women as the physical discomfort and pain.

Is It Right for Me?

Breast reduction surgery is a highly individualized procedure and you should do it for yourself, not to fulfill someone else's desires or to try to fit any sort of ideal image.

Breast reduction is a good option for you if:

- you are physically healthy;

- you have realistic expectations;

- you don't smoke;

- you are bothered by the feeling that your breasts are too large;

- your breasts limit your physical activity;

- you experience back, neck, and shoulder pain caused by the weight of your breasts;

- you have regular indentations from bra straps that support heavy, pendulous breasts;

- you have skin irritation beneath the breast crease;

- your breasts hang low and have stretched skin;

- your nipples rest below the breast crease when your breasts are unsupported;

- you have enlarged areolas caused by stretched skin.

What You Should Know before Your Breast Reduction Surgery

The success and safety of your breast reduction procedure highly depends on your complete candidness during your consultation. You'll be asked a number of questions about your health, desires, and lifestyle.
Be prepared to discuss:

- why you want the surgery, your expectations, and desired outcome;

- medical conditions, drug allergies, and medical treatments;

- use of current medications, vitamins, herbal supplements, alcohol, tobacco, and drugs;

- previous surgeries;

- family history of breast cancer and results of any mammograms or previous biopsies.

Your surgeon may also:

- evaluate your general health status and any pre-existing health conditions or risk factors;

- examine your breasts, and may take detailed measurements of their size and shape, skin quality, placement of your nipples and areolas;

- take photographs for your medical record;

- discuss your options and recommend a course of treatment;

- discuss likely outcomes of your breast reduction procedure and any risks or potential complications;

- discuss the use of anesthesia during your procedure for breast reduction.

Breast Reduction Risks and Safety Information

The decision to have breast reduction surgery is extremely personal. You will have to decide if the benefits will achieve your goals and if the risks of breast reduction surgery and potential complications are acceptable.

Your plastic surgeon and/or plastic surgery staff will explain in detail the risks associated with surgery. You will be asked to sign consent forms to ensure that you fully understand the procedure you will undergo and any risks or potential complications.

The risks of breast reduction and breast reduction complications include:

- unfavorable scarring;
- infection;
- changes in nipple or breast sensation, which may be temporary or permanent;
- anesthesia risks;
- bleeding (hematoma);
- blood clots;
- poor wound healing;
- breast contour and shape irregularities;
- skin discoloration, permanent pigmentation changes, swelling, and bruising;
- damage to deeper structures—such as nerves, blood vessels, muscles, and lungs—can occur and may be temporary or permanent;
- breast asymmetry;
- fluid accumulation;
- excessive firmness of the breast;
- potential inability to breastfeed;
- potential loss of skin/tissue of breast where incisions meet each other;
- potential, partial, or total loss of nipple and areola;
- deep vein thrombosis, cardiac and pulmonary complications;

221

- pain, which may persist;
- allergies to tape, suture materials, and glues, blood products, topical preparations or injectable agents;
- fatty tissue deep in the skin could die (fat necrosis);
- possibility of revisional surgery.

You should know that:

- breast reduction surgery can interfere with certain diagnostic procedures;
- breast and nipple piercing can cause an infection;
- your ability to breastfeed following reduction mammaplasty may be limited—talk to your doctor if you are planning to nurse a baby;
- the breast reduction procedure can be performed at any age, but is best done when your breasts are fully developed;
- changes in the breasts during pregnancy can alter the outcomes of previous breast reduction surgery, as can significant weight fluctuations.

The practice of medicine and surgery is not an exact science. Although good results are expected, there is no guarantee. In some situations, it may not be possible to achieve optimal results with a single breast reduction procedure and another surgery may be necessary.

Where Will My Surgery Be Performed?

Breast reduction procedures may be performed in your plastic surgeon's accredited office-based surgical facility, an ambulatory surgical facility, or a hospital. Your plastic surgeon and the assisting staff will fully attend to your comfort and safety.

When You Go Home

If you experience shortness of breath, chest pains, or unusual heart beats, seek medical attention immediately. Should any of these breast reduction complications occur, you may require hospitalization and additional treatment.

The practice of medicine and surgery is not an exact science. Although good results are expected, there is no guarantee. In some situations, it may not be possible to achieve optimal results with a single surgical procedure and another surgery may be necessary.

Be Careful

Following your physician's instructions is key to the success of your surgery. It is important that the surgical incisions are not subjected to excessive force, abrasion, or motion during the time of healing. Your doctor will give you specific instructions on how to care for yourself and minimize breast reduction surgery risks.

Be sure to ask questions: It's very important to address all your questions directly with your plastic surgeon. It is natural to feel some anxiety, whether excitement for the anticipated outcome or preoperative stress. Discuss these feelings with your plastic surgeon.

Section 25.3

Breast Biopsy

Excerpted from "Having a Breast Biopsy: A Guide for Women and Their Families," by the Agency for Healthcare Research and Quality (AHRQ, www.ahrq.gov), April 2010.

Screening for breast cancer increases the chance of surviving breast cancer. Screening tests can find cancers before they cause symptoms and when they are most treatable. Two common tests are used to screen for breast cancer.

- **Mammogram:** A mammogram is a breast x-ray. It looks for suspicious changes in breast tissue. It can detect cancers even when they are too small to be felt. A mammogram is the best screening test for breast cancer.

- **Breast exam by your doctor or nurse:** This is usually part of a woman's yearly exam. But if you find a breast lump or another change that worries you, don't wait. Make an appointment with your doctor or nurse to have it checked.

When a suspicious area on a mammogram or a lump is found, your doctor will probably send you for more tests. Your doctor might send you for another mammogram or a breast ultrasound. These tests tell your doctor if you need a biopsy. Most women who have further tests do not need a biopsy.

If the test results are still suspicious, your doctor will recommend a biopsy.

What Is a Breast Biopsy?

A biopsy is the only test that can tell for sure if a suspicious area is cancer. During a breast biopsy, the doctor removes a small amount of tissue from the breast.

There are two main kinds of breast biopsies. One is called surgical biopsy. The other is called core-needle biopsy.

The kind of breast biopsy a doctor recommends may depend on what the suspicious area looks like. It also might depend on the size and where it is located in the breast.

After the biopsy, the tissue is sent to a doctor who will look at the tissue under a microscope. This doctor, called a pathologist, looks for tissue changes. The pathology report tells if there is cancer or not. It takes about a week to get the report.

Kinds of Breast Biopsy

Surgical Biopsy

A surgical biopsy is usually done using local anesthesia. Local anesthesia means that the breast will be numbed.

You will have an IV [intravenous therapy] and may have medicine to make you drowsy. The surgeon makes a one- to two-inch cut on the breast and removes part or all of the suspicious tissue. Some of the tissue around it also may be taken out.

A radiologist is a doctor who specializes in medical imaging (like x-rays and mammograms). If the suspicious area can be seen on mammogram or ultrasound but can't be felt, a radiologist usually inserts a thin wire to mark the spot for the surgeon before the biopsy.

Core-Needle Biopsy

A core-needle biopsy is done using local anesthesia. The doctor inserts a hollow needle into the breast and removes a small amount of suspicious tissue. The doctor may place a tiny marker inside the breast. It marks the spot where the biopsy was done.

Radiologists or surgeons usually do core-needle biopsies using special imaging equipment.

Ultrasound-guided core-needle biopsy uses ultrasound to guide the needle to the suspicious area. Ultrasound uses sound waves to create a picture of the inside of the breast. It is like what is used to look at the baby when a woman is pregnant. You will lie on your back or side for this procedure. The doctor will hold the ultrasound device against your breast to guide the needle.

Stereotactic-guided core-needle biopsy uses x-ray equipment and a computer to guide the needle. Usually for this kind of biopsy, you lie on your stomach on a special table. The table will have an opening for your breast. Your breast will be compressed like it is for a mammogram.

Freehand core-needle biopsy does not use ultrasound or x-ray equipment. It is used less often and only for lumps that can be felt through the skin.

Research about Breast Biopsy

Accuracy

Surgical biopsies and core-needle biopsies both work well for finding breast cancer. But biopsies are not 100-percent accurate. In a few cases, a biopsy can miss breast cancer.

Surgical biopsies and ultrasound or stereotactic-guided core-needle biopsies have about the same accuracy. Freehand core-needle biopsies are less accurate.

Out of every 100 women who have breast cancer, the following are true:

- Surgical biopsies will find 98 to 99 of those breast cancers.

- Ultrasound or stereotactic-guided biopsies will find 97 to 99 of those breast cancers.

- Freehand biopsies will find about 86 of those breast cancers.

Side Effects

Bleeding, bruising, and infection can happen after a biopsy. Core-needle biopsies have a much lower risk of these problems than surgical biopsies.

Side effects are rare with any kind of core-needle biopsy.

- Less than 1 out of 100 women who have a core-needle biopsy have a problem like severe bruising, bleeding, or infection. Side effects happen more often with surgical biopsy.

- Up to 10 out of 100 women who have surgical biopsy get severe bruising.

- About 5 out of 100 women who have surgical biopsy get an infection.

Some medicines, including aspirin, increase the risk of bleeding and bruising. Your doctor will ask you about the medicines you take. You may need to stop some medicines a few days before the biopsy.

Pain

Women who have a surgical biopsy sometimes need prescription pain medicine to control pain after the procedure. Women who have a core-needle biopsy rarely need prescription pain medicine.

Biopsy Results

After the biopsy, the pathologist who looked at the tissue will send the pathology report to your doctor. It will tell if the suspicious area is cancer or not. Your doctor will go over the report with you.

Waiting for these results can be difficult. It can take about a week to get the results.

If No Cancer Is Found

If no cancer is found, the biopsy result is called benign. Benign means it is not cancer. Some benign results need follow-up or treatment. Talk to your doctor or nurse about what they recommend.

If Cancer Is Found

If cancer is found, the report will tell you the kind of cancer. It will help you and your doctor talk about the next steps. Usually, you will be referred to a breast cancer specialist. You may need more imaging tests or surgery. All this information will help you and your doctor think through your treatment options.

Take time to think. Most women with breast cancer have time to consider their options.

Make sure to ask your doctor if you don't understand your test results. After going over the results with your doctor, ask for a copy of the pathology report for your records.

Questions for Your Doctor or Nurse

Deciding on a Biopsy

- What kind of biopsy are you recommending?

- Why are you recommending this kind of biopsy?
- Are there any other options?
- What are the possible side effects from my biopsy?
- How long will it take?

Preparing for a Biopsy

- How many days before my biopsy should I stop taking aspirin? Are there other medicines to avoid?
- Can I have someone in the room with me?
- Do I need someone to drive me home?
- Who will give me the results?
- When will I get the results?

When Your Biopsy Is Benign

- What kind of follow-up do I need?
- When should I have my next mammogram?

When Your Biopsy Finds Cancer

- What are the next steps?
- What are my options for treatment?
- Can you tell me about support groups for breast cancer?

Section 25.4

Lumpectomy

Breast lump removal, called lumpectomy, is surgery to remove a breast cancer or other lump in the breast, along with some surrounding tissue from the breast.

This text covers lumpectomy that is done to remove breast cancer. Other reasons to perform a lumpectomy include:

- fibroadenoma;

- other noncancerous tumors of the breast.

Description

If the breast cancer can be seen on a mammogram or ultrasound but the doctor cannot feel the cancer on a physical exam, a wire localization will be done before the surgery:

- A radiologist will use a mammogram or ultrasound to place a needle (or needles) in or near the abnormal breast area.

- This will help the surgeon know where the cancer is so that it can be removed.

Breast lump removal is usually done in an outpatient clinic. You will be given general anesthesia (you will be asleep, but pain free) or local anesthesia (awake, but sedated and pain free). The procedure takes about one hour.

The surgeon makes a small cut on your breast and removes the cancer and some of the breast tissue around it. To make sure the whole lump has been removed, the sample is sent to a pathologist—a specialist who examines it.

- The goal is to remove breast cancer, along with some of the normal breast tissue around it. When no cancer cells are found near the edges of the tissue removed, it is called a clear margin.

- Your surgeon may also remove lymph nodes in your armpit (axilla) to see if cancer has spread to the lymph nodes.

- The surgeon will close the skin with stitches. These may dissolve or need to be removed later. A drain tube may be placed to remove extra fluid.

Your doctor will send the lump to a laboratory for testing.

Why the Procedure Is Performed

Surgery to remove a breast cancer is usually the first step in treatment. The choice of which surgery is best for you can be difficult. Sometimes, it is hard to know whether lumpectomy or mastectomy is best. You and the health care providers who are treating your breast cancer will decide together.

- Lumpectomy is often preferred for smaller breast lumps, because it is a smaller procedure and it has about the same chance of curing breast cancer as a mastectomy.

- Mastectomy, when all breast tissue is removed, may be done if the area of cancer is too large to remove without deforming the breast.

You and your doctor should consider:

- the size of your tumor, where in your breast it is located, whether you have more than one tumor in your breast, how much of your breast the cancer affects, and the size of your breasts;

- your age, family history, whether you have reached menopause, and your overall health.

Risks

Risks for any surgery are:

- bleeding;
- infection;
- reactions to medications.

Risks for this procedure are:

- The appearance of your breast may change. After surgery, you may notice dimpling, a scar, or a difference in shape between the two breasts.

- You may also have numbness in the breast area.

The breast tissue that is removed will be looked at under a microscope after the surgery. If the cancer is too close to the edge of this tissue, you may need another procedure to remove more breast tissue.

Before the Procedure

Always tell your doctor or nurse:

- if you could be pregnant;
- what drugs you are taking, even drugs or herbs you bought without a prescription.

During the days before the surgery:

- You may be asked to stop taking aspirin, ibuprofen (Advil, Motrin), naproxen (Aleve, Naprosyn), clopidogrel (Plavix), warfarin (Coumadin), and any other drugs that make it hard for your blood to clot.
- Ask your doctor which drugs you should still take on the day of the surgery.
- Always try to stop smoking. Your doctor or nurse can help.

On the day of the surgery:

- Follow your doctor's instructions about eating or drinking before surgery.
- Take the drugs your doctor told you to take with a small sip of water.
- Your doctor or nurse will tell you when to arrive for the procedure.

After the Procedure

The recovery period is very short for a simple lumpectomy. You should have little pain. If you do feel pain, you can take pain medicine, such as acetaminophen (Tylenol).

The skin should heal in about a month. You will need to take care of the surgical cut area. Change dressings as your doctor or nurse tells you to. Watch for signs of infection when you get home (such as redness, swelling, or drainage).

You may need to empty a fluid drain a few times a day for one to two weeks. Your doctor will remove the drain later.

Most women can go back to their usual activities in a week or so. Avoid heavy lifting, jogging, or activities that cause pain in the surgical area for one to two weeks.

If cancer is found, you will need to schedule follow-up treatment with your doctor.

Outlook (Prognosis)

The outcome of a lumpectomy for breast cancer depends mostly on the size of the cancer and whether it has spread to lymph nodes underneath your arm.

A lumpectomy for breast cancer is usually followed by radiation therapy and chemotherapy, hormone therapy, or both.

Women usually do not need breast reconstruction after lumpectomy.

Section 25.5

Mastectomy

A mastectomy is surgery to remove the entire breast, including the skin, nipple, and areola. It is usually done to treat breast cancer.

Description

You will be given general anesthesia (you will be asleep and pain-free). There are different types of mastectomy procedures. Which one your surgeon uses depends on the type of breast problem you have.

The surgeon will make a cut in your breast:

- For a subcutaneous mastectomy, the surgeon removes the entire breast but leaves the nipple and areola (the colored circle around the nipple) in place.

- For a total or simple mastectomy, the surgeon cuts breast tissue free from the skin and muscle and removes it. The nipple and the areola are also removed. The surgeon may do a biopsy of lymph nodes in the underarm area to see if the cancer has spread. In some rare breast cancers, a simple mastectomy is performed on both breasts.

- For a modified radical mastectomy, the surgeon removes the entire breast along with some of the lymph nodes underneath the arm.

- For a radical mastectomy, the surgeon removes the skin over the breast, all of the lymph nodes underneath the arm, and the chest muscles. This surgery is rarely done.

- The skin is closed with sutures (stitches).

One or two small plastic drains or tubes are usually left in your chest to remove extra fluid from where the breast tissue used to be.

If all the cancer tissue is removed, a plastic surgeon may be able to reconstruct the breast (with artificial implants or tissue from your own body) during the same operation. You may also choose to have reconstruction later.

Why the Procedure Is Performed

Woman Diagnosed with Breast Cancer

The most common reason for a mastectomy is breast cancer.

If you are diagnosed with breast cancer, talk to your doctor about your choices:

- Lumpectomy is when only the breast cancer and tissue around the cancer are removed. This is also called breast conservation therapy or partial mastectomy. Part of your breast will be left.

- Mastectomy is when all breast tissue is removed. Mastectomy is a better choice if the area of cancer is too large to remove without deforming the breast.

You and your doctor should consider:

- the size of your tumor, where in your breast it is located, whether you have more than one tumor in your breast, how much of your breast the cancer affects, and the size of your breasts;

- your age, family history, overall health, and whether you have reached menopause.

The choice of what is best for you can be difficult. Sometimes, it is hard to know whether lumpectomy or mastectomy is best. You and the health care providers who are treating your breast cancer will decide together what is best.

Women at High Risk for Breast Cancer

Women who have a very high risk of developing breast cancer may choose to have either a subcutaneous or total mastectomy to reduce the risk of breast cancer. This is called prophylactic mastectomy.

You may have a higher risk of getting breast cancer if one or more close family relatives has had breast cancer, especially at an early age. Genetic tests (such as BRCA1 [breast cancer 1 gene] or BRCA2 [breast cancer 2 gene]) may also show that you have a high risk. This surgery should be done only after very careful thought and discussion with your doctor, a genetic counselor, your family, and others.

Mastectomy greatly reduces, but does not eliminate, the risk of breast cancer.

Risks

Risks for any surgery are:

- blood clots in the legs that may travel to the lungs;
- blood loss;
- breathing problems;
- infection, including in the surgical wound, lungs (pneumonia), bladder, or kidney;
- heart attack or stroke during surgery;
- reactions to medications.

Scabbing, blistering, or skin loss along the edge of the surgical cut may occur.

Risks when more invasive surgery, such as a radical mastectomy, is done are:

- Shoulder pain and stiffness: You may also feel pins and needles where the breast used to be and underneath the arm.
- Swelling of the arm (called lymphedema) on the same side as the breast that is removed: This swelling is not common, but it can be an ongoing problem.
- Damage to nerves that go to the muscles of the arm, back, and chest wall.

233

Before the Procedure

You may have many blood and imaging tests (such as CT [computed tomography] scans, bone scans, and chest X-ray) after your doctor finds breast cancer. Your surgeon will want to know whether your cancer has spread to the lymph nodes, liver, lungs, bones, or somewhere else.

Always tell your doctor or nurse if:

- you could be pregnant;
- you are taking any drugs or herbs you bought without a prescription.

During the week before the surgery:

- Several days before your surgery, you may be asked to stop taking aspirin, ibuprofen (Advil, Motrin), naproxen (Aleve, Naprosyn), vitamin E, clopidogrel (Plavix), warfarin (Coumadin), and any other drugs that make it hard for your blood to clot.
- Ask your doctor which drugs you should still take on the day of the surgery.

On the day of the surgery:

- Follow instructions from your doctor or nurse about eating or drinking before surgery.
- Take the drugs your doctor told you to take with a small sip of water.

Your doctor or nurse will tell you when to arrive at the hospital.

After the Procedure

You may stay in the hospital for one to three days, depending on the type of surgery you had. If you have a simple mastectomy, you may go home on the same day. Most women go home after one to two days. You may stay longer if you have breast reconstruction.

Many women go home with drains still in their chest. The doctor will remove them later during an office visit. A nurse will teach you how to look after the drain, or you can have a home care nurse help you.

You may have pain around the site of your cut after surgery. The pain is moderate after the first day and then quickly goes away. You will receive pain medicines before you are released from the hospital.

Fluid may collect in the area of your mastectomy after all the drains are removed. This is called a seroma. It usually goes away on its own, but it may need to be drained using a needle (aspiration).

Outlook (Prognosis)

Most women recover well after mastectomy.

In addition to surgery, you may need other treatments for breast cancer. These treatments may include hormonal therapy, radiation therapy, and chemotherapy. All have their own side effects. Talk to your doctor.

Section 25.6

Prophylactic Mastectomy

Excerpted from "Preventive Mastectomy," by the National Cancer Institute (NCI, www.cancer.gov), part of the National Institutes of Health, July 27, 2006. Reviewed and revised by David A. Cooke, MD, FACP, October 10, 2012.

What is preventive mastectomy, and what types of procedures are used in preventive mastectomy?

Preventive mastectomy (also called prophylactic or risk-reducing mastectomy) is the surgical removal of one or both breasts in an effort to prevent or reduce the risk of breast cancer. Preventive mastectomy involves one of two basic procedures: Total mastectomy and subcutaneous mastectomy. In a total mastectomy, the doctor removes the entire breast and nipple. In a subcutaneous mastectomy, the doctor removes the breast tissue but leaves the nipple intact. Doctors most often recommend a total mastectomy because it removes more tissue than a subcutaneous mastectomy. A total mastectomy provides the greatest protection against cancer developing in any remaining breast tissue.

Why would a woman consider undergoing preventive mastectomy?

Women who are at high risk of developing breast cancer may consider preventive mastectomy as a way of decreasing their risk of this disease. Some of the factors that increase a woman's chance of developing breast cancer are listed in the following text.

Previous breast cancer: A woman who has had cancer in one breast is more likely to develop a new cancer in the opposite breast. Occasionally, such women may consider preventive mastectomy to decrease the chance of developing a new breast cancer.

Family history of breast cancer: Preventive mastectomy may be an option for a woman whose mother, sister, or daughter had breast cancer, especially if they were diagnosed before age 50. If multiple family members have breast or ovarian cancer, then a woman's risk of breast cancer may be even higher.

Breast cancer-causing gene alteration: A woman who tests positive for changes, or mutations, in certain genes that increase the risk of breast cancer (such as the BRCA1 or BRCA2 [breast cancer 1 or breast cancer 2] gene) may consider preventive mastectomy.

Lobular carcinoma in situ: Preventive mastectomy is sometimes considered for a woman with lobular carcinoma in situ, a condition that increases the risk of developing breast cancer in either breast.

Diffuse and indeterminate breast microcalcifications or dense breasts: Rarely, preventive mastectomy may be considered for a woman who has diffuse and indeterminate breast microcalcifications (tiny deposits of calcium in the breast) or for a woman whose breast tissue is very dense. Dense breast tissue is linked to an increased risk of breast cancer and also makes diagnosing breast abnormalities difficult. Multiple biopsies, which may be necessary for diagnosing abnormalities in dense breasts, cause scarring and further complicate examination of the breast tissue, by both physical examination and mammography.

Radiation therapy: A woman who had radiation therapy to the chest (including the breasts) before age 30 is at an increased risk of developing breast cancer throughout her life. This includes women treated for Hodgkin lymphoma.

It is important for a woman who is considering preventive mastectomy to talk with a doctor about her risk of developing breast cancer (with or without a mastectomy), the surgical procedure, and potential complications. All women are different, so preventive mastectomy should be considered in the context of each woman's unique risk factors and her level of concern.

How effective is preventive mastectomy in preventing or reducing the risk of breast cancer?

Existing data suggest that preventive mastectomy may significantly reduce (by about 90 percent) the chance of developing breast cancer in moderate- and high-risk women. However, no one can be certain that this procedure will protect an individual woman from breast cancer. Breast tissue is widely distributed on the chest wall, and can sometimes be found in the armpit, above the collarbone, and as far down as the abdomen. Because it is impossible for a surgeon to remove all breast tissue, breast cancer can still develop in the small amount of remaining tissue.

What are the possible drawbacks of preventive mastectomy?

Like any other surgery, complications such as bleeding or infection can occur. Preventive mastectomy is irreversible and can have psychological effects on a woman due to a change in body image and loss of normal breast functions. A woman should discuss her feelings about mastectomy, as well as alternatives to surgery, with her health care providers. Some women obtain a second medical opinion to help with the decision.

What alternatives to surgery exist for preventing or reducing the risk of breast cancer?

Doctors do not always agree on the most effective way to manage the care of women who have a strong family history of breast cancer and/or have other risk factors for the disease. Some doctors may advise very close monitoring (periodic mammograms, regular checkups that include a clinical breast examination performed by a health care professional, and monthly breast self-examinations) to increase the chance of detecting breast cancer at an early stage. For women who are judged to be at extremely high risk (particularly those with BRCA mutations), breast MRI can further improve early detection. Some doctors may recommend preventive mastectomy, whereas others may prescribe tamoxifen or raloxifene, medications that have been shown to decrease the chances of getting breast cancer in women at high risk of the disease.

Doctors may also encourage women at high risk to limit their consumption of alcohol, eat a low-fat diet, engage in regular exercise, and avoid menopausal hormone use. Although these lifestyle

237

recommendations make sense and are part of an overall healthy way of living, we do not yet have clear and convincing proof that they specifically reduce the risk of developing breast cancer.

What is breast reconstruction?

Breast reconstruction is a plastic surgery procedure in which the shape of the breast is rebuilt. Many women who choose to have preventive mastectomy also decide to have breast reconstruction, either at the time of the mastectomy or at some later time.

Before performing breast reconstruction, the plastic surgeon carefully examines the breasts and discusses the reconstruction options. In one type of reconstructive procedure, the surgeon inserts an implant (a balloon-like device filled with saline or silicone) under the skin and the chest muscles. Another procedure, called tissue flap reconstruction, uses skin, fat, and muscle from the woman's abdomen, back, or buttocks to create the breast shape. The surgeon will discuss with the patient any limitations on exercise or arm motion that might result from these operations.

What type of follow-up care is needed after reconstructive surgery?

Women who have reconstructive surgery are monitored carefully to detect and treat complications, such as infection, movement of the implant, or contracture (the formation of a firm, fibrous shell or scar tissue around the implant caused by the body's reaction to the implant). Women who have tissue flap reconstruction may want to ask their surgeon about physical therapy, which can help them adjust to limitations in activity and exercise after surgery. Routine screening for breast cancer is also part of the postoperative follow-up, because the risk of cancer cannot be completely eliminated. When women with breast implants have mammograms, they should tell the radiology technician about the implant. Special procedures may be necessary to improve the accuracy of the mammogram and to avoid damaging the implant. However, women who have had reconstructive surgery on both breasts should ask their doctors whether mammograms are still necessary.

Section 25.7

Breast Reconstruction

Excerpted from "What You Need to Know about Breast Cancer,"
by the National Cancer Institute (NCI, www.cancer.gov), part of the
National Institutes of Health, October 15, 2009.

Surgery is the most common treatment for breast cancer. Your doctor can explain each type, discuss and compare the benefits and risks, and describe how each will change the way you look:

- Breast-sparing surgery: This is an operation to remove the cancer but not the breast. It's also called breast-conserving surgery. It can be a lumpectomy or a segmental mastectomy (also called a partial mastectomy). Sometimes an excisional biopsy is the only surgery a woman needs because the surgeon removed the whole lump.

- Mastectomy: This is an operation to remove the entire breast (or as much of the breast tissue as possible). In some cases, a skin-sparing mastectomy may be an option. For this approach, the surgeon removes as little skin as possible.

The surgeon usually removes one or more lymph nodes from under the arm to check for cancer cells. If cancer cells are found in the lymph nodes, other cancer treatments will be needed.

You may choose to have breast reconstruction. This is plastic surgery to rebuild the shape of the breast. It may be done at the same time as the cancer surgery or later. If you're considering breast reconstruction, you may wish to talk with a plastic surgeon before having cancer surgery.

In breast-sparing surgery, the surgeon removes the cancer in the breast and some normal tissue around it. The surgeon may also remove lymph nodes under the arm. The surgeon sometimes removes some of the lining over the chest muscles below the tumor.

In total (simple) mastectomy, the surgeon removes the whole breast. Some lymph nodes under the arm may also be removed.

In modified radical mastectomy, the surgeon removes the whole breast and most or all of the lymph nodes under the arm. Often, the lining over the chest muscles is removed. A small chest muscle also may be taken out to make it easier to remove the lymph nodes.

The time it takes to heal after surgery is different for each woman. Surgery causes pain and tenderness. Medicine can help control the pain. Before surgery, you should discuss the plan for pain relief with your doctor or nurse. After surgery, your doctor can adjust the plan if you need more relief.

Any kind of surgery also carries a risk of infection, bleeding, or other problems. You should tell your health care team right away if you develop any problems.

You may feel off balance if you've had one or both breasts removed. You may feel more off balance if you have large breasts. This imbalance can cause discomfort in your neck and back.

Also, the skin where your breast was removed may feel tight. Your arm and shoulder muscles may feel stiff and weak. These problems usually go away. The doctor, nurse, or physical therapist can suggest exercises to help you regain movement and strength in your arm and shoulder. Exercise can also reduce stiffness and pain. You may be able to begin gentle exercise within days of surgery.

Because nerves may be injured or cut during surgery, you may have numbness and tingling in your chest, underarm, shoulder, and upper arm. These feelings usually go away within a few weeks or months. But for some women, numbness does not go away.

Removing the lymph nodes under the arm slows the flow of lymph fluid. The fluid may build up in your arm and hand and cause swelling. This swelling is called lymphedema. It can develop soon after surgery or months or even years later. You'll always need to protect the arm and hand on the treated side of your body from cuts, burns, or other injuries.

You may want to ask your doctor these questions before having surgery:

- What kinds of surgery can I consider? Is breast-sparing surgery an option for me? Is a skin-sparing mastectomy an option? Which operation do you recommend for me? Why?

- Will any lymph nodes be removed? How many? Why?

- How will I feel after the operation? Will I have to stay in the hospital?

- Will I need to learn how to take care of myself or my incision when I get home?

- Where will the scars be? What will they look like?

- If I decide to have plastic surgery to rebuild my breast, how and when can that be done? Can you suggest a plastic surgeon for me to contact?

- Will I have to do special exercises to help regain motion and strength in my arm and shoulder? Will a physical therapist or nurse show me how to do the exercises?

- Is there someone I can talk with who has had the same surgery I'll be having?

- How often will I need checkups?

Breast Reconstruction

Some women who plan to have a mastectomy decide to have breast reconstruction. Other women prefer to wear a breast form (prosthesis) inside their bra. Others decide to do nothing after surgery. All of these options have pros and cons. What is right for one woman may not be right for another. What is important is that nearly every woman treated for breast cancer has choices.

Breast reconstruction may be done at the same time as the mastectomy, or later on. If radiation therapy is part of the treatment plan, some doctors suggest waiting until after radiation therapy is complete.

If you are thinking about breast reconstruction, you should talk to a plastic surgeon before the mastectomy, even if you plan to have your reconstruction later on.

There are many ways for a surgeon to reconstruct the breast. Some women choose to have breast implants, which are filled with saline or silicone gel.

You also may have breast reconstruction with tissue that the plastic surgeon removes from another part of your body. Skin, muscle, and fat can come from your lower abdomen, back, or buttocks. The surgeon uses this tissue to create a breast shape.

The type of reconstruction that is best for you depends on your age, body type, and the type of cancer surgery that you had. The plastic surgeon can explain the risks and benefits of each type of reconstruction.

Chapter 26

Lung Surgery

Lung surgery is surgery to repair or remove lung tissue. Several common lung surgeries are:

- biopsy of an unknown growth;

- lobectomy, to remove one or more lobes of a lung;

- lung transplant;

- pneumonectomy, to remove a lung;

- surgery to prevent the buildup or return of fluid to the chest (pleurodesis);

- surgery to remove an infection or blood in the chest cavity (empyema);

- surgery to remove small balloon-like tissues (blebs) that cause lung collapse (pneumothorax);

- wedge resection, to remove part of a lobe in a lung.

A thoracotomy is a surgical cut that a surgeon makes to open the chest wall.

Description

You will receive general anesthesia before surgery. You will be asleep and unable to feel pain. Two common ways to do surgery on your lungs are thoracotomy and video-assisted thoracoscopic surgery (VATS).

Lung surgery using a thoracotomy is called open surgery. In this surgery:

- You will lie on your side on an operating table. Your arm will be placed above your head.

- Your surgeon will make a surgical cut between two ribs. The cut will go from the front of your chest wall to your back, passing just underneath the armpit. These ribs will be separated.

- Your lung on this side will be deflated so that air will not move in and out of it during surgery. This makes it easier for the surgeon to operate on the lung.

- Your surgeon may not know how much of your lung needs to be removed until your chest is open and the lung can be seen.

- Your surgeon may also remove lymph nodes in this area.

- After surgery, one or more drainage tubes will be placed into your chest area to drain out fluids that build up. These tubes are called chest tubes.

- After the surgery on your lungs, your surgeon will close the ribs, muscles, and skin with sutures.

- Open lung surgery may take from two to six hours.

Video-assisted thoracoscopic surgery:

- Your surgeon will make several small surgical cuts over your chest wall. A videoscope (a tube with a tiny camera on the end) and other small tools will be passed through these cuts.

- Then, your surgeon may remove part or all of your lung, drain fluid or blood that has built up, or do other procedures.

- One or more tubes will be placed into your chest to drain fluids that build up.

- This procedure leads to much less pain and a faster recovery than open lung surgery.

Why the Procedure Is Performed

Thoracotomy or video-assisted thoracoscopic surgery may be done to:

- remove cancer (such as lung cancer);
- treat injuries that cause lung tissue to collapse (pneumothorax or hemothorax);
- treat permanently collapsed lung tissue (atelectasis);
- remove lung tissue that is diseased or damaged from emphysema or bronchiectasis;
- remove blood or blood clots (hemothorax);
- remove tumors, such as solitary pulmonary nodule;
- inflate lung tissue that has collapsed because of disease or an accident;
- remove infection in the chest cavity;
- stop fluid buildup in the chest cavity (pleurodesis);
- biopsy an unknown growth;
- remove a blood clot from the pulmonary artery (pulmonary embolism).

Video-assisted thoracoscopic surgery can be used to treat many of these conditions. However, sometimes video surgery may not be possible, and the surgeon may have to switch to an open surgery.

Risks

Risks for any anesthesia include:

- allergic reactions to medicines;
- breathing problems.

Risks for any surgery include:

- bleeding;
- blood clots in the legs that may travel to the lungs;
- heart attack or stroke during surgery;
- infection, including in the surgical cut, lungs, bladder, or kidney.

Risks of this surgery include:

- failure of the lung to expand;
- injury to the lungs or blood vessels;
- need for a chest tube after surgery;
- pain;
- prolonged air leak;
- repeated fluid buildup in the chest cavity.

Before the Procedure

You will have several visits with your health care provider and undergo medical tests before your surgery. Your health care provider will:

- do a complete physical exam;
- make sure other medical conditions you may have, such as diabetes, high blood pressure, or heart or lung problems are under control;
- perform tests to make sure that you will be able to tolerate the removal of your lung.

If you are a smoker, you should stop smoking several weeks before your surgery. Ask your doctor or nurse for help.

Always tell your doctor or nurse:

- what drugs, vitamins, herbs, and other supplements you are taking, even ones you bought without a prescription;
- if you have been drinking a lot of alcohol, more than one or two drinks a day.

During the week before your surgery:

- You may be asked to stop taking drugs that make it hard for your blood to clot. Some of these are aspirin, ibuprofen (Advil, Motrin), vitamin E, warfarin (Coumadin), clopidogrel (Plavix), or ticlopidine (Ticlid).
- Ask your doctor which drugs you should still take on the day of your surgery.
- Prepare your home for your return from the hospital.

On the day of your surgery:

- Do not eat or drink anything after midnight the night before your surgery.

- Take the medications your doctor prescribed with small sips of water.

- Your doctor or nurse will tell you when to arrive at the hospital.

After the Procedure

Most people stay in the hospital for five to seven days for open thoracotomy and one to three days after video-assisted thoracoscopic surgery. You may spend time in the intensive care unit (ICU) after either surgery.

During your hospital stay, you will:

- be asked to sit on the side of the bed and walk as soon as possible after surgery;

- have tube(s) coming out of the side of your chest to drain fluids;

- wear special stockings on your feet and legs to prevent blood clots;

- receive shots to prevent blood clots;

- receive pain medicine through an IV (a tube that goes into your veins) or by mouth with pills (You may receive your pain medicine through a special machine that gives you a dose of pain medicine when you push a button. This allows you to control how much pain medicine you get.);

- be asked to do a lot of deep breathing to help prevent pneumonia and infection. Deep breathing exercises also help inflate the lung that was operated on. Your chest tube(s) will remain in place until your lung has fully inflated.

Outlook (Prognosis)

The outcome depends on:

- the type of problem being treated;

- how much of the lung is removed;

- your overall health before surgery.

Chapter 27

Heart and Vascular Surgery

Chapter Contents

Section 27.1

Angioplasty

Excerpted from "What Is Coronary Angioplasty?" by the National
Heart, Lung, and Blood Institute (NHLBI, www.nhlbi.nih.gov), part
of the National Institutes of Health, February 1, 2012.

Coronary angioplasty is a procedure used to open narrow or blocked
coronary (heart) arteries. The procedure restores blood flow to the
heart muscle.

Your doctor may recommend coronary angioplasty if you have narrow
or blocked coronary arteries as a result of coronary heart disease (CHD).

Angioplasty is one treatment for CHD. Other treatments include
medicines and coronary artery bypass grafting (CABG). CABG is a
type of surgery in which a healthy artery or vein from the body is connected, or grafted, to a blocked coronary artery.

The grafted artery or vein bypasses (that is, goes around) the blocked
portion of the coronary artery. This improves blood flow to the heart.

Compared with CABG, some advantages of angioplasty are that it:

* doesn't require open-heart surgery;

* doesn't require general anesthesia (that is, you won't be given
  medicine to make you sleep during the procedure);

* has a shorter recovery time.

However, angioplasty isn't for everyone. For some people, CABG
might be a better option. For example, CABG might be used to treat
people who have severe CHD, narrowing of the left main coronary
artery, or poor function in the lower left heart chamber.

Your doctor will consider many factors when deciding which
treatment(s) to recommend.

Angioplasty also is used as an emergency treatment for heart attack. As plaque builds up in the coronary arteries, it can rupture. This
can cause a blood clot to form on the surface of the plaque and block
blood flow to the heart muscle.

Quickly opening the blockage restores blood flow and reduces heart
muscle damage during a heart attack.

How Is Coronary Angioplasty Done?

Before you have coronary angioplasty, your doctor will need to know the location and extent of the blockages in your coronary (heart) arteries. To find this information, your doctor will use coronary angiography. This test uses dye and special X-rays to show the insides of your arteries.

During angiography, a small tube (or tubes) called a catheter is inserted into an artery, usually in the groin (upper thigh). The catheter is threaded to the coronary arteries.

Special dye, which is visible on X-ray pictures, is injected through the catheter. The X-ray pictures are taken as the dye flows through your coronary arteries. The dye shows whether blockages are present and their location and severity.

For the angioplasty procedure, another catheter with a balloon at its tip (a balloon catheter) is inserted in the coronary artery and placed in the blockage. Then, the balloon is expanded. This pushes the plaque against the artery wall, relieving the blockage and improving blood flow.

A small mesh tube called a stent usually is placed in the artery during angioplasty. The stent is wrapped around the deflated balloon catheter before the catheter is inserted into the artery.

When the balloon is inflated to compress the plaque, the stent expands and attaches to the artery wall. The stent supports the inner artery wall and reduces the chance of the artery becoming narrow or blocked again.

Some stents are coated with medicine that is slowly and continuously released into the artery. They are called drug-eluting stents. The medicine helps prevent scar tissue from blocking the artery following angioplasty.

What to Expect before Coronary Angioplasty

Coronary angioplasty is done in a hospital. A cardiologist will perform the procedure. A cardiologist is a doctor who specializes in diagnosing and treating heart diseases and conditions.

If angioplasty isn't done as an emergency treatment, you'll meet with your cardiologist beforehand. He or she will go over your medical history (including the medicines you take), do a physical exam, and talk to you about the procedure.

Your doctor also may recommend tests, such as blood tests, an EKG (electrocardiogram), and a chest X-ray.

Once the angioplasty is scheduled, your doctor will advise you of the following:

- When to begin fasting (not eating or drinking) before the procedure (Often, you have to stop eating and drinking six to eight hours before the procedure.)
- What medicines you should and shouldn't take on the day of the procedure
- When to arrive at the hospital and where to go

Even though angioplasty takes only one to two hours, you'll likely need to stay in the hospital overnight. Your doctor may advise you to not drive for a certain amount of time after the procedure. Thus, you'll probably need to arrange a ride home.

What to Expect during Coronary Angioplasty

Coronary angioplasty is done in a special part of the hospital called the cardiac catheterization laboratory. The "cath lab" has special video screens and X-ray machines.

Your doctor will use this equipment to see enlarged pictures of the blockages in your coronary arteries.

Preparation

In the cath lab, you'll lie down. An intravenous (IV) line will be placed in your arm to give you fluids and medicines. The medicines will relax you and help prevent blood clots from forming.

The area where your doctor will insert the catheter will be shaved. The catheter usually is inserted in your groin (upper thigh). The shaved area will be cleaned and then numbed. The numbing medicine may sting as it's going in.

The Procedure

During angioplasty, you'll be awake but sleepy.

Your doctor will use a needle to make a small hole in an artery in your arm or groin. A thin, flexible guide wire will be inserted into the artery through the small hole. Then, your doctor will remove the needle and place a tapered tube called a sheath over the guide wire and into the artery.

Next, your doctor will put a long, thin, flexible tube called a guiding catheter through the sheath and slide it over the guide wire. The catheter is moved to the opening of a coronary artery, and the guide wire is removed.

Your doctor will inject special dye through the catheter. The dye will help show the inside of the coronary artery and any blockages on an X-ray picture called an angiogram.

Another guide wire is then put through the catheter into the coronary artery and threaded past the blockage. A thin catheter with a balloon at its tip (a balloon catheter) is threaded over the wire and through the guiding catheter.

The balloon catheter is positioned in the blockage. Then, the balloon is inflated. This pushes the plaque against the artery wall, relieving the blockage and improving blood flow through the artery. Sometimes the balloon is inflated and deflated more than once to widen the artery.

Your doctor may put a stent (small mesh tube) in your artery to help keep it open. If so, the stent will be wrapped around the balloon catheter.

When your doctor inflates the balloon, the stent will expand against the wall of the artery. When the balloon is deflated and pulled out of the artery with the catheter, the stent remains in place in the artery.

After angioplasty is done, the sheath, guide wires, and catheters are removed from your artery. Pressure is applied to stop bleeding at the catheter insertion site. Sometimes a special device is used to seal the hole in the artery.

During angioplasty, you'll receive strong antiplatelet medicines through your IV line. These medicines help prevent blood clots from forming in the artery or on the stent. Your doctor may start you on antiplatelet medicines before the angioplasty.

What to Expect after Coronary Angioplasty

After coronary angioplasty, you'll be moved to a special care unit. You'll stay there for a few hours or overnight. You must lie still for a few hours to allow the blood vessel in your arm or groin (upper thigh) to seal completely.

While you recover, someone on your health care team will check your blood pressure, heart rate, oxygen level, and temperature. The site where the catheters were inserted also will be checked for bleeding. That area may feel sore or tender for a while.

Going Home

Most people go home the day after the procedure. When your doctor thinks you're ready to leave the hospital, you'll get instructions to follow at home, such as the following:

- How much activity or exercise you can do (Most people are able to walk the day after the angioplasty.)

- When you should follow up with your doctor

- What medicines you should take

- What you should look for daily when checking for signs of infection around the catheter insertion site (Signs of infection include redness, swelling, and drainage.)

- When you should call your doctor (For example, you may need to call if you have shortness of breath; a fever; or signs of infection, pain, or bleeding.)

- When you should call 911 (for example, if you have any chest pain)

Your doctor will prescribe medicine to help prevent blood clots from forming. Take all of your medicine as your doctor prescribes.

If you got a stent during angioplasty, the medicine reduces the risk that blood clots will form in the stent. Blood clots in the stent can block blood flow and cause a heart attack.

Recovery and Recuperation

Most people recover from angioplasty and return to work within a week of leaving the hospital.

Your doctor will want to check your progress after you leave the hospital. During the followup visit, your doctor will examine you, make changes to your medicines (if needed), do any necessary tests, and check your overall recovery.

Use this time to ask questions you may have about activities, medicines, or lifestyle changes, or to talk about any other issues that concern you.

Complications from Stents

Restenosis

Another problem that can occur after angioplasty is too much tissue growth within the treated portion of the artery. This can cause the artery to become narrow or blocked again, often within six months. This complication is called restenosis.

When a stent (small mesh tube) isn't used during angioplasty, 30 percent of people have restenosis. When a stent is used, 15 percent of people have restenosis.

Stents coated with medicine (drug-eluting stents) reduce the growth of scar tissue around the stent. These stents further reduce the risk of restenosis. When these stents are used, about 10 percent of people have restenosis.

Other treatments, such as radiation, can help prevent tissue growth within a stent. For this procedure, a wire is put through a catheter to where the stent is placed. The wire releases radiation to stop any tissue growth that may block the artery.

Blood Clots

Studies suggest that there's a higher risk of blood clots forming in medicine-coated stents compared with bare metal stents. However, no firm evidence shows that these stents increase the chance of having a heart attack or dying if used as recommended. Researchers continue to study medicine-coated stents.

Taking medicine as prescribed by your doctor can lower your risk of blood clots. People who have medicine-coated stents usually are advised to take antiplatelet medicines, such as clopidogrel and aspirin, for up to a year or longer.

As with all procedures, you should talk with your doctor about your treatment options, including the risks and benefits.

Section 27.2

Coronary Artery Bypass Grafting Surgery

Excerpted from "What Is Coronary Artery Bypass Grafting?" by the
National Heart, Lung, and Blood Institute (NHLBI, www.nhlbi.nih.gov),
part of the National Institutes of Health, February 23, 2012.

Coronary artery bypass grafting (CABG) is a type of surgery that
improves blood flow to the heart. Surgeons use CABG to treat people
who have severe coronary heart disease (CHD).

CHD is a disease in which a waxy substance called plaque builds
up inside the coronary arteries. These arteries supply oxygen-rich
blood to your heart.

Over time, plaque can harden or rupture (break open). Hardened
plaque narrows the coronary arteries and reduces the flow of oxygen-rich
blood to the heart. This can cause chest pain or discomfort called angina.

If the plaque ruptures, a blood clot can form on its surface. A large
blood clot can mostly or completely block blood flow through a coronary
artery. This is the most common cause of a heart attack. Over time,
ruptured plaque also hardens and narrows the coronary arteries.

CABG is one treatment for CHD. During CABG, a healthy artery
or vein from the body is connected, or grafted, to the blocked coronary
artery. The grafted artery or vein bypasses (that is, goes around) the
blocked portion of the coronary artery. This creates a new path for
oxygen-rich blood to flow to the heart muscle.

Surgeons can bypass multiple coronary arteries during one surgery.

Types of Coronary Artery Bypass Grafting

There are several types of coronary artery bypass grafting (CABG).
Your doctor will recommend the best option for you based on your needs.

Traditional Coronary Artery Bypass Grafting

Traditional CABG is used when at least one major artery needs to
be bypassed. During the surgery, the chest bone is opened to access
the heart.

Medicines are given to stop the heart; a heart-lung bypass machine keeps blood and oxygen moving throughout the body during surgery. This allows the surgeon to operate on a still heart.

After surgery, blood flow to the heart is restored. Usually, the heart starts beating again on its own. Sometimes mild electric shocks are used to restart the heart.

Off-Pump Coronary Artery Bypass Grafting

This type of CABG is similar to traditional CABG because the chest bone is opened to access the heart. However, the heart isn't stopped, and a heart-lung bypass machine isn't used. Off-pump CABG sometimes is called beating heart bypass grafting.

Minimally Invasive Direct Coronary Artery Bypass Grafting

This type of surgery differs from traditional CABG because the chest bone isn't opened to reach the heart. Instead, several small cuts are made on the left side of the chest between the ribs. This type of surgery mainly is used to bypass blood vessels at the front of the heart.

Minimally invasive bypass grafting is a fairly new procedure. It isn't right for everyone, especially if more than one or two coronary arteries need to be bypassed.

What to Expect before Coronary Artery Bypass Grafting

You may have tests to prepare you for coronary artery bypass grafting (CABG). For example, you may have blood tests, an EKG (electrocardiogram), echocardiography, a chest X-ray, cardiac catheterization, and coronary angiography.

Your doctor will tell you how to prepare for CABG surgery. He or she will advise you about what you can eat or drink, which medicines to take, and which activities to stop (such as smoking). You'll likely be admitted to the hospital on the same day as the surgery.

If tests for coronary heart disease show that you have severe blockages in your coronary (heart) arteries, your doctor may admit you to the hospital right away. You may have CABG that day or the day after.

What to Expect during Coronary Artery Bypass Grafting

Coronary artery bypass grafting (CABG) requires a team of experts. A cardiothoracic surgeon will do the surgery with support from an anesthesiologist, perfusionist (heart-lung bypass machine specialist), other surgeons, and nurses.

There are several types of CABG. They range from traditional surgery to newer, less-invasive methods.

Traditional Coronary Artery Bypass Grafting

This type of surgery usually lasts 3–6 hours, depending on the number of arteries being bypassed. Many steps take place during traditional CABG.

You'll be under general anesthesia for the surgery. The term "anesthesia" refers to a loss of feeling and awareness. General anesthesia temporarily puts you to sleep.

During the surgery, the anesthesiologist will check your heartbeat, blood pressure, oxygen levels, and breathing. A breathing tube will be placed in your lungs through your throat. The tube will connect to a ventilator (a machine that supports breathing).

The surgeon will make an incision (cut) down the center of your chest. He or she will cut your chest bone and open your rib cage to reach your heart.

You'll receive medicines to stop your heart. This allows the surgeon to operate on your heart while it's not beating. You'll also receive medicines to protect your heart function during the time that it's not beating.

A heart-lung bypass machine will keep oxygen-rich blood moving throughout your body during the surgery.

The surgeon will take an artery or vein from your body—for example, from your chest or leg—to use as the bypass graft. For surgeries with several bypasses, both artery and vein grafts are commonly used.

- Artery grafts: These grafts are much less likely than vein grafts to become blocked over time. The left internal mammary artery most often is used for an artery graft. This artery is located inside the chest, close to the heart. Arteries from the arm or other places in the body also are used.

- Vein grafts: Although veins are commonly used as grafts, they're more likely than artery grafts to become blocked over time. The saphenous vein—a long vein running along the inner side of the leg—typically is used.

When the surgeon finishes the grafting, he or she will restore blood flow to your heart. Usually, the heart starts beating again on its own. Sometimes mild electric shocks are used to restart the heart.

You'll be disconnected from the heart-lung bypass machine. Then, tubes will be inserted into your chest to drain fluid.

The surgeon will use wire to close your chest bone (much like how a broken bone is repaired). The wire will stay in your body permanently. After your chest bone heals, it will be as strong as it was before the surgery.

Stitches or staples will be used to close the skin incision. The breathing tube will be removed when you're able to breathe without it.

Nontraditional Coronary Artery Bypass Grafting

Nontraditional CABG includes off-pump CABG and minimally invasive CABG.

Off-Pump Coronary Artery Bypass Grafting

Surgeons can use off-pump CABG to bypass any of the coronary (heart) arteries. Off-pump CABG is similar to traditional CABG because the chest bone is opened to access the heart.

However, the heart isn't stopped and a heart-lung-bypass machine isn't used. Instead, the surgeon steadies the heart with a mechanical device.

Off-pump CABG sometimes is called beating heart bypass grafting.

Minimally Invasive Direct Coronary Artery Bypass Grafting

There are several types of minimally invasive direct coronary artery bypass (MIDCAB) grafting. These types of surgery differ from traditional bypass surgery because the chest bone isn't opened to reach the heart. Also, a heart-lung bypass machine isn't always used for these procedures.

MIDCAB procedure: This type of surgery mainly is used to bypass blood vessels at the front of the heart. Small incisions are made between your ribs on the left side of your chest, directly over the artery that needs to be bypassed.

The incisions usually are about three inches long. (The incision made in traditional CABG is at least six to eight inches long.) The left internal mammary artery most often is used for the graft in this procedure. A heart-lung bypass machine isn't used during MIDCAB grafting.

Port-access coronary artery bypass procedure: The surgeon does this procedure through small incisions (ports) made in your chest.

Artery or vein grafts are used. A heart-lung bypass machine is used during this procedure.

Robot-assisted technique: This type of procedure allows for even smaller, keyhole-sized incisions. A small video camera is inserted in one incision to show the heart, while the surgeon uses remote-controlled surgical instruments to do the surgery. A heart-lung bypass machine sometimes is used during this procedure.

What to Expect after Coronary Artery Bypass Grafting

Recovery in the Hospital

After surgery, you'll typically spend one or two days in an intensive care unit (ICU). Your health care team will check your heart rate, blood pressure, and oxygen levels regularly during this time.

An intravenous (IV) line will likely be inserted into a vein in your arm. Through the IV line, you may get medicines to control blood flow and blood pressure. You also will likely have a tube in your bladder to drain urine and a tube in your chest to drain fluid.

You may receive oxygen therapy (oxygen given through nasal prongs or a mask) and a temporary pacemaker while in the ICU. A pacemaker is a small device that's placed in the chest or abdomen to help control abnormal heart rhythms.

Your doctor also might recommend that you wear compression stockings on your legs. These stockings are tight at the ankle and become looser as they go up the legs. This creates gentle pressure that keeps blood from pooling and clotting.

While in the ICU, you'll also have bandages on your chest incision (cut) and on the areas where arteries or veins were removed for grafting.

After you leave the ICU, you'll be moved to a less intensive care area of the hospital for three to five days before going home.

Section 27.3

Transmyocardial Laser Revascularization (TMR)

Transmyocardial revascularization (TMR) is a surgical procedure for patients who have inoperable coronary artery disease and angina (chest pain).

Patients with coronary artery disease are treated with interventional procedures (angioplasty and stenting), coronary artery bypass grafting (surgery), and medications to improve blood flow to the heart muscle. If these procedures do not eliminate the symptoms of angina, TMR is another possible treatment option.

How Does TMR Work?

TMR is a treatment aimed at improving blood flow to areas of the heart that were not treated by angioplasty or surgery. A special carbon dioxide (CO_2) laser is used to create small channels in the heart muscle, improving blood flow in the heart. TMR is a surgical procedure. The procedure is performed through a small left chest incision or through a midline incision. Frequently, it is performed with coronary artery bypass surgery, but occasionally it is performed independently.

Once the incision is made, the surgeon exposes the heart muscle. A laser handpiece is then positioned on the area of the heart to be treated. A special high-energy, computerized CO_2 laser, called the CO_2 Heart Laser 2 1, is used to create between 20 to 40 one-millimeter-wide channels (about the width of the head of a pin) in the oxygen-poor left ventricle (left lower pumping chamber) of the heart. The doctor determines how many channels to create during the procedure. The outer areas of the channels close, but the inside of the channels remain open inside the heart to improve blood flow.

261

The CO_2 Heart Laser 2 1 uses a computer to direct laser beams to the appropriate area of the heart in between heartbeats, when the ventricle is filled with blood and the heart is relatively still. This helps to prevent electrical disturbances in the heart.

Clinical evidence suggests blood flow is improved in two ways:

1. The channels act as bloodlines. When the ventricle pumps or squeezes oxygen-rich blood out of the heart, it sends blood through the channels, restoring blood flow to the heart muscle.

2. The procedure may promote angiogenesis, or growth of new capillaries (small blood vessels) that help supply blood to the heart muscle.

TMR usually takes one to two hours. The procedure may last longer if it is combined with other heart procedures.

How Do You Get Evaluated for TMR?

Talk to your cardiologist about whether TMR surgery is an option for you.

Resources

http://www.plcmed.com

Section 27.4

Valve Repair and Replacement

Excerpted from "How Is Heart Valve Disease Treated?" by the National
Heart, Lung, and Blood Institute (NHLBI, www.nhlbi.nih.gov), part of
the National Institutes of Health, November 16, 2011.

Your doctor may recommend repairing or replacing your heart valve(s), even if your heart valve disease isn't causing symptoms. Repairing or replacing a valve can prevent lasting damage to your heart and sudden death.

Having heart valve repair or replacement depends on many factors, including:

- the severity of your valve disease;

- your age and general health;

- whether you need heart surgery for other conditions, such as bypass surgery to treat CHD.

Bypass surgery and valve surgery can be done at the same time.

When possible, heart valve repair is preferred over heart valve replacement. Valve repair preserves the strength and function of the heart muscle. People who have valve repair also have a lower risk of IE after the surgery, and they don't need to take blood-thinning medicines for the rest of their lives.

However, heart valve repair surgery is harder to do than valve replacement. Also, not all valves can be repaired. Mitral valves often can be repaired. Aortic and pulmonary valves often have to be replaced.

Repairing Heart Valves

Heart surgeons can repair heart valves by doing the following:

- Separating fused valve flaps

- Removing or reshaping tissue so the valve can close tighter

- Adding tissue to patch holes or tears or to increase the support at the base of the valve

Sometimes cardiologists repair heart valves using cardiac catheterization. Although catheter procedures are less invasive than surgery, they may not work as well for some patients.

Work with your doctor to decide whether repair is appropriate. If so, your doctor can advise you on the best procedure for doing it.

Balloon Valvuloplasty

Heart valves that don't fully open (stenosis) can be repaired with surgery or with a less invasive catheter procedure called balloon valvuloplasty. This procedure also is called balloon valvotomy.

During the procedure, a catheter (thin tube) with a balloon at its tip is threaded through a blood vessel to the faulty valve in your heart. The balloon is inflated to help widen the opening of the valve. Your doctor then deflates the balloon and removes both it and the tube.

You're awake during the procedure, which usually requires an overnight stay in a hospital.

Balloon valvuloplasty relieves many of the symptoms of heart valve disease, but it may not cure it. The condition can worsen over time. You still may need medicines to treat symptoms or surgery to repair or replace the faulty valve.

Balloon valvuloplasty has a shorter recovery time than surgery. The procedure may work as well as surgery for some patients who have mitral valve stenosis. Thus, for these people, balloon valvuloplasty often is preferred over surgical repair or replacement.

Balloon valvuloplasty doesn't work as well as surgery for adults who have aortic valve stenosis.

Doctors often use balloon valvuloplasty to repair valve stenosis in infants and children.

Replacing Heart Valves

Sometimes heart valves can't be repaired and must be replaced. This surgery involves removing the faulty valve and replacing it with a man-made or biological valve.

Biological valves are made from pig, cow, or human heart tissue and may have man-made parts as well. These valves are specially treated, so you won't need medicines to stop your body from rejecting the valve.

Man-made valves last longer than biological valves and usually don't have to be replaced. Biological valves usually have to be replaced after about 10 years, although newer ones may last 15 years or longer.

Unlike biological valves, however, man-made valves require you to take blood-thinning medicines for the rest of your life. These medicines prevent blood clots from forming on the valve. Blood clots can cause a heart attack or stroke. Man-made valves also raise your risk of IE.

You and your doctor will decide together whether you should have a man-made or biological replacement valve.

If you're a woman of childbearing age or if you're athletic, you may prefer a biological valve so you don't have to take blood-thinning medicines. If you're elderly, you also may prefer a biological valve, as it will likely last for the rest of your life.

Other Approaches for Repairing and Replacing Heart Valves

Some newer forms of heart valve repair and replacement surgery are less invasive than traditional surgery. These procedures use smaller incisions (cuts) to reach the heart valves. Hospital stays for these newer types of surgery usually are three to five days, compared with 5-day stays for traditional heart valve surgery.

New surgeries tend to cause less pain and have a lower risk of infection. Recovery time also tends to be shorter—two to four weeks versus six to eight weeks for traditional surgery.

Some cardiologists and surgeons are exploring catheter procedures that involve threading clips or other devices through blood vessels to faulty heart valves. The clips or devices are used to reshape the valves and stop the backflow of blood.

People who receive these clips recover more easily than people who have surgery. However, the clips may not treat backflow as well as surgery. Researchers are still studying this treatment method.

Doctor also may use catheters to replace faulty aortic valves. This procedure is called transcatheter aortic valve implantation (TAVI).

For this procedure, the catheter usually is inserted into an artery in the groin (upper thigh) and threaded to the heart. At the end of the catheter is a deflated balloon with a folded replacement valve around it.

Once the replacement valve is properly placed, the balloon is used to expand the new valve so it fits securely within the old valve. The balloon is then deflated, and the balloon and catheter are removed.

A replacement valve also can be inserted in an existing replacement valve that is failing. This is called a valve-in-valve procedure.

Catheter procedures may be an option for patients who have conditions that make open-heart surgery too risky. Only a few medical centers have experience with these fairly new procedures.

Doctors also treat faulty aortic valves with a procedure called the Ross operation. During this operation, your doctor removes your faulty aortic valve and replaces it with your pulmonary valve. Your pulmonary valve is then replaced with a pulmonary valve from a deceased human donor.

This is more involved surgery than typical valve replacement, and it has a greater risk of complications.

The Ross operation may be especially useful for children because the surgically replaced valves continue to grow with the child. Also, lifelong treatment with blood-thinning medicines isn't required.

But in some patients, one or both valves fail to work well within a few years of the surgery. Experts continue to debate and study the usefulness of this procedure.

Serious risks from all types of heart valve surgery vary according to your age, health, the type of valve defect(s) you have, and the surgical procedures used.

Section 27.5

Arrhythmia Surgery

Excerpted from "What Is an Arrhythmia?" by the National Heart, Lung, and Blood Institute (NHLBI, www.nhlbi.nih.gov), part of the National Institutes of Health, July 1, 2011.

What Is an Arrhythmia?

An arrhythmia is a problem with the rate or rhythm of the heartbeat. During an arrhythmia, the heart can beat too fast, too slow, or with an irregular rhythm.

A heartbeat that is too fast is called tachycardia. A heartbeat that is too slow is called bradycardia.

Most arrhythmias are harmless, but some can be serious or even life threatening. During an arrhythmia, the heart may not be able to pump enough blood to the body. Lack of blood flow can damage the brain, heart, and other organs.

Types of Arrhythmia

The four main types of arrhythmia are premature (extra) beats, supraventricular arrhythmias, ventricular arrhythmias, and bradyarrhythmias.

Premature (Extra) Beats

Premature beats are the most common type of arrhythmia. They're harmless most of the time and often don't cause any symptoms.

When symptoms do occur, they usually feel like fluttering in the chest or a feeling of a skipped heartbeat. Most of the time, premature beats need no treatment, especially in healthy people.

Premature beats that occur in the atria (the heart's upper chambers) are called premature atrial contractions, or PACs. Premature beats that occur in the ventricles (the heart's lower chambers) are called premature ventricular contractions, or PVCs.

In most cases, premature beats happen naturally. However, some heart diseases can cause premature beats. They also can happen because of stress, too much exercise, or too much caffeine or nicotine.

Supraventricular Arrhythmias

Supraventricular arrhythmias are tachycardias (fast heart rates) that start in the atria or atrioventricular (AV) node. The AV node is a group of cells located between the atria and the ventricles.

Types of supraventricular arrhythmias include atrial fibrillation (AF), atrial flutter, paroxysmal supraventricular tachycardia (PSVT), and Wolff-Parkinson-White (WPW) syndrome.

Atrial Fibrillation

AF is the most common type of serious arrhythmia. It involves a very fast and irregular contraction of the atria.

In AF, the heart's electrical signals don't begin in the SA node. Instead, they begin in another part of the atria or in the nearby pulmonary veins.

The signals don't travel normally. They may spread throughout the atria in a rapid, disorganized way. This causes the walls of the atria to quiver very fast (fibrillate) instead of beating normally. As a result, the atria aren't able to pump blood into the ventricles the way they should.

In AF, electrical signals can travel through the atria at a rate of more than 300 per minute. Some of these abnormal signals can travel to the ventricles, causing them to beat too fast and with an irregular rhythm. AF usually isn't life threatening, but it can be dangerous if it causes the ventricles to beat very fast.

AF has two major complications—stroke and heart failure.

In AF, blood can pool in the atria, causing blood clots to form. If a clot breaks off and travels to the brain, it can cause a stroke. Blood-thinning medicines that reduce the risk of stroke are an important part of treatment for people who have AF.

Heart failure occurs if the heart can't pump enough blood to meet the body's needs. AF can lead to heart failure because the ventricles are beating very fast and can't completely fill with blood. Thus, they may not be able to pump enough blood to the lungs and body.

Damage to the heart's electrical system causes AF. The damage most often is the result of other conditions that affect the health of the heart, such as high blood pressure, coronary heart disease, and rheumatic heart disease. Inflammation also is thought to play a role in the development of AF.

Other conditions also can lead to AF, including an overactive thyroid gland (too much thyroid hormone produced) and heavy alcohol use. The risk of AF increases with age.

Sometimes AF and other supraventricular arrhythmias can occur for no obvious reason.

Atrial Flutter

Atrial flutter is similar to AF. However, the heart's electrical signals spread through the atria in a fast and regular—instead of irregular—rhythm. Atrial flutter is much less common than AF, but it has similar symptoms and complications.

Paroxysmal Supraventricular Tachycardia

PSVT is a very fast heart rate that begins and ends suddenly. PSVT occurs because of problems with the electrical connection between the atria and the ventricles.

In PSVT, electrical signals that begin in the atria and travel to the ventricles can reenter the atria, causing extra heartbeats. This type of arrhythmia usually isn't dangerous and tends to occur in young people. It can happen during vigorous physical activity.

A special type of PSVT is called Wolff-Parkinson-White syndrome. WPW syndrome is a condition in which the heart's electrical signals travel along an extra pathway from the atria to the ventricles.

This extra pathway disrupts the timing of the heart's electrical signals and can cause the ventricles to beat very fast. This type of arrhythmia can be life threatening.

Ventricular Arrhythmias

These arrhythmias start in the heart's lower chambers, the ventricles. They can be very dangerous and usually require medical care right away.

Ventricular arrhythmias include ventricular tachycardia and ventricular fibrillation (v-fib). Coronary heart disease, heart attack, a weakened heart muscle, and other problems can cause ventricular arrhythmias.

Ventricular Tachycardia

Ventricular tachycardia is a fast, regular beating of the ventricles that may last for only a few seconds or for much longer.

A few beats of ventricular tachycardia often don't cause problems. However, episodes that last for more than a few seconds can be dangerous. Ventricular tachycardia can turn into other, more serious arrhythmias, such as v-fib.

Ventricular Fibrillation

V-fib occurs if disorganized electrical signals make the ventricles quiver instead of pump normally. Without the ventricles pumping blood to the body, sudden cardiac arrest and death can occur within a few minutes.

To prevent death, the condition must be treated right away with an electric shock to the heart called defibrillation.

V-fib may occur during or after a heart attack or in someone whose heart is already weak because of another condition.

Torsades de pointes (torsades) is a type of v-fib that causes a unique pattern on an EKG (electrocardiogram) test. Certain medicines or imbalanced amounts of potassium, calcium, or magnesium in the bloodstream can cause this condition.

People who have long QT syndrome are at increased risk for torsades. People who have this condition need to be careful about taking certain antibiotics, heart medicines, and over-the-counter products.

Bradyarrhythmias

Bradyarrhythmias occur if the heart rate is slower than normal. If the heart rate is too slow, not enough blood reaches the brain. This can cause you to pass out.

In adults, a heart rate slower than 60 beats per minute is considered a bradyarrhythmia. Some people normally have slow heart rates, especially people who are very physically fit. For them, a heartbeat slower than 60 beats per minute isn't dangerous and doesn't cause symptoms. But in other people, serious diseases or other conditions may cause bradyarrhythmias.

Bradyarrhythmias can be caused by:

- heart attacks;

- conditions that harm or change the heart's electrical activity, such as an underactive thyroid gland or aging;

- an imbalance of chemicals or other substances in the blood, such as potassium;

- medicines such as beta blockers, calcium channel blockers, some antiarrhythmia medicines, and digoxin.

How Are Arrhythmias Treated?

Common arrhythmia treatments include medicines, medical procedures, and surgery. Your doctor may recommend treatment if your arrhythmia causes serious symptoms, such as dizziness, chest pain, or fainting.

Your doctor also may recommend treatment if the arrhythmia increases your risk for problems such as heart failure, stroke, or sudden cardiac arrest.

Surgery

Doctors treat some arrhythmias with surgery. This may occur if surgery is already being done for another reason, such as repair of a heart valve.

One type of surgery for AF is called maze surgery. During this surgery, a surgeon makes small cuts or burns in the atria. These cuts or burns prevent the spread of disorganized electrical signals.

If coronary heart disease is the cause of your arrhythmia, your doctor may recommend coronary artery bypass grafting. This surgery improves blood flow to the heart muscle.

Section 27.6

Carotid Endarterectomy

"What Is Carotid Endarterectomy?" by the National Heart, Lung, and Blood Institute (NHLBI, www.nhlbi.nih.gov), part of the National Institutes of Health, December 1, 2010.

Carotid endarterectomy, or CEA, is a type of surgery that is used to prevent strokes in people who have carotid artery disease.

Carotid artery disease occurs if plaque builds up in the two large arteries on each side of your neck (the carotid arteries). The carotid arteries supply your brain with oxygen-rich blood.

Plaque is made up of fat, cholesterol, calcium, and other substances found in the blood. Over time, plaque hardens and narrows the carotid arteries. This limits or blocks the flow of oxygen-rich blood to your brain, which can lead to a stroke.

A stroke also can occur if the plaque in a carotid artery cracks or ruptures (bursts). Blood cell fragments called platelets stick to the site of the injury and may clump together to form blood clots. Blood clots can partly or fully block a carotid artery.

A piece of plaque or a blood clot also can break away from the wall of the carotid artery. The plaque or clot can travel through the bloodstream and get stuck in one of the brain's smaller arteries. This can block blood flow in the artery and cause a stroke.

Overview

During CEA, a surgeon makes an incision (cut) in the neck and removes plaque buildup from a carotid artery. This helps restore normal blood flow through the artery.

CEA can lower the risk of stroke in people who have narrowed or blocked carotid arteries and stroke or transient ischemic attack (TIA) symptoms. During a TIA, or "mini-stroke," you may have some or all of the symptoms of a stroke. However, the symptoms usually last less than 1–2 hours (although they may last up to 24 hours).

CEA also can lower the risk of stroke in people who have severely blocked carotid arteries but no stroke symptoms.

Carotid angioplasty is another common treatment for carotid artery disease. For this procedure, a thin tube with a balloon on the end is threaded to the narrowed or blocked carotid artery.

Once in place, the balloon is inflated to push the plaque outward against the wall of the artery. Usually, the doctor then places a small metal stent (tube) in the artery. The stent lowers the risk of the artery becoming blocked again.

People who have carotid artery disease also may be given anticlotting medicines. These medicines help reduce blood clotting and lower the risk of stroke.

What to Expect during Carotid Endarterectomy

Carotid endarterectomy (CEA) is done in a hospital. The surgery usually takes about two hours.

You will have anesthesia during the surgery so you don't feel pain. The term anesthesia refers to a loss of feeling and awareness. General anesthesia temporarily puts you to sleep. Local anesthesia numbs only certain areas of your body.

Your surgeon may choose to give you local anesthesia so he or she can talk to you during the surgery. This allows the surgeon to check your brain's reaction to the decrease in blood flow that occurs during the surgery.

During CEA, your surgeon will make an incision (cut) in your neck to expose the blocked section of the carotid artery. He or she will put a clamp on your artery to stop blood from flowing through it.

During the procedure, your brain gets blood from the carotid artery on the other side of your neck. However, your surgeon also may use a tube called a shunt to move blood around the narrowed or blocked carotid artery.

Next, your surgeon will make a cut in the blocked part of the artery. To remove the plaque, he or she will remove the inner lining of the artery around the blockage.

Finally, your surgeon will close the artery with stitches and stop any bleeding. He or she will then close the incision in your neck.

If you have small arteries or have already had a CEA, your surgeon might place a patch over the cut in the artery before closing the incision in your neck. The patch may reduce the risk of stroke for some patients.

Some surgeons use another technique called eversion carotid endarterectomy. For this surgery, one of the branches of the carotid artery is cut and turned inside out. The plaque is then cleaned out and the artery is reattached.

What to Expect after Carotid Endarterectomy

After carotid endarterectomy (CEA), you may stay in the hospital for one to two days. This allows you to safely recover from the procedure.

If your surgery takes place early in the day and you're doing well, you may be able to go home the same day.

Recovery

For a few days after the surgery, your neck may hurt. You also may find it hard to swallow. Your doctor may advise you to eat soft foods that are easy to swallow until your neck isn't as sore. Your doctor may prescribe medicine to help control any pain or discomfort.

Talk with your doctor about when it's safe for you to go back to your normal activities after having CEA.

Section 27.7

Aneurysm Repair

"Abdominal aortic aneurysm repair—open,"
© 2012 A.D.A.M., Inc. Reprinted with permission.

Open abdominal aortic aneurysm repair is surgery to fix a widened part (aneurysm) in your aorta, the large artery that carries blood to your belly (abdomen), pelvis, and legs.

An aortic aneurysm is when part of this artery becomes too large or balloons outward.

Your surgeon opens up your belly and replaces the aortic aneurysm with a man-made, cloth-like material.

Description

The surgery will take place in an operating room. You will be given general anesthesia (you will be asleep and pain-free).

- In one approach, you will lie on your back. The surgeon will make a cut in the middle of your belly, from just below the breastbone to below the navel. Rarely, the cut goes across the belly.

- In another approach, you will lie slightly tilted on your right side. The surgeon will make a five- to six-inch cut from the left side of your belly, ending a little below your belly button.

- Your surgeon will then replace the part of the aorta that has the aneurysm with a long tube graft. This tube graft is made from man-made (synthetic) cloth and is sewn in with sutures.

- In some cases, the ends of the tube graft will be tunneled through each groin and attached to the leg vessels.

- Once the surgery is done, your legs will be examined to make sure that there is a pulse.

- The cut is closed with sutures or staples.

Surgery for aortic aneurysm replacement may take two to four hours. Most patients recover in the intensive care unit (ICU) after the surgery.

Why the Procedure Is Performed

Open surgery to repair an abdominal aortic aneurysm is sometimes done as an emergency procedure when there is any bleeding inside your body from the aneurysm.

You may also have an abdominal aortic aneurysm that is not causing any symptoms or problems. Your doctor may have found out about this problem from tests called ultrasound or CT [computed tomography] scan. There is a risk that this aneurysm may suddenly break open (rupture) if you do not have surgery to repair it. However, surgery to repair the aneurysm may also be risky, depending on your overall health.

You and your doctor must decide whether the risk of having this surgery is smaller than the risk of rupture if you do not have the surgery. The doctor is more likely to recommend surgery if the aneurysm is:

- larger (about two inches or five centimeters); or

- growing more quickly (a little less than 1/4 inch over the last 6 to 12 months).

Risks

The risks for this surgery are higher if you have:

- heart disease;
- kidney failure;
- lung disease;
- past stroke;
- other serious medical problems.

Risks of problems or complications are also higher for older people. Risks for any surgery are:

- blood clots in the legs that may travel to the lungs;
- breathing problems;
- heart attack or stroke;
- infection, including in the lungs (pneumonia), urinary tract, and belly;
- reactions to medicines.

Risks for this surgery are:

- bleeding before or after surgery;

- damage to a nerve, causing pain or numbness in the leg;

- damage to your intestines or other nearby organs;

- infection of the graft;

- injury to the ureter, the tube that carries urine from your kidneys to your bladder;

- lower sex drive or inability to get an erection;

- poor blood supply to your legs, your kidneys, or other organs;

- spinal cord injury;

- wound breaks open;

- wound infections.

Before the Procedure

Your doctor will do a thorough physical exam and tests before you have surgery.

Always tell your doctor or nurse what drugs you are taking, even drugs, supplements, or herbs you bought without a prescription.

If you are a smoker, you should stop smoking at least four weeks before your surgery. Your doctor or nurse can help.

During the two weeks before your surgery:

- You will have visits with your doctor to make sure medical problems such as diabetes, high blood pressure, and heart or lung problems are being treated well.

- You may be asked to stop taking drugs that make it harder for your blood to clot. These include aspirin, ibuprofen (Advil, Motrin), clopidogrel (Plavix), Naprosyn (Aleve, Naproxen), and other drugs like these.

- Ask your doctor which drugs you should still take on the day of your surgery.

- Always let your doctor know about any cold, flu, fever, herpes breakout, or other illness you may have before your surgery.

Do not drink anything after midnight the day before your surgery, including water.

On the day of your surgery take the drugs your doctor told you to take with a small sip of water. Your doctor or nurse will tell you when to arrive at the hospital.

After the Procedure

Most people stay in the hospital for 5 to 10 days. During a hospital stay, you will:

- Be in the intensive care unit (ICU), where you will be monitored very closely right after surgery. You may need a breathing machine during the first day.

- Have a urinary catheter

- Have a tube that goes through your nose into your stomach to help drain fluids for one or two days. You will then slowly begin drinking, then eating.

- Receive medicine to keep your blood thin

- Be encouraged to sit on the side of the bed and then walk

- Wear special stockings to prevent blood clots in your legs

- Be asked to use a breathing machine to help clear your lungs

- Receive pain medicine into your veins or into the space that surrounds your spinal cord (epidural)

Outlook (Prognosis)

Full recovery for open surgery to repair an aortic aneurysm may take two or three months. Most people make a full recovery from this surgery.

Most people who have an aneurysm repaired before it breaks open (ruptures) have a good outlook.

Chapter 28

Implantable Devices for Heart Problems

Chapter Contents

Section 28.1

Cardioverter Defibrillator

Excerpted from "What Is an Implantable Cardioverter Defibrillator?"
by the National Heart, Lung, and Blood Institute (NHLBI, www.nhlbi
.nih.gov), part of the National Institutes of Health, November 9, 2011.

An implantable cardioverter defibrillator (ICD) is a small device
that's placed in the chest or abdomen. Doctors use the device to help
treat irregular heartbeats called arrhythmias.

An ICD uses electrical pulses or shocks to help control life-
threatening arrhythmias, especially those that can cause sudden cardiac arrest (SCA).

SCA is a condition in which the heart suddenly stops beating. If the
heart stops beating, blood stops flowing to the brain and other vital
organs. SCA usually causes death if it's not treated within minutes.

How Does an Implantable Cardioverter Defibrillator Work?

An implantable cardioverter defibrillator (ICD) has wires with electrodes on the ends that connect to one or more of your heart's chambers.
These wires carry the electrical signals from your heart to a small
computer in the ICD. The computer monitors your heart rhythm.

If the ICD detects an irregular rhythm, it sends low-energy electrical pulses to prompt your heart to beat at a normal rate. If the low-
energy pulses restore your heart's normal rhythm, you might avoid the
high-energy pulses or shocks of the defibrillator (which can be painful).

Single-chamber ICDs have a wire that goes to either the right atrium or right ventricle. The wire senses electrical activity and corrects
faulty electrical signaling within that chamber.

Dual-chamber ICDs have wires that go to both an atrium and a
ventricle. These ICDs provide low-energy pulses to either or both chambers. Some dual-chamber ICDs have three wires. They go to an atrium
and both ventricles.

The wires on an ICD connect to a small metal box implanted in
your chest or abdomen. The box contains a battery, pulse generator,

and small computer. When the computer detects irregular heartbeats, it triggers the ICD's pulse generator to send electrical pulses. Wires carry these pulses to the heart.

The ICD also can record the heart's electrical activity and heart rhythms. The recordings can help your doctor fine-tune the programming of your ICD so it works better to correct irregular heartbeats.

The type of ICD you get is based on your heart's pumping abilities, structural defects, and the type of irregular heartbeats you've had. Your ICD will be programmed to respond to the type of arrhythmia you're most likely to have.

What to Expect during Implantable Cardioverter Defibrillator Surgery

Placing an implantable cardioverter defibrillator (ICD) requires minor surgery, which usually is done in a hospital. You'll be given medicine right before the surgery that will help you relax and might make you fall asleep.

Your doctor will give you medicine to numb the area where he or she will put the ICD. He or she also may give you antibiotics to prevent infections.

First, your doctor will thread the ICD wires through a vein to the correct place in your heart. An x-ray "movie" of the wires as they pass through your vein and into your heart will help your doctor place them.

Once the wires are in place, your doctor will make a small cut into the skin of your chest or abdomen. He or she will then slip the ICD's small metal box through the cut and just under your skin. The box contains the battery, pulse generator, and computer.

Once the ICD is in place, your doctor will test it. You'll be given medicine to help you sleep during this testing so you don't feel any electrical pulses. Then your doctor will sew up the cut. The entire surgery takes a few hours.

What to Expect after Implantable Cardioverter Defibrillator Surgery

Expect to stay in the hospital one to two days after implantable cardioverter defibrillator (ICD) surgery. This allows your health care team to check your heartbeat and make sure your ICD is working well.

You'll need to arrange for a ride home from the hospital because you won't be able to drive for at least a week while you recover from the surgery.

For a few days to weeks after the surgery, you may have pain, swelling, or tenderness in the area where your ICD was placed. The pain usually is mild, and over-the-counter medicines can help relieve it. Talk to your doctor before taking any pain medicines.

Your doctor may ask you to avoid high-impact activities and heavy lifting for about a month after ICD surgery. Most people return to their normal activities within a few days of having the surgery.

Risks of Implantable Cardioverter Defibrillators

Unnecessary Electrical Pulses

Implantable cardioverter defibrillators (ICDs) can sometimes give electrical pulses or shocks that aren't needed.

A damaged wire or a very fast heart rate due to extreme physical activity may trigger unnecessary pulses. These pulses also can occur if you forget to take your medicines.

Children tend to be more physically active than adults. Thus, younger people who have ICDs are more likely to receive unnecessary pulses than older people.

Pulses sent too often or at the wrong time can damage the heart or trigger an irregular, sometimes dangerous heartbeat. They also can be painful and upsetting.

If needed, your doctor can reprogram your ICD or prescribe medicine so unnecessary pulses occur less often.

Risks Related to Surgery

Although rare, some ICD risks are related to the surgery used to place the device. These risks include the following:

- Swelling, bruising, or infection at the area where the ICD was placed

- Bleeding from the site where the ICD was placed

- Blood vessel, heart, or nerve damage

- A collapsed lung

- A bad reaction to the medicine used to make you relax or sleep during the surgery

Other Risks

People who have ICDs may be at higher risk for heart failure. Heart failure is a condition in which your heart can't pump enough blood to meet your body's needs. It's not clear whether an ICD increases the risk of heart failure, or whether heart failure is just more common in people who need ICDs.

Although rare, an ICD may not work properly. This will prevent the device from correcting irregular heartbeats. If this happens, your doctor may be able to reprogram the device. If that doesn't work, you doctor might have to replace the ICD.

The longer you have an ICD, the more likely it is that you'll have some of the related risks.

Section 28.2

Pacemaker

Excerpted from "What Is a Pacemaker?" by the National Heart, Lung, and Blood Institute (NHLBI, www.nhlbi.nih.gov), part of the National Institutes of Health, February 28, 2012.

A pacemaker is a small device that's placed in the chest or abdomen to help control abnormal heart rhythms. This device uses electrical pulses to prompt the heart to beat at a normal rate.

Pacemakers are used to treat arrhythmias. Arrhythmias are problems with the rate or rhythm of the heartbeat. During an arrhythmia, the heart can beat too fast, too slow, or with an irregular rhythm.

A heartbeat that's too fast is called tachycardia. A heartbeat that's too slow is called bradycardia.

During an arrhythmia, the heart may not be able to pump enough blood to the body. This can cause symptoms such as fatigue (tiredness), shortness of breath, or fainting. Severe arrhythmias can damage the body's vital organs and may even cause loss of consciousness or death.

A pacemaker can relieve some arrhythmia symptoms, such as fatigue and fainting. A pacemaker also can help a person who has abnormal heart rhythms resume a more active lifestyle.

How Does a Pacemaker Work?

A pacemaker consists of a battery, a computerized generator, and wires with sensors at their tips. (The sensors are called electrodes.) The battery powers the generator, and both are surrounded by a thin metal box. The wires connect the generator to the heart.

A pacemaker helps monitor and control your heartbeat. The electrodes detect your heart's electrical activity and send data through the wires to the computer in the generator.

If your heart rhythm is abnormal, the computer will direct the generator to send electrical pulses to your heart. The pulses travel through the wires to reach your heart.

Newer pacemakers can monitor your blood temperature, breathing, and other factors. They also can adjust your heart rate to changes in your activity.

The pacemaker's computer also records your heart's electrical activity and heart rhythm. Your doctor will use these recordings to adjust your pacemaker so it works better for you.

Your doctor can program the pacemaker's computer with an external device. He or she doesn't have to use needles or have direct contact with the pacemaker.

Pacemakers have one to three wires that are each placed in different chambers of the heart.

- The wires in a single-chamber pacemaker usually carry pulses from the generator to the right ventricle (the lower right chamber of your heart).

- The wires in a dual-chamber pacemaker carry pulses from the generator to the right atrium (the upper right chamber of your heart) and the right ventricle. The pulses help coordinate the timing of these two chambers' contractions.

- The wires in a biventricular pacemaker carry pulses from the generator to an atrium and both ventricles. The pulses help coordinate electrical signaling between the two ventricles. This type of pacemaker also is called a cardiac resynchronization therapy (CRT) device.

What to Expect during Pacemaker Surgery

Placing a pacemaker requires minor surgery. The surgery usually is done in a hospital or special heart treatment laboratory.

Before the surgery, an intravenous (IV) line will be inserted into one of your veins. You will receive medicine through the IV line to help you relax. The medicine also might make you sleepy.

Your doctor will numb the area where he or she will put the pacemaker so you don't feel any pain. Your doctor also may give you antibiotics to prevent infection.

First, your doctor will insert a needle into a large vein, usually near the shoulder opposite your dominant hand. Your doctor will then use the needle to thread the pacemaker wires into the vein and to correctly place them in your heart.

An x-ray "movie" of the wires as they pass through your vein and into your heart will help your doctor place them. Once the wires are in place, your doctor will make a small cut into the skin of your chest or abdomen.

He or she will slip the pacemaker's small metal box through the cut, place it just under your skin, and connect it to the wires that lead to your heart. The box contains the pacemaker's battery and generator.

Once the pacemaker is in place, your doctor will test it to make sure it works properly. He or she will then sew up the cut. The entire surgery takes a few hours.

What to Expect after Pacemaker Surgery

Expect to stay in the hospital overnight so your health care team can check your heartbeat and make sure your pacemaker is working well. You'll likely have to arrange for a ride to and from the hospital because your doctor may not want you to drive yourself.

For a few days to weeks after surgery, you may have pain, swelling, or tenderness in the area where your pacemaker was placed. The pain usually is mild; over-the-counter medicines often can relieve it. Talk to your doctor before taking any pain medicines.

Your doctor may ask you to avoid vigorous activities and heavy lifting for about a month after pacemaker surgery. Most people return to their normal activities within a few days of having the surgery.

Chapter 29

Joint, Bone, and Spine Surgery

Chapter Contents

Section 29.1

Carpal Tunnel Surgery

"Carpal Tunnel Syndrome Fact Sheet," by the National Institute on
Neurological Disorders and Stroke (NINDS, www.ninds.nih.gov), part of
the National Institutes of Health, September 18, 2012.

You're working at your desk, trying to ignore the tingling or numbness you've had for months in your hand and wrist. Suddenly, a sharp, piercing pain shoots through the wrist and up your arm. Just a passing cramp? More likely you have carpal tunnel syndrome, a painful progressive condition caused by compression of a key nerve in the wrist.

What is carpal tunnel syndrome?

Carpal tunnel syndrome occurs when the median nerve, which runs from the forearm into the palm of the hand, becomes pressed or squeezed at the wrist. The median nerve controls sensations to the palm side of the thumb and fingers (although not the little finger), as well as impulses to some small muscles in the hand that allow the fingers and thumb to move. The carpal tunnel—a narrow, rigid passageway of ligament and bones at the base of the hand—houses the median nerve and tendons. Sometimes, thickening from irritated tendons or other swelling narrows the tunnel and causes the median nerve to be compressed. The result may be pain, weakness, or numbness in the hand and wrist, radiating up the arm. Although painful sensations may indicate other conditions, carpal tunnel syndrome is the most common and widely known of the entrapment neuropathies in which the body's peripheral nerves are compressed or traumatized.

How is carpal tunnel syndrome treated?

Treatments for carpal tunnel syndrome should begin as early as possible, under a doctor's direction. Underlying causes such as diabetes or arthritis should be treated first. Initial treatment generally involves resting the affected hand and wrist for at least two weeks, avoiding activities that may worsen symptoms, and immobilizing the wrist in a splint to avoid further damage from twisting or bending. If there is inflammation, applying cool packs can help reduce swelling.

Carpal tunnel release is one of the most common surgical procedures in the United States. Generally recommended if symptoms last for six months, surgery involves severing the band of tissue around the wrist to reduce pressure on the median nerve. Surgery is done under local anesthesia and does not require an overnight hospital stay. Many patients require surgery on both hands.

Open release surgery, the traditional procedure used to correct carpal tunnel syndrome, consists of making an incision up to two inches in the wrist and then cutting the carpal ligament to enlarge the carpal tunnel. The procedure is generally done under local anesthesia on an outpatient basis, unless there are unusual medical considerations.

Endoscopic surgery may allow faster functional recovery and less postoperative discomfort than traditional open release surgery. The surgeon makes two incisions (about half an inch each) in the wrist and palm, inserts a camera attached to a tube, observes the tissue on a screen, and cuts the carpal ligament (the tissue that holds joints together). This two-portal endoscopic surgery, generally performed under local anesthesia, is effective and minimizes scarring and scar tenderness, if any. Single portal endoscopic surgery for carpal tunnel syndrome is also available and can result in less postoperative pain and a minimal scar. It generally allows individuals to resume some normal activities in a short period of time.

Although symptoms may be relieved immediately after surgery, full recovery from carpal tunnel surgery can take months. Some patients may have infection, nerve damage, stiffness, and pain at the scar. Occasionally the wrist loses strength because the carpal ligament is cut. Patients should undergo physical therapy after surgery to restore wrist strength. Some patients may need to adjust job duties or even change jobs after recovery from surgery.

Recurrence of carpal tunnel syndrome following treatment is rare. The majority of patients recover completely.

Section 29.2

Hip Replacement Surgery

"Questions and Answers about Hip Replacement," by the National Institute of Arthritis and Musculoskeletal and Skin Diseases (NIAMS, www.niams.nih.gov), part of the National Institutes of Health, updated April 2012.

Hip replacement, or arthroplasty, is a surgical procedure in which the diseased parts of the hip joint are removed and replaced with new, artificial parts. These artificial parts are called the prosthesis. The goals of hip replacement surgery include increasing mobility, improving the function of the hip joint, and relieving pain.

Who should have hip replacement surgery?

People with hip joint damage that causes pain and interferes with daily activities despite treatment may be candidates for hip replacement surgery. Osteoarthritis is the most common cause of this type of damage. However, other conditions, such as rheumatoid arthritis (a chronic inflammatory disease that causes joint pain, stiffness, and swelling), osteonecrosis (or avascular necrosis, which is the death of bone caused by insufficient blood supply), injury, fracture, and bone tumors also may lead to breakdown of the hip joint and the need for hip replacement surgery.

In the past, doctors reserved hip replacement surgery primarily for people over 60 years of age. The thinking was that older people typically are less active and put less stress on the artificial hip than do younger people. In more recent years, however, doctors have found that hip replacement surgery can be very successful in younger people as well. New technology has improved the artificial parts, allowing them to withstand more stress and strain and last longer.

Today, a person's overall health and activity level are more important than age in predicting a hip replacement's success. Hip replacement may be problematic for people with some health problems, regardless of their age. For example, people who have chronic disorders such as Parkinson disease, or conditions that result in severe muscle weakness, are more likely than people without chronic diseases to damage or dislocate an artificial hip. People who are at high risk for infections or in poor health are less likely to recover successfully. Therefore they may not be good candidates for this surgery. Recent studies also suggest that people who elect to have surgery before advanced joint deterioration occurs tend to recover more easily and have better outcomes.

What does hip replacement surgery involve?

The hip joint is located where the upper end of the femur, or thigh bone, meets the pelvis, or hip bone. A ball at the end of the femur, called the femoral head, fits in a socket (the acetabulum) in the pelvis to allow a wide range of motion.

During a traditional hip replacement, which lasts from one to two hours, the surgeon makes a six- to eight-inch incision over the side of the hip through the muscles and removes the diseased bone tissue and cartilage from the hip joint, while leaving the healthy parts of the joint intact. Then the surgeon replaces the head of the femur and acetabulum with new, artificial parts. The new hip is made of materials that allow a natural gliding motion of the joint.

In recent years, some surgeons have begun performing what is called a minimally invasive, or mini-incision, hip replacement, which requires smaller incisions and a shorter recovery time than traditional hip replacement. Candidates for this type of surgery are usually age 50 or younger, of normal weight based on body mass index, and healthier than candidates for traditional surgery. Joint resurfacing is also being used.

Regardless of whether you have traditional or minimally invasive surgery, the parts used to replace the joint are the same and come in two general varieties: Cemented and uncemented.

Cemented parts are fastened to existing, healthy bone with a special glue or cement. Hip replacement using these parts is referred to as a cemented procedure. Uncemented parts rely on a process called biologic fixation, which holds them in place. This means that the parts are made with a porous surface that allows your own bone to grow into the pores and hold the new parts in place. Sometimes a doctor will use a cemented femur part and uncemented acetabular part. This combination is referred to as a hybrid replacement.

What can be expected immediately after surgery?

You will be allowed only limited movement immediately after hip replacement surgery. When you are in bed, pillows or a special device are usually used to brace the hip in the correct position. You may receive fluids through an intravenous tube to replace fluids lost during surgery. There also may be a tube located near the incision to drain fluid, and a type of tube called a catheter may be used to drain urine until you are able to use the bathroom. The doctor will prescribe medicine for pain or discomfort.

On the day after surgery or sometimes on the day of surgery, therapists will teach you exercises to improve recovery. A respiratory therapist may ask you to breathe deeply, cough, or blow into a simple device that measures lung capacity. These exercises reduce the collection of fluid in the lungs after surgery.

As early as one to two days after surgery, you may be able to sit on the edge of the bed, stand, and even walk with assistance.

While you are still in the hospital, a physical therapist may teach you exercises such as contracting and relaxing certain muscles, which can strengthen the hip. Because the new, artificial hip has a more limited range of movement than a natural, healthy hip, the physical therapist also will teach you the proper techniques for simple activities of daily living, such as bending and sitting, to prevent injury to your new hip.

Section 29.3

Knee Replacement Surgery

"Knee joint replacement," © 2012 A.D.A.M., Inc.
Reprinted with permission.

Knee joint replacement is surgery to replace a knee joint with a man-made (artificial) joint. The artificial joint is called a prosthesis.

Description

During knee joint replacement surgery, damaged cartilage and bone are removed from the knee joint. Man-made (artificial) pieces, called prostheses, are then placed in the knee. These pieces may be placed in up to three surfaces in the knee joint:

- Lower end of the thigh bone: This bone is called the femur. The replacement part is usually made of metal.

- Upper end of the shin bone—the large bone in your lower leg: This bone is called the tibia. The replacement part is usually made from metal and a strong plastic.

- Back side of your kneecap: Your kneecap is called the patella. The replacement part is usually made from a strong plastic.

You will not feel any pain during the surgery because you will have one of these two types of anesthesia:

- General anesthesia: This means you will be asleep and unable to feel pain.

- Regional (spinal or epidural) anesthesia: Medicine is put into your back to make you numb below your waist. You will also get medicine to make you sleepy. And you may get medicine that will make you forget about the procedure, even though you are not fully asleep.

After you receive anesthesia, your surgeon will make a cut over your knee to open it up. This cut is often 8 to 10 inches long. Then your surgeon will:

293

- Move your kneecap (patella) out of the way, then cut the ends of your thigh bone and shin (lower leg) bone to fit the replacement part.

- Cut the underside of your kneecap to prepare it for the new pieces that will be attached there.

- Fasten the two parts of the prosthesis to your bones. One part will be attached to the end of your thigh bone and the other part will be attached to your shin bone.

- Attach both parts to the underside of your kneecap. A special bone cement is used to attach these parts.

- Repair your muscles and tendons around the new joint and close the surgical cut.

The surgery usually takes around two hours.

Usually, artificial knees have both metal and plastic parts. Some surgeons now use different materials, including metal on metal, ceramic on ceramic, or ceramic on plastic.

Why the Procedure Is Performed

The most common reason to have a knee joint replaced is to relieve severe arthritis pain. Your doctor may recommend knee joint replacement if:

- you're having symptoms of knee arthritis, such as:
  - you can't sleep through the night because of knee pain;
  - your knee pain limits or keeps you from doing your normal activities, such as bathing, preparing meals, and household chores;
  - you can't walk and take care of yourself;
- your knee pain has not improved with other treatment;
- you understand what surgery and recovery will be like.

Knee joint replacement is usually done in people ages 60 and older. Younger people who have a knee joint replaced may put extra stress on the artificial knee and cause it to wear out early.

Risks

Risks of any surgery are:

- bleeding;

- blood clots that may travel from your legs to your lungs;

- breathing problems;

- heart attack or stroke during surgery;

- infection, including in the lungs, urinary tract, and chest.

Before the Procedure

Always tell your doctor or nurse what drugs you are taking, even drugs, supplements, or herbs you bought without a prescription.
During the two weeks before your surgery:

- Prepare your home.

- Two weeks before surgery you may be asked to stop taking drugs that make it harder for your blood to clot. These include aspirin, ibuprofen (Advil, Motrin), naproxen (Naprosyn, Aleve), and other drugs.

- You may also need to stop taking medicines that can make your body more likely to get an infection. These include methotrexate, Enbrel, or other medicines that suppress your immune system.

- Ask your doctor which drugs you should still take on the day of your surgery.

- If you have diabetes, heart disease, or other medical conditions, your surgeon will ask you to see the doctor who treats you for these conditions.

- Tell your doctor if you have been drinking a lot of alcohol, more than one or two drinks a day.

- If you smoke, you need to stop. Ask your doctor or nurse for help. Smoking will slow down wound and bone healing. Your recovery may not be as good if you keep smoking.

- Always let your doctor know about any cold, flu, fever, herpes breakout, or other illness you have before your surgery.

- You may want to visit a physical therapist to learn some exercises to do before surgery.

- Set up your home to make everyday tasks easier.

- Practice using a cane, walker, crutches, or a wheelchair correctly to:
  - get in and out of the shower;
  - go up and down stairs;

- sit down to use the toilet and stand up after using the toilet;
- use the shower chair.

On the day of your surgery:

- You will usually be asked not to drink or eat anything for 6 to 12 hours before the procedure.
- Take the drugs your doctor told you to take with a small sip of water.
- Your doctor or nurse will tell you when to arrive at the hospital.

After the Procedure

You will stay in the hospital for three to five days. During that time you will recover from your anesthesia and from the surgery itself. You will be asked to start moving and walking as soon as the first day after surgery.

Full recovery will take three months to a year.

Some people need a short stay in a rehabilitation center after they leave the hospital and before they go home. At a rehab center, you will learn how to safely do your daily activities on your own.

Outlook (Prognosis)

The results of a total knee replacement are often excellent. The operation relieves pain for most people. Most people do not need help walking after they fully recover.

Most artificial knee joints last 10 to 15 years. Some last as long as 20 years before they loosen and need to be replaced again.

Section 29.4

Shoulder Replacement Surgery

The shoulder is a ball and socket joint. The ball portion of the joint is called the humeral head, and is part of the humerus (upper arm bone). The socket portion is called the glenoid, and is part of the scapula (shoulder blade). The humeral head (ball) fits into the glenoid (socket) and the two bones rub together as the shoulder moves.

Ball and Socket of Healthy Shoulder Joint Surfaces

In a healthy shoulder joint, the surfaces of these bones where the ball and socket rub together are very smooth and covered with a tough protective tissue called cartilage. Arthritis causes damage to the bone surfaces and cartilage. These damaged surfaces eventually become painful as they rub together.

Arthritic Shoulder Joint Surfaces

There are many ways to treat the pain caused by arthritis. One way is total shoulder replacement surgery. The decision to have total shoulder replacement surgery should be made very carefully after consulting your doctor and learning as much as you can about the shoulder joint, arthritis, and the surgery. In total shoulder replacement surgery, the ball and socket that have been damaged by arthritis are removed and replaced with artificial parts made of metal and a very durable plastic material. We call these artificial parts implants. These implants are shaped so that the shoulder joint will move in a way that is very similar to the way the joint moved when it was healthy.

What to Bring to the Hospital

In the following text is a list of things you may want to bring with you to the hospital in preparation for your surgery. Talk with your physician as he/she may have additional information about preparing for your hospital stay.

- Your personal belongings should be left in the car until after surgery. Tell your family that your room will be assigned when you are in surgery or in recovery, at which point they can bring your personal items to your room.

- Personal grooming items that you may want to pack include a toothbrush, toothpaste, hairbrush, eyeglasses/contacts, comb, deodorant, shaving cream/electric razor, shampoo, lotion, undergarments, and a robe.

- Bring slippers or flat rubber-soled shoes for walking in the hallways.

- Bring loose fitting clothing for your trip home.

- Bring any medications you are currently taking. You should also write down your medication information to be given to the hospital staff. Be sure to include the name, strength, and how often you take the medications. Please communicate any allergies you might have to your doctors and the nursing staff.

- If you use a breathing exerciser (IBE), be sure to bring it with you from home, as you will probably need this right after surgery. Leave jewelry, credit cards, car and house keys, checkbooks, and items of personal value at home. Bring only enough pocket money for items such as newspapers, magazines, etc.

Getting to the Joint

The patient is first taken into the operating room and positioned on a special operating table as though lounging in a beach chair. The arm is placed on a board that will allow the surgeon to move it up or down as necessary during the surgery. Anesthesia is given and, when it has taken effect, the skin around the shoulder and upper arm is thoroughly scrubbed and sterilized with an antiseptic liquid.

An incision about six inches long is then made over the shoulder joint. The incision is gradually made deeper through muscle and other tissue until the bones of the shoulder joint are exposed.

Replacing the Socket Portion of the Joint

The implant that replaces the socket consists of a durable plastic insert with a very smooth, cupped surface.

Removing the Surface of the Socket

The arm is maneuvered until the humeral head is dislocated from the socket.

Special precision instruments are then used to remove the damaged cartilage and bone surface from the glenoid, and to shape the socket so it will match the shape of the implant that will be inserted. Holes are then drilled into the socket to accommodate the fixation pegs on the implant. These pegs help stabilize the implant.

Inserting the Implant

The socket implant is attached by using a special kind of cement for bones. The cement is pressed into the holes. The implant is then inserted.

Replacing the Ball Portion of the Joint

The implant that replaces the ball consists of a long metal stem that fits down into the humerus. A metal head in the shape of a partial sphere is mounted on top of this stem. This head contacts the socket implant in the shoulder blade.

Preparing the Humeral Canal

The upper arm bone has relatively soft, porous bone tissue in the center. This part of the bone is called the canal.

Special instruments are used to clear some of this soft bone from the canal.

Using a precision guide and saw, the damaged rounded portion (ball) of the humerus is removed.

Inserting the Implant

The metal stem implant may be held in place by either using the special bone cement, or by making it fit very tightly in the canal. The surgeon will choose the best method, depending on the patient's age and expected activity level.

If cement is used, it is injected into the canal first, and then the implant is inserted into the canal. If cement is not used, the implant is simply inserted into the canal.

On some implants, the stem and partial sphere are one piece. On others, they may be two separate pieces. If the partial sphere is a separate piece, it is usually secured to the top of the stem after the stem has been inserted.

Closing the Wound

When all the implants are in place, the surgeon places the new ball that is now part of the upper arm bone into the new socket that is part of the shoulder blade. If necessary, the surgeon may adjust the ligaments that surround the shoulder to achieve the best possible shoulder function.

When the ligaments are properly adjusted, the surgeon sews the layers of tissue back into their proper position. A plastic tube may be inserted into the wound to allow liquids to drain from the site during the first few hours after surgery. After the tube is inserted, the edges of the skin are sewn together, and a sterile bandage is applied to the shoulder. Then, the patient is taken to the recovery room.

Section 29.5

Spinal Stenosis Surgery

Excerpted from "Spinal Stenosis," by the National Institute on Arthritis and Musculoskeletal and Skin Diseases (NIAMS, www.niams.nih.gov), part of the National Institutes of Health, April 2009.

Spinal stenosis is a narrowing of spaces in the spine (backbone) that results in pressure on the spinal cord and/or nerve roots. This disorder usually involves the narrowing of one or more of three areas of the spine: (1) the canal in the center of the column of bones (vertebral or spinal column) through which the spinal cord and nerve roots run, (2) the canals at the base or roots of nerves branching out from the spinal cord, or (3) the openings between vertebrae (bones of the spine) through which nerves leave the spine and go to other parts of the body. The narrowing may involve a small or large area of the spine. Pressure on the lower part of the spinal cord or on nerve roots branching out from that area may give rise to pain or numbness in the legs. Pressure on the upper part of the spinal cord (that is, the neck area) may produce similar symptoms in the shoulders, or even the legs.

Surgery

In many cases, the conditions causing spinal stenosis cannot be permanently altered by nonsurgical treatment, even though these measures may relieve pain for a period of time. To determine how much nonsurgical treatment will help, a doctor may recommend such treatment first. However, surgery might be considered immediately if a patient has numbness or weakness that interferes with walking, impaired bowel or bladder function, or other neurological involvement. The effectiveness of nonsurgical treatments, the extent of the patient's pain, and the patient's preferences may all factor into whether or not to have surgery.

The purpose of surgery is to relieve pressure on the spinal cord or nerves and restore and maintain alignment and strength of the spine. This can be done by removing, trimming, or adjusting diseased parts that are causing the pressure or loss of alignment. The most common surgery is called decompressive laminectomy: Removal of the lamina (roof) of one or more vertebrae to create more space for the nerves. A surgeon may perform a laminectomy with or without fusing vertebrae or removing part of a disk. Various devices may be used to enhance fusion and strengthen unstable segments of the spine following decompression surgery.

Patients with spinal stenosis caused by spinal trauma or achondroplasia may need surgery at a young age. When surgery is required in patients with achondroplasia, laminectomy (removal of the roof) without fusion is usually sufficient.

Major Risks of Surgery

All surgery, particularly that involving general anesthesia and older patients, carries risks. The most common complications of surgery for spinal stenosis are a tear in the membrane covering the spinal cord at the site of the operation, infection, or a blood clot that forms in the veins. These conditions can be treated but may prolong recovery. The presence of other diseases and the physical condition of the patient are also significant factors to consider when making decisions about surgery.

Long-Term Outcomes of Surgical Treatment

Removal of the obstruction that has caused the symptoms usually gives patients some relief; most patients have less leg pain and are able to walk better following surgery. However, if nerves were badly damaged before surgery, there may be some remaining pain or numbness or no improvement. Also, the degenerative process will likely continue, and pain or limitation of activity may reappear after surgery. The largest trial to date comparing surgical and non-surgical interventions for the treatment of low back and associated leg pain caused by spinal stenosis found that for patients with spinal stenosis, surgical treatment was more effective than non-surgical treatment in relieving symptoms and improving function. However, the functional status of patients who received non-surgical therapies also improved somewhat during the study.

Section 29.6

Low Back Surgery

Excerpted from "Low Back Pain Fact Sheet," by the National Institute on Neurological Disorders and Stroke (NINDS, www.ninds.nih.gov), part of the National Institutes of Health, September 19, 2012.

If you have lower back pain, you are not alone. Nearly everyone at some point has back pain that interferes with work, routine daily activities, or recreation. Americans spend at least $50 billion each year on low back pain, the most common cause of job-related disability and a leading contributor to missed work. Back pain is the second most common neurological ailment in the United States—only headache is more common. Fortunately, most occurrences of low back pain go away within a few days. Others take much longer to resolve or lead to more serious conditions.

Acute or short-term low back pain generally lasts from a few days to a few weeks. Most acute back pain is mechanical in nature—the result of trauma to the lower back or a disorder such as arthritis. Pain from trauma may be caused by a sports injury, work around the house or in the garden, or a sudden jolt such as a car accident or other stress on spinal bones and tissues. Symptoms may range from muscle ache to shooting or stabbing pain, limited flexibility and/or range of motion, or an inability to stand straight. Occasionally, pain felt in one part of the body may radiate from a disorder or injury elsewhere in the body. Some acute pain syndromes can become more serious if left untreated.

Chronic back pain is measured by duration—pain that persists for more than three months is considered chronic. It is often progressive and the cause can be difficult to determine.

Surgical Treatment for Low Back Pain

In the most serious cases, when low back pain does not respond to other therapies, surgery may relieve pain caused by back problems or serious musculoskeletal injuries. Some surgical procedures may be performed in a doctor's office under local anesthesia, whereas others require hospitalization. It may be months following surgery before the patient is fully healed, and he or she may suffer permanent loss of flexibility. Since invasive back surgery is not always successful, it should be performed only in patients with progressive neurologic disease or damage to the peripheral nerves.

Diskectomy is one of the more common ways to remove pressure on a nerve root from a bulging disk or bone spur. During the procedure the surgeon takes out a small piece of the lamina (the arched bony roof of the spinal canal) to remove the obstruction below.

Foraminotomy is an operation that cleans out or enlarges the bony hole (foramen) where a nerve root exits the spinal canal. Bulging disks or joints thickened with age can cause narrowing of the space through which the spinal nerve exits and can press on the nerve, resulting in pain, numbness, and weakness in an arm or leg. Small pieces of bone over the nerve are removed through a small slit, allowing the surgeon to cut away the blockage and relieve the pressure on the nerve.

Intradiscal Electrothermal Therapy (IDET) uses thermal energy to treat pain resulting from a cracked or bulging spinal disk. A special needle is inserted via a catheter into the disk and heated to a high temperature for up to 20 minutes. The heat thickens and seals the disk wall and reduces inner disk bulge and irritation of the spinal nerve.

Nucleoplasty uses radiofrequency energy to treat patients with low back pain from contained, or mildly herniated, disks. Guided by X-ray imaging, a wand-like instrument is inserted through a needle into the disk to create a channel that allows inner disk material to be removed. The wand then heats and shrinks the tissue, sealing the disk wall. Several channels are made depending on how much disk material needs to be removed.

Radiofrequency lesioning is a procedure using electrical impulses to interrupt nerve conduction (including the conduction of pain signals) for 6 to12 months. Using X-ray guidance, a special needle is inserted into nerve tissue in the affected area. Tissue surrounding the needle tip is heated for 90–120 seconds, resulting in localized destruction of the nerves.

Spinal fusion is used to strengthen the spine and prevent painful movements. The spinal disk(s) between two or more vertebrae is removed and the adjacent vertebrae are fused by bone grafts and/or metal devices secured by screws. Spinal fusion may result in some loss of flexibility in the spine and requires a long recovery period to allow the bone grafts to grow and fuse the vertebrae together.

Spinal laminectomy (also known as spinal decompression) involves the removal of the lamina (usually both sides) to increase the size of the spinal canal and relieve pressure on the spinal cord and nerve roots.

Other surgical procedures to relieve severe chronic pain include rhizotomy, in which the nerve root close to where it enters the spinal cord is cut to block nerve transmission and all senses from the area of the body experiencing pain; cordotomy, where bundles of nerve fibers on one or both sides of the spinal cord are intentionally severed to stop the transmission of pain signals to the brain; and dorsal root entry zone operation, or DREZ, in which spinal neurons transmitting the patient's pain are destroyed surgically.

Chapter 30

Gastrointestinal Surgery

Chapter Contents

Section 30.1

Appendectomy

The Condition

Appendectomy is the surgical removal of the appendix. The operation is done to remove an infected appendix. An infected appendix, called appendicitis, can burst and release bacteria and stool into the abdomen.

What are the common symptoms?

- Abdominal pain that starts around the navel
- Not wanting to eat
- Low fever
- Nausea and sometimes vomiting
- Diarrhea or constipation

Treatment Options

Surgery

Laparoscopic appendectomy: The appendix is removed with instruments placed into small abdominal incisions.

Open appendectomy: The appendix is removed through an incision in the lower right abdomen.

Nonsurgical

Surgery is the only option for an acute (sudden) infection of the appendix.

Benefits and Risks

An appendectomy will remove the infected organ and relieve pain. Once the appendix is removed, appendicitis will not happen again. The risk of not having surgery is the appendix can burst resulting in an abdominal infection called peritonitis.

Possible complications include abscess, infection of the wound or abdomen, intestinal blockage, hernia at the incision, pneumonia, risk of premature delivery (if you are pregnant), and death.

Expectations

Before your operation: Evaluation usually includes blood work, urinalysis, and an abdominal CT [computed tomography] scan, or abdominal ultrasound. Your surgeon and anesthesia provider will review your health history, medications, and options for pain control.

The day of your operation: You will not be allowed to eat or drink while you are being evaluated for an emergency appendectomy.

Your recovery: If you have no complications you usually can go home in one or two days after laparoscopic or open procedures.

Call your surgeon if you are in severe pain, have stomach cramping, a high fever, odor or increased drainage from your incision, or no bowel movements for three days.

The Conditions, Signs and Symptoms, and Diagnostic Tests

Keeping You Informed

Appendicitis pain: Pain can be different for each person because the appendix can touch different organs. This can be confusing and make it difficult to diagnose appendicitis.

Most often pain starts around the navel and then moves to the right lower abdomen. The pain is often worse with walking or talking. During pregnancy, the appendix sits higher in the abdomen so the pain may seem to come from the upper abdomen. In the elderly, symptoms are often not as noticeable because there is less swelling.[1,2]

Other medical disorders have symptoms similar to appendicitis, such as inflammatory bowel disease, pelvic inflammatory disease, gastroenteritis, urinary tract infection, right lower lobe pneumonia, Meckel's diverticulum, intussusception, and constipation.

Table 30.1. Risks of Appendectomy

The Risk	What Happens	Keeping You Informed
Infection	For simple acute appendicitis, wound infection is reported as 0 to 34 per 1,000 patients for laparoscopic and 1 to 70 per 1,000 for open procedures. The risk increases for a perforated appendix and abdominal infection.[2,3,8–11]	Antibiotics are typically given right before the operation. Your health care team should wash their hands before examining you.
Abscess	An abscess is reported as 0 to 24 per 1,000 patients for laparoscopic and 0 to 10 per 1,000 for open procedures.[2,3,8]	Call your surgeon if your wound is red or draining pus. Antibiotics are used to treat an abscess.
Intestinal obstruction	Swelling of the tissue around the intestine can stop stool and fluid from passing through your intestine. Short-term intestinal obstruction is reported as 38 per 1,000 patients.[8]	Your abdomen will be checked for bowel sounds, and you will be asked if you are passing gas. If you have a temporary block, a nasogastric tube may be placed through your nose into your stomach for one to two days to remove fluid from your stomach.
Pneumonia	Pneumonia is reported as 25 per 1,000 patients.[3,8]	Deep-breathing exercises and movement can help expand your lungs and decrease this risk.
Heart problems	Heart problems are rare. Heart attacks are reported as 4 per 1,000 patients and stroke as 2 per 1,000.[8]	Call your surgeon if you have chest pain. Your anesthesia provider is always prepared in advanced cardiac life support. Special leg compression stockings and blood thinning medication may be given.
Kidney problems	Urinary tract infections are reported as 11 per 1,000 patients and decreased renal flow as 4 per 1,000.[8]	Let your nurse know when you urinate. Call your surgeon if you have signs of a urinary tract infection (pain with urination, fever, cloudy urine). Blood work may be done to check for renal flow.

Table 30.1. Risks of Appendectomy *continued*

The Risk	What Happens	Keeping You Informed
Deep vein thrombosis (blood clots)	No movement during the operation can lead to blood clots forming in the legs. In rare cases, the clot can travel to the lungs.	Your surgeon or nurse will place support or compression (squeezing) stockings on your legs and may give you blood thinning medication. Your job is to get up and moving after the operation.
Bleeding	Bleeding is extremely rare.[2,3]	A blood transfusion is usually not required.
Pregnancy risks	Premature labor is reported as 83 per 1,000 patients and fetal loss as 26 per 1,000.[7]	The risk of fetal loss increases to 109 per 1,000 patients with peritonitis (infection of the abdominal cavity).
Pediatric risks	Complications are rare and range from 0 to 5 per 1,000 patients for simple appendectomy. There are no deaths reported in current studies for simple appendectomy.[5,9–11]	Children with gangrenous or perforated appendices have increased wound infection rates (26 per 1,000) and abdominal infections (44 per 1,000). There is an increased rate of abscess (90 per 1,000) with laparoscopic surgery.[5]
Elderly risks	The complication rate is higher in the elderly, with 143 to 208 per 1,000 patients. Death is reported as 3 to 20 per 1,000 elderly patients.[6]	Complications, lengths of stay, and deaths are lower with laparoscopic versus open procedure in the elderly, while the cost is higher.[6]
Death	Death is extremely rare in healthy people for appendectomy without peritonitis, with mortality reported as 0 to 18 per 1,000 patients.[2,8]	The risk of death increases with having another severe disease, total dependence on others to function, a contaminated wound, and chronic pulmonary disease.[8]

The Condition

The appendix: The appendix is a small pouch that hangs from the large intestine where the small and large intestine join. If the appendix becomes blocked and swollen, bacteria can grow in the pouch. The cause of infection can be from an illness, thick mucus or hard stool trapped in the opening of the appendix, or parasites.

Appendicitis: Appendicitis is an infection of the appendix. The infection and swelling can decrease the blood supply to the wall of the appendix. This leads to tissue death, and the appendix can rupture or burst causing bacteria and stool to release into the abdomen. This is called a ruptured appendix. A ruptured appendix can lead to peritonitis, which is an infection of your entire abdomen. Appendicitis affects 1 in 1,000 people, most often between the ages of 10 and 30 years old. It is a common reason for an operation in children, and it is the most common surgical emergency in pregnancy.

Appendectomy is the surgical removal of the appendix.

Symptoms

Stomach pain that usually starts around the navel and then often moves to the lower right side of the abdomen.

- Loss of appetite

- Low fever, usually below 100.3 degrees Fahrenheit

- Nausea and sometimes vomiting

- Diarrhea or constipation

Common Diagnostic Tests

History and physical: The focus will be on your abdominal pain.

Tests:

- Abdominal ultrasound: Checks for an enlarged appendix

- Computed tomography (CT) scan: Checks for an enlarged appendix and infection

- Complete blood count (CBC): A blood test to check for infection

- Rectal exam: Checks for tenderness on the right side and for any rectal problems that could be causing the abdominal pain

- Pelvic exam: May be done in young women to check for pain from gynecological problems like pelvic inflammation or infection

- Urinalysis: Checks for an infection in your urine, which can cause abdominal pain

- Electrocardiogram (ECG): Sometimes done in the older adult to make sure heart problems are not the cause of pain

Surgical and Nonsurgical Treatment

Surgical Treatment

An operation is the only option for acute infection of the appendix.

Laparoscopic Appendectomy

This technique is the most common for simple appendicitis. The surgeon will make one to three small incisions in the abdomen. A port (nozzle) is inserted into one of the slits, and carbon dioxide gas inflates the abdomen. This process allows the surgeon to see the appendix more easily. A laparoscope is inserted through another port. It looks like a telescope with a light and camera on the end so the surgeon can see inside the abdomen. Surgical instruments are placed in the other small openings and used to remove the appendix. The area is washed with sterile fluid to decrease the risk of further infection. The carbon dioxide comes out through the slits, and then the sites are closed with sutures or staples or covered with a glue-like bandage and Steri-Strips. Your surgeon may start with a laparoscopic technique and need to change to an open technique. This change is done for your safety.

Open Appendectomy

The surgeon makes an incision about two to four inches long in the lower right side of the abdomen and cuts through fat and muscle layers to the appendix. The appendix is removed from the intestine. The area is washed with sterile fluid to decrease the risk of further infection. A small drainage tube may be placed going from the inside to the outside of the abdomen. The drain is usually removed in the hospital. The site is closed with sutures or staples or covered with glue-like bandage and Steri-Strips.

Nonsurgical Treatment

If you only have some of the signs of appendicitis, your surgeon may monitor you to see if the symptoms get any worse. If you have an abscess (a collection of pus), your surgeon may treat you with antibiotics first and may have you come back for elective surgery in four to six weeks.

Keeping You Informed

Conversion rates: Conversion rates from a laparoscopic to an open procedure average 110 per 1,000 patients.[2] Conversion to an open technique is most commonly due to adhesions (bands of scar-like tissue sticking on organs), followed by perforation (bursting) and peritonitis.[3,4]

Pediatric considerations: There is no reported difference in the length of hospital stay for laparoscopic versus open procedures for non-ruptured (2.3 versus 2.0 days) and ruptured (5.5 versus 6.2 days) appendices.[5]

Ruptured appendix: Unfortunately, many people do not know they have appendicitis until the appendix bursts. If this happens, it causes more serious problems. The incidence of ruptured appendix is 270 per 1,000 patients. This is higher in the very young and very old and also higher during pregnancy because the symptoms (nausea, vomiting, right-sided pain) may be similar to other pregnancy conditions.[1,7]

Risks of This Procedure

Your surgeon will do everything possible to minimize risks, but appendectomy, like all operations, has risks. See Table 30.1.

Expectations: Preparation for Your Operation

Preparing for Your Operation

Appendectomy is usually an emergency procedure. You can help prepare for your operation by telling your surgeon about other medical problems that you have and all of the medications that you are taking.

Be sure to tell your surgeon if you are taking blood thinners (Plavix, Coumadin, aspirin).

Home Preparation

You can often go home in one or two days. Your hospital stay may be longer for a ruptured appendix.

Anesthesia

You will meet with your anesthesia provider before the operation. Let him or her know if you have allergies, neurologic disease (epilepsy or stroke), heart disease, stomach problems, lung disease (asthma, emphysema), endocrine disease (diabetes, thyroid conditions), loose teeth, or if you smoke, drink alcohol, use drugs, or take any herbs or vitamins.

Don't Eat or Drink

You will not be allowed to eat or drink while you are being evaluated for your emergency appendectomy. Not eating or drinking reduces your risk of complications from anesthesia.

What to Bring

- Insurance card and identification
- Advance directive
- List of medicines
- Personal items such as eyeglasses and dentures
- Loose-fitting comfortable clothes
- Leave jewelry and valuables at home

What You Can Expect

A bracelet with your name and identification number will be placed on your wrist. Your wristband should be checked by all health care team members before providing any procedures or giving you medication. If you have any allergies, an allergy bracelet should also be placed on your wrist.

An intravenous line (IV) will be started to give you fluids and medication. The medication will make you feel sleepy.

A tube will be placed down your throat to help you breathe during the operation.

Your surgeon will perform your operation and then close your incisions. A drain may be placed from the inside of your incision out your abdomen.

After your operation, you will be moved to a recovery room.

Preventing Pneumonia

Movement and deep breathing after your operation can help prevent fluid in your lungs and pneumonia.[10]

Preventing Blood Clots

When you have an operation, you are at risk of getting blood clots because of not moving during anesthesia. The longer and more complicated your operation, the greater the risk. Your doctor will know your risk for blood clots, and steps will be taken to prevent them. This may include blood thinning medication and support or compression (squeezing) stockings.

Preventing Infection

The risk of infection can be lowered if antibiotics are given right before the operation and hair is removed at the surgical site with clippers versus shaving.

All health care providers should wash their hands before examining you.

Questions to Ask

Ask about the risks, problems, and side effects of general anesthesia.

Keeping You Informed

Anesthesia: The most frequent option for general anesthesia is called balanced anesthesia, where a combination of different drugs is used. Common drugs are:

- inhaled gases—nitrous oxide;
- barbiturates—thiopental;
- benzodiazepines—midazolam;
- opioids—fentanyl, morphine;
- other agent—Propofol.

Deep Breathing

Take 5 to 10 deep breaths every hour while you are awake. Breathe deeply and hold for three to five seconds. Young children can do deep breathing by blowing bubbles.

Your Recovery and Discharge

Thinking Clearly

The anesthesia may cause you to feel different for one or two days. Do not drive, drink alcohol, or make any big decisions for at least two days.

Nutrition

- When you wake up, you will be able to drink small amounts of liquid. If you are not nauseous, you can begin eating regular foods.
- Continue to drink lots of fluids, usually about 8 to 10 glasses per day.

Activity

- You will be helped by getting out of bed and walking.
- Slowly increase your activity.
- Do not lift or participate in strenuous activity for three to five days for laparoscopic and 10 to 14 days for open procedures.
- Avoid driving until your pain is under control without narcotics.
- You can have sex when you feel ready, usually after your sutures or staples are removed.
- It is normal to feel tired. You may need more sleep than usual.

Work and Return to School

- You can go back to work when you feel well enough. Discuss the timing with your surgeon.
- Children can usually go to school one week or less after an operation for an unruptured appendix and up to two weeks after a ruptured appendix.
- Most children will not return to gym class, sports, and climbing games for two to four weeks after the operation.

Wound Care

- Always wash your hands before and after touching near your incision site.
- Do not soak in a bathtub until your stitches, Steri-Strips, or staples are removed. You may take a shower after the second postoperative day unless you are told not to.
- Follow your surgeon's instructions on when to change your bandages.
- A small amount of drainage from the incision is normal. If the drainage is thick and yellow or the site is red, you may have an infection, so call your surgeon.

- If you have a drain in one of your incisions, it will be taken out when the drainage stops.

- Surgical staples will be removed during your first office visit.

- Steri-strips will fall off in 7 to 10 days or they will be removed during your first office visit.

- Avoid wearing tight or rough clothing. It may rub your incisions and make it harder for them to heal.

- Protect the new skin, especially from the sun. The sun can burn and cause darker scarring.

- Your scar will heal in about four to six weeks and will become softer and continue to fade over the next year. Keep the wound site out of the sun or use sunscreen.

- Sensation around your incision will return in a few weeks or months.

Bowel Movements

- After intestinal surgery, you may have loose watery stools for several days. If watery diarrhea lasts longer than three days, contact your surgeon.

- Pain medication (narcotics) can cause constipation. Increase the fiber in your diet with high-fiber foods if you are constipated. Your surgeon may also give you a prescription for a stool softener.

- Foods high in fiber include beans, bran cereals and whole grain breads, peas, dried fruit (figs, apricots, and dates), raspberries, blackberries, strawberries, sweet corn, broccoli, baked potatoes with skin, plums, pears, apples, greens, and nuts.

Pain

The amount of pain is different for each person. Some people need only one to three doses of pain control medication, while others use narcotics for a full week.

Home Medications

The medicine you need after your operation is usually related to pain control.

When to Contact Your Surgeon

If you have:

- Pain that will not go away
- Pain that gets worse
- A fever of more than 101 degrees Fahrenheit (38.3 degrees Celsius)
- Vomiting
- Swelling, redness, bleeding, or bad-smelling drainage from your wound site
- Strong abdominal pain
- No bowel movement or unable to pass gas for three days
- Watery diarrhea lasting longer than three days

Pain Control

Everyone reacts to pain in a different way. A scale from 0 to 10 is often used to measure pain. At a "0," you do not feel any pain. A "10" is the worst pain you have ever felt.

Common Medicines to Control Pain

Narcotics or opioids are used for severe pain. Some side effects of narcotics are sleepiness; lowered blood pressure, heart rate, and breathing rate; skin rash and itching; constipation; nausea; and difficulty urinating. Some examples of narcotics include morphine, oxycodone, and hydromorphone. Medications are available to control many of the side effects of narcotics.

Non-Narcotic Pain Medication

Most nonopioid pain medications are nonsteroidal antiinflammatory drugs (NSAIDs). They are used to treat mild pain or combined with a narcotic to treat severe pain. They also can reduce inflammation. Some side effects of NSAIDs are stomach upset, bleeding in the stomach or intestines, and fluid retention. These side effects usually are not seen with short-term use. Examples of NSAIDs include ibuprofen and naproxen.

Non-Medicine Pain Control

Distraction helps you focus on other activities instead of your pain. Music, games, and other engaging activities are especially helpful with children in mild pain.

Splinting your stomach by placing a pillow over your abdomen with firm pressure before coughing or movement can help reduce the pain.

Guided imagery helps you direct and control your emotions. Close your eyes and gently inhale and exhale. Picture yourself in the center of somewhere beautiful. Feel the beauty surrounding you and your emotions coming back to your control. You should feel calmer.

Keeping You Informed

Extreme pain puts extra stress on your body at a time when your body needs to focus on healing. Do not wait until your pain has reached a level "10" or is unbearable before telling your doctor or nurse. It is much easier to control pain before it becomes severe.

Laparoscopic Pain

Following a laparoscopic procedure, pain is sometimes felt in the shoulder. This is due to the gas inserted into your abdomen during the procedure. Moving and walking helps to decrease the gas and the right shoulder pain.[2,3]

Glossary of Terms and More Information

Glossary of Terms

Abdominal ultrasound: Sound waves are used to determine the location of deep structures in the body. A hand roller is placed on top of clear gel and rolled across the abdomen.

Abscess: Localized collection of pus.

Advance directives: Documents signed by a competent person giving direction to health care providers about treatment choices. They give you the chance to tell your feelings about health care decisions.

Adhesion: A fibrous band or scar tissue that causes internal organs to adhere or stick together.

Complete blood count (CBC): A blood test that measures red blood cells (RBCs) and white blood cells (WBCs). WBCs increase with inflammation. The normal range for WBCs is 8,000 to 12,000.

Computed tomography (CT) scan: A specialized X-ray and computer that show a detailed, three-dimensional picture of your abdomen. A CT scan normally takes about one and a half to 2 hours.

318

Electrocardiogram (ECG): Measures the rate and regularity of heartbeats, the size of the heart chambers, and any damage to the heart.

Nasogastric tube: A soft plastic tube inserted in the nose and down to the stomach.

Radiographic barium contrast enema: A special X-ray of the large intestines. Pictures are taken of the abdomen after barium dye is inserted into the rectum.

Urinalysis: A visual and chemical examination of the urine most often used to screen for urinary tract infections and kidney disease.

For More Information

For more information, please go to the American College of Surgeons Patient Education Website at www.facs.org/patienteducation.

References

The information provided is chosen from clinical research. The research in the following text does not represent all of the information available about your operation.

1. Anderson B, Nielsen TF. Appendicitis in pregnancy: Diagnosis, management and complications. *ACTA Obstetricia Gynecologica Scandinavica.* 1999; 78(9):758–762.

2. Ho H. Appendectomy. In: *ACS Surgery: Principles and Practice* 2004. New York, NY: WebMD, 2004.

3. Sauerland S, Lefering R, Neugebauer EAM. Laparoscopic versus open surgery for suspected appendicitis (Review). *The Cochrane Database of Systematic Reviews* 2004, Issue 4 Art No: CD001546. pgb2.DOI: 10.1002/14651858.CD001546.pub2.

4. Liu SI, Siewart B, Raptopoulos V, Hodin RA. Factors associated with conversion to laparotomy in patients undergoing laparoscopic appendectomy. *Journal of the American College of Surgeons.* 2002;194(3):298–305.

5. Paik PS, Towson JA, Anthone GF, et al. Intra-abdominal abscesses following laparoscopic and open appendectomies. *Journal of Gastrointestinal Surgery.* 1997;1(2):188–193.

6. Harrell AG, Lincourt AE, Novitsky YW, et al. Advantages of laparoscopic appendectomy in the elderly. *American Surgeon.* 2006;72(6):474–480.

7. Cohen-Kerem R, Railton C, Oren D, Lishner M, Koren G. Pregnancy outcome following non-obstetric surgical intervention. *American Journal of Surgery*. 2005;190(3):467–473.

8. Margenthaler JA, Longo WE, Virgo KS, Johnson FE, Oprian CA, Henderson WG, Daley J, Khuri SF. Risk factors for adverse outcomes after the surgical treatment of appendicitis in adults. *Annals of Surgery*. 2003;238(1):59–66.

9. Emil S, Laberge JM, Mikhail P, Baican L, Flageole H, Nguyen L, Shaw K. Appendicitis in children: A ten-year update of therapeutic recommendations. *Journal of Pediatric Surgery*. 2003;38(2):236–242.

10. Newman K, Ponsky T, Kittle K, et al. Appendicitis 2000: Variability in practice, outcomes and resources utilization at 30 pediatric hospitals. *Journal of Pediatric Surgery*. 2003;38(3):372–379.

11. Chen C, Botelho C, Cooper A, et al. Current practice patterns in the treatment of perforated appendicitis in children. *Journal of the American College of Surgeons*. 2003;196(2):212–221.

12. Overend TJ, Anderson CM, Lucy SD, et al. The effect of incentive spirometry on post-operative complications. *Chest*. 2001;120:971–978.

Health Reference Series *Medical Advisor's Notes and Updates*

Appendectomy has long been accepted to be only treatment for acute appendicitis. In the past few years, this assertion has been questioned. Several studies have shown that appendectomy can be treated with antibiotic therapy, rather than by surgery, in at least some cases. This topic remains highly controversial, and it is not yet clear whether the outcomes of antibiotic therapy are superior, inferior, or equal to surgery for appendicitis. Additional research will be required to determine whether the traditional wisdom should hold or be overturned.

Section 30.2

Bowel Diversion Surgeries: Ileostomy, Colostomy, Ileoanal Reservoir, and Continent Ileostomy

Excerpted from "Bowel Diversion Surgeries: Ileostomy, Colostomy, Ileoanal Reservoir, and Continent Ileostomy," by the National Institute of Diabetes and Digestive and Kidney Diseases (NIDDK, www.niddk.nih.gov), part of the National Institutes of Health, April 23, 2012.

Bowel diversion surgery allows stool to safely leave the body when—because of disease or injury—the large intestine is removed or needs time to heal. Bowel is a general term for any part of the small or large intestine.

Some bowel diversion surgeries—those called ostomy surgery—divert the bowel to an opening in the abdomen where a stoma is created. A surgeon forms a stoma by rolling the bowel's end back on itself, like a shirt cuff, and stitching it to the abdominal wall. An ostomy pouch is attached to the stoma and worn outside the body to collect stool.

Other bowel diversion surgeries reconfigure the intestines after damaged portions are removed. For example, after removing the colon, a surgeon can create a colon-like pouch out of the last part of the small intestine, avoiding the need for an ostomy pouch.

Cancer, trauma, inflammatory bowel disease (IBD), bowel obstruction, and diverticulitis are all possible reasons for bowel diversion surgery.

Bowel diversion surgeries affect the large intestine and often the small intestine.

The small intestine runs from the stomach to the large intestine and has three main sections: The duodenum, which is the first 10 inches; the jejunum, which is the middle 8 feet; and the ileum, which is the final 12 feet. Bowel diversion surgeries only affect the ileum.

The large intestine is about five feet long and runs from the small intestine to the anus. The colon and rectum are the two main sections of the large intestine. Semisolid digestive waste enters the colon from the small intestine. Gradually, the colon absorbs moisture and forms stool as digestive waste moves toward the rectum. The rectum is about six inches long and is located right before the anus. The rectum stores stool, which leaves the body through the anus. The rectum and anus control bowel movements.

Different Types of Bowel Diversion Surgery

Several surgical options exist for bowel diversion.

- Ileostomy diverts the ileum to a stoma. Semisolid waste flows out of the stoma and collects in an ostomy pouch, which must be emptied several times a day. An ileostomy bypasses the colon, rectum, and anus and has the fewest complications.

- Colostomy is similar to an ileostomy, but the colon—not the ileum—is diverted to a stoma. As with an ileostomy, stool collects in an ostomy pouch.

- Ileoanal reservoir surgery is an option when the large intestine is removed but the anus remains intact and disease-free. The surgeon creates a colon-like pouch, called an ileoanal reservoir, from the last several inches of the ileum. The ileoanal reservoir is also called a pelvic pouch or J-pouch. Stool collects in the ileoanal reservoir and then exits the body through the anus during a bowel movement. People who have undergone ileoanal reservoir surgery initially have about 6 to 10 bowel movements a day. Two or more surgeries are usually required, including a temporary ileostomy, and an adjustment period lasting several months is needed for the newly formed ileoanal reservoir to stretch and adjust to its new function. After the adjustment period, bowel movements decrease to as few as four to six a day.

- Continent ileostomy is an option for people who are not good candidates for ileoanal reservoir surgery because of damage to the rectum or anus but do not want to wear an ostomy pouch. As with ileoanal reservoir surgery, the large intestine is removed and a colon-like pouch, called a Kock pouch, is made from the end of the ileum. The surgeon connects the Kock pouch to a stoma. A Kock pouch must be drained each day by inserting a tube through the stoma. An ostomy pouch is not needed and the stoma is covered by a patch when it is not in use.

Some people only need a temporary bowel diversion; others need permanent bowel diversion.

Which Bowel Diversion Surgery Is Appropriate?

The type, degree, and location of bowel damage, and personal preference, are all factors in determining which surgery is most appropriate. For example, people whose disease affects the ileum are poor candidates for ileoanal reservoir surgery or continent ileostomy because of the increased risk of disease recurrence and the need for pouch removal.

Discussing treatment options with a doctor and seeking the advice of an ostomy nurse—a specialist who cares for people with bowel diversions—are highly recommended.

Concerns Related to Bowel Diversion

Although bowel diversion surgery can bring great relief, many people fear the practical, social, and psychological issues related to bowel diversion. An ostomy nurse is trained to help patients deal with these issues both before and after surgery. People living with an ostomy or who need bowel diversion surgery may also find useful advice and information through local or online support groups.

Section 30.3

Colectomy

Large bowel resection is surgery to remove all or part of your large bowel. This surgery is also called colectomy. The large bowel is also called the large intestine or colon.

- Removal of the entire colon and the rectum is called a proctocolectomy.

- Removal of part or all of the colon but not the rectum is called subtotal colectomy.

The large bowel connects the small intestine to the anus. Normally, stool passes through the large bowel before leaving the body through the anus.

Description

You will get general anesthesia before your surgery. This will make you asleep and pain-free. The surgery can be performed laparoscopically or with open surgery.

Depending on what type of procedure you have, your surgeon will make one or more cuts in your belly.

In a laparoscopic colectomy, the surgeon uses a camera to see inside your belly and small instruments to remove part of your large bowel. You will have three to five small cuts in your lower belly. The surgeon passes the medical instruments through these cuts.

- You may also have a cut of about two to three inches if your surgeon needs to put a hand inside your belly to feel or remove the diseased bowel.

- During laparoscopy, your belly will be filled with gas to expand it. This makes the area easier to see and work in.

- Your surgeon will remove the diseased part of your large bowel.

- The surgeon will then sew the healthy ends of the bowel back together. This is called anastomosis.

- Then the cuts on the skin will be closed with stitches.

For open colectomy, your surgeon will make a 6- to 8-inch cut in your lower belly.

- The surgeon will find the part of your colon that is diseased.

- The surgeon will put clamps on both ends of this part to close it off.

- Then the surgeon will remove the diseased part.

- If there is enough healthy large intestine left, your surgeon will sew or staple the healthy ends back together. Most patients have this done.

- If you do not have enough healthy large intestine to reconnect, you may have a colostomy.

In most cases, the colostomy is short-term. It can be closed with another operation later. But, if a large part of your bowel is removed, the colostomy may be permanent.

Your surgeon may also look at lymph nodes and other organs, and may remove some of them.

Colectomy surgery usually takes between one and four hours.

Why the Procedure Is Performed

Large bowel resection is used to treat many conditions, including:

- a block in the intestine due to scar tissue;

- colon cancer;

- diverticular disease (disease of the large bowel).

Other reasons to perform bowel resection are:

- familial polyposis;

- injuries that damage the large bowel;

- intussusception (when one part of the intestine pushes into another);

- precancerous polyps (nodes);

- severe gastrointestinal bleeding;

- twisting of the bowel (volvulus);
- ulcerative colitis.

Risks

Talk with your doctor about these possible risks and complications. Risks for any anesthesia are:

- reactions to medicines;
- breathing problems.

Risks for any surgery are:

- blood clots in the legs that may travel to the lungs;
- breathing problems;
- heart attack or stroke;
- infection, including in the lungs, urinary tract, and belly.

Risks for this surgery are:

- bleeding inside your belly;
- bulging tissue through the surgical cut, called an incisional hernia;
- damage to nearby organs in the body;
- damage to the ureter or bladder;
- problems with the colostomy;
- scar tissue that forms in the belly and causes a blockage of the intestines;
- the edges of your intestines that are sewn together come open (anastomotic leak—this may be life-threatening);
- wound breaks open (dehiscence);
- wound infections.

Before the Procedure

Always tell your doctor or nurse what drugs you are taking, even drugs, supplements, or herbs you bought without a prescription.

Talk with your doctor or nurse about these things before you have surgery:

- Intimacy and sexuality
- Pregnancy
- Sports
- Work

During the two weeks before your surgery:

- Two weeks before surgery you may be asked to stop taking drugs that make it harder for your blood to clot. These include aspirin, ibuprofen (Advil, Motrin), Naprosyn (Aleve, Naproxen), and others.
- Ask your doctor which drugs you should still take on the day of your surgery.
- If you smoke, try to stop. Ask your doctor for help.
- Always let your doctor know about any cold, flu, fever, herpes breakout, or other illness you may have before your surgery.
- Eat high fiber foods and drink six to eight glasses of water every day.

The day before your surgery:

- A few days before surgery, you will be given a bowel prep that includes drinking fluids and taking laxatives and enemas. This is done to make sure that the colon is free of any stool.
- You may be asked to drink only clear liquids such as broth, clear juice, and water after noon.
- Do not drink anything after midnight, including water. Sometimes you will not be able to drink anything for up to 12 hours before surgery.

On the day of your surgery:

- Take the drugs your doctor told you to take with a small sip of water.
- Your doctor or nurse will tell you when to arrive at the hospital.

After the Procedure

You will be in the hospital for three to seven days. You may have to stay longer if your colectomy was an emergency operation.

You may also need to stay longer if a large amount of your small intestine was removed or you develop any complications. By the second or third day, you will probably be able to drink clear liquids. Your doctor or nurse will slowly add thicker fluids and then soft foods as your bowel begins to work again.

Outlook (Prognosis)

Most people who have a large bowel resection recover fully. Even with a colostomy, most people are able to do most activities they were doing before their surgery. This includes most sports, travel, gardening, hiking, and other outdoor activities, and most types of work.

If you have a long-term (chronic) condition, such as cancer, Crohn disease, or ulcerative colitis, you may need ongoing medical treatment.

Section 30.4

Colon and Rectal Cancer Surgery

Excerpted from "What You Need to Know about Cancer of the Colon and Rectum," by the National Cancer Institute (NCI, www.cancer.gov), part of the National Institutes of Health, May 26, 2006. Reviewed by David A. Cooke, MD, FACP, October 11, 2012.

Many people with colorectal cancer want to take an active part in making decisions about their medical care. It is natural to want to learn all you can about your disease and treatment choices. However, shock and stress after the diagnosis can make it hard to think of everything you want to ask your doctor. It often helps to make a list of questions before an appointment.

To help remember what your doctor says, you may take notes or ask whether you may use a tape recorder. You may also want to have a family member or friend with you when you talk to your doctor—to take part in the discussion, to take notes, or just to listen.

You do not need to ask all your questions at once. You will have other chances to ask your doctor or nurse to explain things that are not clear and to ask for more details.

Your doctor may refer you to a specialist who has experience treating colorectal cancer, or you may ask for a referral. Specialists who treat colorectal cancer include gastroenterologists (doctors who specialize in diseases of the digestive system), surgeons, medical oncologists, and radiation oncologists. You may have a team of doctors.

Treatment Methods

The choice of treatment depends mainly on the location of the tumor in the colon or rectum and the stage of the disease. Treatment for colorectal cancer may involve surgery, chemotherapy, biological therapy, or radiation therapy. Some people have a combination of treatments.

Colon cancer sometimes is treated differently from rectal cancer. Treatments for colon and rectal cancer are described separately below.

Your doctor can describe your treatment choices and the expected results. You and your doctor can work together to develop a treatment plan that meets your needs.

Cancer treatment is either local therapy or systemic therapy.

Local therapy: Surgery and radiation therapy are local therapies. They remove or destroy cancer in or near the colon or rectum. When colorectal cancer has spread to other parts of the body, local therapy may be used to control the disease in those specific areas.

Systemic therapy: Chemotherapy and biological therapy are systemic therapies. The drugs enter the bloodstream and destroy or control cancer throughout the body.

Because cancer treatments often damage healthy cells and tissues, side effects are common. Side effects depend mainly on the type and extent of the treatment. Side effects may not be the same for each person, and they may change from one treatment session to the next. Before treatment starts, your health care team will explain possible side effects and suggest ways to help you manage them.

At any stage of disease, supportive care is available to relieve the side effects of treatment, to control pain and other symptoms, and to ease emotional concerns.

Surgery

Surgery is the most common treatment for colorectal cancer.

Colonoscopy: A small malignant polyp may be removed from your colon or upper rectum with a colonoscope. Some small tumors in the lower rectum can be removed through your anus without a colonoscope.

Laparoscopy: Early colon cancer may be removed with the aid of a thin, lighted tube (laparoscope). Three or four tiny cuts are made into your abdomen. The surgeon sees inside your abdomen with the laparoscope. The tumor and part of the healthy colon are removed. Nearby lymph nodes also may be removed. The surgeon checks the rest of your intestine and your liver to see if the cancer has spread.

Open surgery: The surgeon makes a large cut into your abdomen to remove the tumor and part of the healthy colon or rectum. Some nearby lymph nodes are also removed. The surgeon checks the rest of your intestine and your liver to see if the cancer has spread.

When a section of your colon or rectum is removed, the surgeon can usually reconnect the healthy parts. However, sometimes reconnection is not possible. In this case, the surgeon creates a new path for waste to leave your body. The surgeon makes an opening (stoma) in the wall of the abdomen, connects the upper end of the intestine to the stoma, and closes the other end. The operation to create the stoma is called a colostomy. A flat bag fits over the stoma to collect waste, and a special adhesive holds it in place.

For most people, the stoma is temporary. It is needed only until the colon or rectum heals from surgery. After healing takes place, the surgeon reconnects the parts of the intestine and closes the stoma. Some people, especially those with a tumor in the lower rectum, need a permanent stoma.

People who have a colostomy may have irritation of the skin around the stoma. Your doctor, your nurse, or an enterostomal therapist can teach you how to clean the area and prevent irritation and infection.

The time it takes to heal after surgery is different for each person. You may be uncomfortable for the first few days. Medicine can help control your pain. Before surgery, you should discuss the plan for pain relief with your doctor or nurse. After surgery, your doctor can adjust the plan if you need more pain relief.

It is common to feel tired or weak for a while. Also, surgery sometimes causes constipation or diarrhea. Your health care team monitors you for signs of bleeding, infection, or other problems requiring immediate treatment.

Treatment for Colon Cancer

Most patients with colon cancer are treated with surgery. Some people have both surgery and chemotherapy. Some with advanced disease get biological therapy.

A colostomy is seldom needed for people with colon cancer.

Although radiation therapy is rarely used to treat colon cancer, sometimes it is used to relieve pain and other symptoms.

Treatment for Rectal Cancer

For all stages of rectal cancer, surgery is the most common treatment. Some patients receive surgery, radiation therapy, and chemotherapy. Some with advanced disease get biological therapy.

About one out of eight people with rectal cancer needs a permanent colostomy.

Radiation therapy may be used before and after surgery. Some people have radiation therapy before surgery to shrink the tumor, and some have it after surgery to kill cancer cells that may remain in the area. At some hospitals, patients may have radiation therapy during surgery. People also may have radiation therapy to relieve pain and other problems caused by the cancer.

Section 30.5

Gallbladder Removal Surgery (Cholecystectomy)

Overview

Cholecystectomy is the surgical removal of the gallbladder. The operation is done to remove gallstones or to remove an infected or inflamed gallbladder.

Common symptoms:

- Sharp pain in the upper center or right abdomen

- Low fever

- Nausea and feeling bloated

Treatment Options

Surgery:

- Laparoscopic cholecystectomy: The gallbladder is removed with instruments placed into four small slits in the abdomen.

- Open cholecystectomy: The gallbladder is removed through an incision on the right side under the rib cage.

Nonsurgical:

- Stone retrieval

For gallstones without symptoms:

- Watchful waiting

- Increased exercise

- Diet changes

Benefits and Risks

Gallbladder removal will relieve pain, treat infection, and in most cases stop gallstones from coming back. The risks of not having surgery are the possibility of worsening symptoms, infection, or bursting of the gallbladder.

Possible complications include bleeding, bile duct injury, fever, liver injury, infection, numbness, raised scars, hernia at the incision, anesthesia complications, puncture of the intestine, and death.

Expectations

- Before your operation: Evaluation usually includes blood work, an abdominal ultrasound, and an evaluation by your surgeon and anesthesia provider to review your health history and medications and to discuss pain control options.

- The day of your operation: You will not eat or drink for at least four hours before the operation. Most often you will take your normal medication with a sip of water.

- Your recovery: If you have no complications, you are often discharged home the same day after a laparoscopic procedure and in two to three days after an open procedure. Call your surgeon if you are in severe pain, have stomach cramping, a high fever or chills, your skin turns yellow, or there is odor and increased drainage from your incision.

The Condition, Signs and Symptoms, and Diagnostic Tests

Keeping You Informed

Most people with gallstones do not have symptoms. Eighty percent of people with gallstones go 20 years or longer without symptoms.[1,2]

Gallstones are more common in people who:

- are Native American;
- have a family history of gallstones;
- are overweight;
- eat a lot of sugar;
- are pregnant;
- do not exercise regularly;
- lose weight rapidly; or
- use estrogen to manage menopause.[3,4]

Gallbladder pain or biliary colic is usually temporary. It starts in the middle or right side of the abdomen and can last from 30 minutes to 24 hours. The pain may occur after eating a fatty meal.

- Acute cholecystitis pain lasts longer than six hours, and there is abdominal tenderness and fever.
- Pain on the right side of the abdomen can also be from ulcers, liver problems, and heart pain.

Standard treatment of acute cholecystitis is intravenous fluids, antibiotics, pain medication, and cholecystectomy.[5]

The Condition

The gallbladder: The gallbladder is a small pear-shaped organ under the liver.

The liver makes about three to five cups of bile every day. Bile is stored in the gallbladder, and when food is eaten, especially fatty foods, the gallbladder squeezes bile out through the cystic duct and into the small intestine.

Gallstones: The medical term for gallstone formation is cholelithiasis. A gallstone in the common bile duct is called choledocholithiasis.

Gallstones in the ducts can block the flow of bile and cause swelling of the gallbladder.

Cholecystitis is inflammation of the gallbladder, which can happen suddenly (acute) or over a longer period of time (chronic).

Perforated gallbladder is a condition when the gallbladder bursts or leaks, which happens only in rare cases but can be life threatening.

Cholecystectomy is the surgical removal of the gallbladder. The most common reason for a cholecystectomy is to remove gallstones that cause biliary colic (acute pain in the abdomen caused by spasm or blockage of the cystic or bile duct).

Symptoms

The most common symptoms of cholecystitis are:

- sharp pain in the right abdomen;
- low fever;
- nausea and bloating; and
- jaundice (yellowing of the skin) may occur if gallstones are in the common bile duct.

Common Diagnostic Tests

- Abdominal ultrasounds: This is the most common test to check for gallstones. You may be asked not to eat for eight hours before the test.
- Blood tests:
  - Complete blood count
  - Liver function tests
  - Coagulation profile
- HIDA [hepatobiliary iminodiacetic acid] scan, cholescintigraphy
- Endoscopic retrograde cholangiogram
- Magnetic resonance cholangiopancreatography

Surgical and Nonsurgical Treatment

Surgical Treatment

An operation is the recommended treatment for gallbladder pain from gallstones, and it is the only treatment for acute cholecystitis.

Laparoscopic cholecystectomy: This technique is the most common for simple cholecystectomy. The surgeon will make four small slits in the abdomen. A port (nozzle) is inserted into one of the slits, and carbon dioxide gas inflates the abdomen. This process allows the surgeon to see the gallbladder more easily. A laparoscope is inserted through another port. It looks like a telescope with a light and video camera on the end so the surgeon can see inside the abdomen. Surgical instruments are placed into the other small openings and used to remove the gallbladder.

The surgeon removes the gallbladder through the incision. The carbon dioxide comes out through the small slits and then the sites are closed with sutures, metal clips called staples, or Steri-Strips. Your surgeon may start with a laparoscopic technique and need to change to an open technique.

The procedure takes about one to two hours.

Open cholecystectomy: The surgeon makes an incision approximately six inches long in the upper right side of the abdomen and cuts through the fat and muscle to the gallbladder. The gallbladder is removed, and any ducts are clamped off.

The site is stapled or sutured closed, and a small drain may be placed going from the inside to the outside of the abdomen. The drain is usually removed in the hospital. The procedure takes about one to two hours.

Procedure Options

Procedures may be done to remove gallstones from the common bile duct.

Laparoscopic transcystic common bile duct stone extraction is performed with insertion of instruments into the abdomen similar to laparoscopic cholecystectomy. The bile duct is entered, and stones are removed directly or with a wire basket.

Endoscopic retrograde cholangiopancreatography is done by inserting an endoscope into your mouth and continuing to pass it through your stomach and then into the common bile duct. Gallstones are removed directly or with a balloon or basket.

Complication rates range from 0 to 9.1 per 1,000 procedures.[6]

Nonsurgical Treatment

- Watchful waiting: If gallstones are seen on your ultrasound but you do not have symptoms, watchful waiting is recommended.

- Gallstones only, without cholecystitis:
  - Increase your exercise. Exercising two to three hours a week reduces the risk of gallstones.[7,8]
  - Eat more fruits and vegetables, and eat fewer foods high in sugars and carbohydrates like donuts, pastry, and white bread.
  - Alternative medicine options are available.[9]

Keeping You Informed

Conversion rates from a laparoscopic to an open technique are less than 1% for young healthy people.

The need to convert from a laparoscopic to an open procedure can increase significantly if you are over 65 years, are male, have a history of acute cholecystitis, past abdominal operations, high fever, high bilirubin, repeated gallbladder attacks, and diseases that limit your activity.[5]

Questions You Should Ask

- What type of procedure is right for me and why?
- How much experience do you have with this procedure?
- Has the procedure been done often at this center?
- Do you know the approximate cost of the procedure?

Risks of This Procedure

Your surgeon will do everything possible to minimize risks, but cholecystectomy, like all operations, has risks. See Table 30.2.

Expectations: Preparation for Your Operation

Preparing for Your Operation

Tell your surgeon about other medical problems that you have. Bring a list of all of the medications that you are taking, and show that list to your surgeon and anesthesia provider.

Most often you will take your morning medication with a sip of water. If you are taking blood thinners (Plavix, Coumadin, aspirin), your surgeon may ask you to stop taking these.

Home preparation: You can often go home the same day after a laparoscopic procedure. Your hospital stay will be longer (two to three days) for an open procedure.

Anesthesia: You will meet with your anesthesia provider before the operation. Let him or her know if you have allergies, neurologic disease (epilepsy or stroke), heart disease, stomach problems, lung disease (asthma, emphysema), endocrine disease (diabetes, thyroid conditions), loose teeth, or if you smoke, abuse alcohol or drugs, or take any herbs or vitamins.

The Day of Your Operation

Don't eat or drink. Not eating or drinking for at least four hours before the operation reduces your risk of complications from anesthesia.
What to bring:

- Insurance card and identification
- Advance directive
- List of medicines
- Personal items such as eyeglasses and dentures
- Loose-fitting comfortable clothes
- Leave jewelry and valuables at home

What You Can Expect

A bracelet with your name and identification number will be placed on your wrist. Your wristband should be checked by all health care team members before providing any procedures or giving you medication. If you have any allergies, an allergy bracelet should also be placed on your wrist.

An intravenous line (IV) will be started to give your fluids and medication. The medication will make you feel sleepy.

A tube will be placed down your throat to help you breathe during the operation.

Your surgeon will perform your operation and then close your incisions. If you have an open operation, a drain may be placed from the inside of your incision out your abdomen.

After your operation, you will be moved to a recovery room.

Preventing pneumonia: Movement and deep breathing after your operation can help prevent fluid in your lungs and pneumonia.[10]

Preventing blood clots: When you have surgery, you are at risk of getting blood clots because of not moving during anesthesia. The longer and more complicated your surgery, the greater the risk. Your doctor will know your risk for blood clots, and steps will be taken to prevent them. This may include blood thinning medication and support or compression (squeezing) stockings.

Preventing infection: The risk of infection can be lowered if antibiotics are given right before surgery and hair is removed at the surgical site with clippers versus shaving.

All health care providers should wash their hands before examining you.

Table 30.2. Risks of Cholecystectomy

The Risk	What Happens	Keeping You Informed
Infection	Infections occur in less than 1 per 1,000 patients who have laparoscopic procedures.[5,6,13,14]	Your health care team should wash their hands before examining you. Antibiotics are given right before the operation.[5]
Common bile duct injury	Injury to the bile duct is reported in 1 per 1,000 patients for open cholecystectomy and in 1 to 5 per 1,000 for laparoscopic cholecystectomy.[5,6,14]	Your surgeon and nurse will watch for jaundice, fever, and abnormal blood tests.[5] Further testing or surgery may be needed.
Bleeding	Bleeding is rare. If you have chronic biliary disease, your liver may not form clotting factors.[5,6,13]	Your surgeon will check a coagulation profile to monitor for bleeding problems. A blood transfusion usually is not required for cholecystectomy.
Bile leakage	Bile leakage after surgery is very rare.	Your surgeon will check for fever, monitor labs, and may need to perform other tests such as sonography or endoscopic retrograde cholangiopancreatography (ERCP).
Retained common bile duct stone	A gallstone may pass after surgery and block the bile from draining.[5]	Your surgeon will check blood tests for your liver function.
Pneumonia	General anesthesia, lack of deep breathing and movement are possible causes.	Deep breathing exercises can help expand your lungs and prevent complications after surgery.[10]
Heart problems	Heart problems are rare. Cardiac arrhythmias were reported in about 5 per 1,000 patients and heart attack in 1 per 1,000.[6,13]	Your surgeon may have you see a heart specialist before your operation. Your anesthesia provider is always prepared in advanced cardiac life support.

Keeping You Informed

An effective way to do deep breathing is to breathe deeply and hold for three to five seconds. Take 5 to 10 deep breaths every hour while you are awake. Young children can do deep breathing by blowing bubbles.

Questions You Should Ask

- What medications should I stop taking before my operation?

Table 30.2. Risks of Cholecystectomy *continued*

The Risk	What Happens	Keeping You Informed
Kidney problems	Kidney or urinary problems have been reported in 5 per 1,000 patients. Dehydration and liver problems can increase this risk.[6,13]	Your surgeon may give you extra fluids before your operation.[5] Let your nurse know when you urinate.
Deep vein thrombosis (blood clots)	No movement during surgery can lead to blood clots forming in the legs. In rare cases the clot can travel to the lungs.	Your surgeon or nurse will place support or compression (squeezing) stockings on your legs and may give you blood thinning medication. Your job is to get up and walk after surgery.
Premature labor and fetal loss	Fetal loss is reported as 40 per 1,000 patients for uncomplicated cholecystectomy and as high as 600 per 1,000 when pancreatitis is present. The risk of preterm labor also increases.[11,12]	These risks increase with peritonitis (infection of the abdominal cavity).
Injury to the intestines or abdominal organs	Instrument insertion and use during laparoscopic technique can injure the intestines	The surgeon will use extreme care and continuously watch for any bleeding or bowel contents during the procedure. Patients who are obese or who have a history of past abdominal operations or adhesions make it more difficult to move and manipulate instruments.[5]
Death	Death is extremely rare in healthy people and is reported as 0 to 1 per 1,000 patients. The risk of death increases with gangrene, a burst gallbladder, or severe diseases that limit your activity.[1,6]	Your entire surgical team will review for possible complications and be prepared to decrease all risks.

- When should I stop taking them?

- Should I take any medicines on the day of my operation?

- What are the risks, problems, and side effects of general anesthesia?

- Do I need antibiotics before surgery?

- What will you do to prevent blood clots?

- If hair has to be removed on my abdomen, how will it be done?

- Did you wash your hands?

Your Recovery and Discharge

Thinking Clearly

The anesthesia may cause you to feel different for two or three days. Do not drive, drink alcohol, or make any big decisions for at least two days.

Nutrition

- When you wake up, you will be able to drink small amounts of liquid. If you are not nauseous, you can begin eating regular foods.

- Continue to drink lots of fluids, usually about 8 to 10 glasses per day.

Activity

- You will be helped getting out of bed and walking.

- Slowly increase your activity.

- Do not lift or participate in strenuous activity for 3–5 days for laparoscopic and 10–14 days for open procedure.

- Avoid driving until your pain is under control without narcotics.

- You can have sex when you feel ready, usually after your sutures or staples are removed.

- It is normal to feel tired. You may need more sleep than usual.

Work

You can go back to work when you feel well enough. Discuss the timing with your surgeon.

Wound Care

- Always wash your hands before and after touching near your incision site.

- Do not soak in a bathtub until your stitches, Steri-Strips, or staples are removed. You may take a shower after the second postoperative day unless you are told not to.

- Follow your surgeon's instructions on when to change your bandages.

- A small amount of drainage from the incision is normal. If the drainage is thick and yellow or the site is red, you may have an infection so call your surgeon.

- If you have a drain in one of your incisions, it will be taken out when the drainage stops.

- Surgical staples will be removed during your first office visit.

- Steri-strips will fall off in 7 to 10 days or they will be removed during your first office visit.

- Avoid wearing tight or rough clothing. It may rub your incisions and make it harder for them to heal.

- Protect the new skin, especially from the sun. The sun can burn and cause darker scarring.

- Your scar will heal in about four to six weeks and will become softer and continue to fade over the next year. Keep the wound site out of the sun or use sunscreen.

- Sensation around your incision will return in a few weeks or months.

Bowel Movements

- After intestinal surgery, you may have loose watery stools for several days. If watery diarrhea lasts longer than three days, contact your surgeon.

- Pain medication (narcotics) can cause constipation. Increase the fiber in your diet with high-fiber foods if you are constipated. Your surgeon may also give you a prescription for a stool softener.

High-Fiber Foods

Food high in fiber include beans, bran cereals and whole-grain breads, peas, dried fruit (figs, apricots, and dates), raspberries, blackberries, strawberries, sweet corn, broccoli, baked potatoes with skin, plums, pears, apples, greens, and nuts.

Pain

The amount of pain is different for each person. Some people need only two to three doses of pain control medication, while others use narcotics for a full week.

Home Medications

The medicine you need after your operation is usually related to pain control.

When to Contact Your Surgeon

If you have:

- Pain that will not go away

- Pain that gets worse

- A fever of more than 101 degrees Fahrenheit (38.3 degrees Celsius)

- Vomiting

- Swelling, redness, bleeding, or bad-smelling drainage from your wound site

- Strong abdominal pain

- Jaundice or yellow skin

- No bowel movement or unable to pass gas for three days

- Water diarrhea lasting longer than three days

Pain Control

Everyone reacts to pain in a different ways. A scale from 0 to 10 is often used to measure pain. At a "0," you do not feel any pain. A "10" is the worst pain you have ever felt.

Common Medicines to Control Pain

Narcotics or opioids are used for severe pain. Some side effects of narcotics are sleepiness; lowered blood pressure, heart rate, and breathing rate; skin rash and itching; constipation; nausea; and difficulty urinating. Some examples of narcotics include morphine, oxycodone, and hydromorphone. Medications are available to control many of the side effects of narcotics.

Non-Narcotic Pain Medication

Most nonopioid pain medications are nonsteroidal anti-inflammatory drugs (NSAIDs). They are used to treat mild pain or combined with a narcotic to treat severe pain. They also can reduce inflammation. Some side effects of NSAIDs are stomach upset, bleeding in the stomach or intestines, and fluid retention. These side effects usually are not seen with short-term use. Examples of NSAIDs include ibuprofen and naproxen.

Non-Medicine Pain Control

Distraction helps you focus on other activities instead of your pain. Music, games, and other engaging activities are especially helpful with children in mild pain.

Splinting your stomach by placing a pillow over your abdomen with firm pressure before coughing or movement can help reduce the pain.

Guided imagery helps you direct and control your emotions. Close your eyes and gently inhale and exhale. Picture yourself in the center of somewhere beautiful. Feel the beauty surrounding you and your emotions coming back to your control. You should feel calmer.

Keeping You Informed

Extreme pain puts extra stress on your body at a time when your body needs to focus on healing. Do not wait until your pain has reached a level "10" or is unbearable before telling your doctor or nurse. It is much easier to control pain before it becomes severe.

Glossary of Terms and for More Information

Glossary of Terms

Abdominal ultrasound: This test uses sound waves to determine the location of deep structures in the body. A hand roller is placed on top of clear gel and rolled across the abdomen.

Advance directives: Documents signed by a competent person giving direction to health care providers about treatment choices. They give you the chance to tell your feelings about health care decisions.

Adhesions: A fibrous band or scar tissue that causes internal organs to adhere or stick together.

Bilirubin: A blood test used to determine liver and gallbladder dysfunction.

Complete blood count (CBC): A blood test that measures red blood cells (RBCs) and white blood cells (WBCs). WBCs increase with inflammation. The normal range for WBCs is 8,000 to 12,000.

Endoscopic retrograde cholangiogram: An endoscope with a camera on the end is passed through your mouth, stomach, and intestines into the bile duct to check for and remove gallstones.

HIDA (hepatobiliary iminodiacetic acid scan): A scan that images the liver, gallbladder, and bile ducts following the injection of radiolabeled dye into the veins.

Hernia: A bulge through an abnormal opening in the abdominal wall.

Magnetic resonance cholangiopancreatography: A scan that uses powerful magnets and radio waves to show pictures of the body.

For More Information

For more information, please go to the American College of Surgeons Patient Education Web site at www.facs.org/patienteducation.

The information provided in this brochure is chosen from recent clinical research. The research listed below does not represent all of the information that is available about your operation.

1. Society for Surgery of the Alimentary Tract. Treatment of gallstones and gallbladder disease. (2003).

2. National Institutes of Health. Gallstones and laparoscopic cholecystectomy. NIH Consensus Statement (1992)12:1–28.

3. Nakeeb A, Cumuzzie AG, Martin L, et al. Gallstone: Genetics versus environment. *Annals of Surgery* (2002)235:842–849.

4. Weinsier RL, Wilson LJ, Lee J. Medically safe rate of weight loss for the treatment of obesity: A guideline based on risk of gallstone formation. *American Journal of Medicine* (1995)98: 115–117.

5. Souba W, Fink M, Jurkovich G, et al. *ACS Surgery: Principles and Practice.* New York, NY: WebMD, 2004.

6. Petelin J. Laparoscopic common bile duct exploration. *Surgical Endoscopy* (2003)17:1705–1715.

7. Leitzmann MF, Giovannucci EL, Rimm EB, et al. The relation of physical activity to risk for symptomatic gallstone disease in men. *Annals of Internal Medicine* (1998)128:417–425.

8. Leitzmann MF, Rimm EB, Willet WC, et al. Recreational physical activity and the risk of cholecystectomy in women. *New England Journal of Medicine* (1999)341:777–784.

9. Moga MM. Alternative treatment of gallbladder disease. *Medical Hypothesis* (2003)60:143–147.

10. Overend TJ, Anderson CM, Lucy SD, et al. The effect of incentive spirometry on post-operative complications. *Chest* (2001)120:971–978.

11. Graham G, Baxi L, Tharakan T. Laparoscopic cholecystectomy during pregnancy: A case series and review of the literature. *Obstetrics and Gynecology Survival* (1998)53:566–574.

12. Al-Fozan H, Tulandi T. Safety and risks of laparoscopy in pregnancy. *Current Opinion in Obstetrics and Gynecology* (2002)14:375–379.

13. Khaitan L, Apelgren K, Hunter L, et al. A report on the Society of American Gastrointestinal Endoscopic Surgeons (SAGES) outcome initiative. *Surgical Endoscopy* (2003)17:365–370.

14. Giger UF, Michel JM, Opitz I, et al. Risk factors for perioperative complications in patients undergoing laparoscopic cholecystectomy: analysis of 22,953 consecutive cases from the Swiss Association of Laparoscopic and Thoracoscopic Surgery database. *Journal of the American College of Surgeons* (2006)203:723–728.

Section 30.6

Hemorrhoid Surgery

© 2012 A.D.A.M., Inc. Reprinted with permission.

Description

Hemorrhoid surgery is often done in an outpatient clinic or your doctor's office, with little or no anesthesia.

Hemorrhoids can be surgically removed using a special stapler or sutures (stiches). After the hemorrhoid is removed, you may have stitches that dissolve on their own and gauze packing to reduce bleeding.

Other treatments may include:

- a shot into the hemorrhoid to reduce swelling (sclerotherapy);

- a rubber band around the hemorrhoid to cut off its blood supply;

- shrinking the hemorrhoid with heat, or freezing it with liquid nitrogen;

- minor surgery to treat the hemorrhoid (hemorrhoidectomy).

Smaller hemorrhoids may not need surgery.

Why the Procedure Is Performed

Most small hemorrhoids can be managed with lifestyle changes and diet.

Your doctor may recommend hemorrhoid surgery if lifestyle and diet changes and medicines have not worked.

Risks

Risks for any surgery are:

- bleeding;

- infection.

Risks for any anesthesia are:

- reactions to medications;
- breathing problems, pneumonia;
- heart problems.

Risks for hemorrhoid surgery are:

- leaking a small amount of stool (long-term problems are rare);
- problems passing urine because of the pain.

Before the Procedure

Always tell your doctor or nurse:

- if you could be pregnant;
- what medicines you are taking, even those you bought without a prescription.

Several days before surgery, you may be asked to stop taking aspirin, ibuprofen Advil, Motrin, naproxen (Aleve, Naprosyn), warfarin (Coumadin), and any other drugs that make it hard for your blood to clot.

On the day of the surgery:

- If you are having general anesthesia, you will usually be asked not to drink or eat anything after midnight the night before the surgery.
- Take any medicines your doctor told you to take with a small sip of water.

After the Procedure

You may have a lot of pain after surgery as the area tightens and relaxes. You may be given medications to relieve pain.

Gradually return to your normal activities. Avoid lifting, pulling, or strenuous activity until your bottom has healed. This includes straining during bowel movements or urination. To avoid straining, you will need to use stool softeners. Eat more fiber to ease bowel movements. Drink 8 to 10 glasses of water a day.

Soaking in a warm bath (sitz bath) can help relieve pain. Sit in three to four inches of warm water a few times a day.

You should have a complete recovery in about two weeks.

Outlook (Prognosis)

Most people do very well after hemorrhoid surgery. You will still need to take steps to help prevent the hemorrhoids from coming back. Eating a high-fiber diet, drinking plenty of water, and avoiding constipation may help.

Section 30.7

Hernia Repair Surgery

The Condition

A hernia occurs when a small tissue bulges out through an opening in the muscles. Any part of the abdominal wall can weaken and develop a hernia, but the most common sites are the groin (inguinal), the navel (umbilical), and a previous surgical incision site.

What Are the Common Symptoms?

- Visible bulge in the scrotum or groin area, especially with coughing or straining
- Pain or pressure at the hernia site

Treatment Options

Surgical Procedure

Open hernia repair: An incision is made over the site and the hernia is repaired with mesh or, less often, by suturing the muscle closed.

Laparoscopic hernia repair: The hernia is repaired with mesh or sutures using instruments placed into small incisions in the abdomen.

Nonsurgical

Watchful waiting is an option for adults with hernias that are not uncomfortable.[1] This is not recommended for femoral hernias or for infants.[2-6]

Benefits and Risks

Benefits: An operation is the only way to repair a hernia. You can return to your normal activities and, in most cases, will not have further discomfort.

Risk of not having an operation: Your hernia pain and the size can increase. If your intestine becomes trapped in the hernia pouch, you will have sudden pain, vomiting, and require an immediate operation.

Possible complications include: Return of the hernia; infection; injury to the bladder, blood vessels, intestines, or nerves; difficulty passing urine; continued pain; and swelling of the testes or groin area.

Expectations

Before your operation: Evaluation may include blood work and urinalysis. Your surgeon and anesthesia provider will discuss your health history, which home medications you should take the day of your operation, and options for pain control.

The day of your operation: You will not eat or drink for six hours before the operation. Most often you will take your normal medication with a sip of water. You will need someone to drive you home.

Your recovery: If you do not have complications you usually will go home the same day.

Call your surgeon if you have severe pain, stomach cramping, chills, a high fever (over 101 degrees Fahrenheit), odor or increased drainage from your incision, or do not have bowel movements for three days.

The Condition, Signs and Symptoms, and Diagnostic Tests

Keeping You Informed: Who Gets Hernias?

There may be no cause for a hernia. Some risk factors are:[3-4]

- older age: muscles become weaker;
- obesity: increased weight places pressure on abdominal muscle;
- sudden twist, pulls, or strains;
- chronic straining;
- family history;
- connective tissue disorders;
- pregnancy: 1 in 2,000 women develop a hernia during pregnancy.

Pediatric Considerations

Inguinal hernias occur in up to 50 of 1,000 full-term and 300 of 1,000 preterm infants. Inguinal hernias are five times more common in boys.[5]

Infants or children always have surgical repair because of the high risk of incarceration. Incarceration can occur in up to 100 of 1,000 children and up to 400 of 1,000 premature infants. In females, 150 of 1,000 have an ovary in their hernia sac.[5–7]

Other medical disorders that have symptoms similar to hernias include enlarged lymph nodes, cysts, and testicular problems such as scrotal hydrocele.[3–4]

The Condition: The Hernia

An inguinal hernia occurs when the abdominal cavity bulges through the opening in the muscle. A reducible hernia can be pushed back into the opening. When intestine or abdominal tissue fills the hernia sac and cannot be pushed back, it is called irreducible or incarcerated. A hernia is strangulated when the blood supply to the intestine or hernia sac is decreased.[3–4]

There are two types of groin hernias.

An inguinal hernia appears as a bulge in the groin or scrotum. Inguinal hernias account for 80% of all hernias and are more common in men.

A femoral hernia appears as a bulge in the groin, upper thigh, or labia (skin folds surrounding the vaginal opening). Femoral hernias are more common in women. They are always repaired because of a high risk of strangulation.[1–2,6]

Herniorrhaphy is a surgical term for repair of a hernia.

Symptoms

The most common symptoms are:

- bulge in the groin, scrotum, or abdominal area that often increases in size with coughing or straining;

- hernia pain or pressure.

Sharp abdominal pain and vomiting may mean that the intestine has slipped through the hernia sac and is strangulated. This is a medical emergency and immediate treatment is needed.

Common Diagnostic Tests

History and physical: The area is checked for a bulge.

Additional Tests

A physical exam is the best way to determine an inguinal hernia.[3] Other tests may include:

- digital exam;

- blood tests;

- urinalysis;

- electrocardiogram (EKG) only if a high risk for heart problems;

- ultrasound;

- computerized tomography (CT) scan.

Surgical and Nonsurgical Treatment

Surgical Treatment

The type of operation depends on the hernia size and location, your health, age, anesthesia risk, and the surgeon's expertise.

An operation is the only treatment for incarcerated/strangulated and femoral hernias.

Open Hernia Repair

The surgeon makes an incision near the hernia site. The weak muscle area is repaired. An open repair can be done with local anesthesia.

Mesh can be sutured (sewn) or stapled to strong tissues next to the hernia site. Mesh plugs can also be placed into the inguinal or femoral hernia space. The mesh plug fills the open site and sutures may not be needed.

In non-mesh hernia repair the hernia opening is sutured together and the tissue around the site is used to strengthen the weak area.

Open repair without mesh is used mainly to repair strangulated or infected hernias, for single small hernias (less than 3 cm), or for simple infant and pediatric hernias. If needed an orchidopexy (moving down the undescended testicle into the scrotum) may be done with infant hernia repair.[3-4]

Laparoscopic Hernia Repair

The surgeon will make several small punctures or incisions in the abdomen. Ports (hollow tubes) are inserted into the openings. The abdomen is inflated with carbon dioxide gas to make it easier for the surgeon to see the internal organs. Surgical tools and a laparoscopic light are placed into the ports. The hernia is repaired with mesh, sutured, or stapled in place. The repair is done as a TransAbdominal PrePeritoneal (TAPP) procedure, meaning the peritoneum (the sac that contains all of the abdominal organs) is entered, or as a Totally ExtraPeritoneal (TEP) procedure.[3-4]

Pediatric variations: Pediatric repair is usually done without mesh. For laparoscopic repair smaller ports are used, and it may be referred to as needlescopic repair.

Nonsurgical Treatment

Watchful waiting is an option if you have an inguinal hernia without symptoms. Hernia incarceration occurred in less than 2% of men who waited longer than two years to have a repair.[1-2] Femoral hernias should always be repaired because of the high risk (30–40%) of incarceration and bowel strangulation within two years of diagnosis.[1]

Trusses or belts made to apply pressure on a hernia require correct fitting. Complications include testicular nerve damage and incarceration.[4]

Keeping You Informed: Open Versus Laparoscopic Repair

Initially there is quicker return to usual activities and less pain and numbness with the laparoscopic procedure. There is no difference in long-term outcomes.

Risk of Complications

The risk of complications increases for both the open and the laparoscopic procedure if the hernia extends into the scrotum.[8] See Table 30.3.

Table 30.3. Risks of Hernia Repair (continued on next pages)

The Risk	What Happens	Keeping You Informed
Long-term pain	Pain lasting more than 3 months is reported in 74 of 1,000 patients who have laparoscopic repair and 127 of 1,000 for open mesh procedures. Severe pain occurs in 17 of 1,000 adults.[8]	Pain is usually less with laparoscopic procedures than open procedures. Pain continues to decrease over time. Pain can be treated with non-steroidal anti-inflammatory medications.
Recurrence	Recurrence is reported in 37 of 1000 adults and an average of 24 of 1,000 children. Mesh is not routinely used in infant hernia repair.[3-8] (Recurrence occurs half as often when mesh is used versus non-mesh repair.)	There is no difference between mesh plugs, flat mesh, and open mesh. Laparoscopic repair is often recommended for recurrent hernias because the surgeon avoids previous scar tissue.[3-4] There is a higher rate of recurrence in older men with laparoscopic repair.
Urinary retention	Having trouble urinating occurs in 22 of 1,000 patients receiving general or regional anesthesia and 4 of 1,000 patients for local anesthesia.[7-8]	General or regional anesthesia, older age, and enlarged prostate are associated with urinary retention. A temporary urinary catheter may be inserted.[3-4]
Seroma	A seroma (collection of clear/yellow fluid) can occur in 80 of 1,000 mesh repairs and 31 of 1,000 for non-mesh procedures.	Seromas can form around the former hernia site. Most disappear on their own. Removal of fluid with a needle may be required.[3-4] Seromas are rare for infants/children.[5,7]
Injury to internal organs—bowel, bladder, blood vessels	Injury can be caused by instruments inserted with laparoscopic repair. Bowel/bladder injury is reported as 1 in 1,000 and blood vessel injury is less than 1 in 1,000.[7-8]	For bladder injury, a Foley catheter remains in place to drain the urine until the bladder is healed, or surgical repair may be needed. For a bowel injury, the site is repaired and/or a nasogastric tube is placed to keep the stomach empty. Any injury to a blood vessel is repaired.[3-4]
Infection	Wound infection occurs an average of 5 of 1,000 laparoscopic patients; 25 of 1,000 in open mesh and open non-mesh procedures. Pediatric wound infection is reported as 12 of 1,000 patients.[7-8]	Antibiotics are typically not given for inguinal or femoral hernia repair. Smoking and having other diseases can increase the infection rate.[3]

Table 30.3. Risks of Hernia Repair (continued from previous page)

The Risk	What Happens	Keeping You Informed
Hematoma	Hematoma (collection of blood in the wound site or scrotum) is reported as 122 of 1,000 for mesh procedures and 70 of 1,000 when mesh is not used. There is no difference between open mesh and non-mesh procedures.[7–8]	Hematomas are treated with anti-inflammatory medications and rest. Rarely blood replacement or further testing for a blood vessel injury is needed.[4]
Testicular pain/ swelling	There is no difference in testicular problems for open vs. laparoscopic procedures. Testicular pain is reported in 8 of 1,000 patients for mesh repair. Less than 1 of 1,000 men reported decreased libido following repair.[7–8]	Postoperative testicular swelling (orchitis) may be due to manipulation of the veins near the testes. The swelling often appears 2–5 days after the operation and can last 6–12 weeks. Treatment includes anti-inflammatory medications.[3]
Hernia at port site	Hernia at the site where the laparoscopic trochar (tube) was inserted occurs in less than 4 of 1,000.[4]	This risk is reduced with the use of smaller trochars and instruments.[3–4]
Nerve pain (tingling or numbness)	Tingling and numbness in the groin or scrotum is reported less for laparoscopic procedures (74 of 1,000) than for open procedures (107 of 1,000). A trapped nerve is reported in 2 of 1,000 patients.[7–8]	Pressure, staples, stitches, or a trapped nerve in the surgical area can cause the nerve pain. Inform your doctor if you feel severe, sharp, or tingling pain in the groin and leg immediately after your procedure. An operation may be required if the nerve is trapped.[3]

Expectations: Preparation for Your Operation

Home Medication

Bring a list of all of the medications and vitamins that you are taking. Most often you will take your morning medication with a sip of water. If you are taking blood thinners (Plavix, Coumadin, aspirin, non-steroidal anti-inflammatory medication), your surgeon may ask you to stop taking these.

Home Preparation

You may go home the same day of your procedure. If you have nausea, vomiting, are unable to pass urine, or if the hernia was

Table 30.3. Risks of Hernia Repair (continued from previous pages)

The Risk	What Happens	Keeping You Informed
Pediatric risks	Reported risks include: Testicular atrophy (decreased size of the testes) 1.6 of 1,000 children; hydrocele (fluid around the testes) 12 of 1,000; wound infection 12 of 1,000; apnea (periods of not breathing) right after the operation 47 of 1,000 for premature infants.[5,10–12]	The open procedure is more common in pediatric hernia repair. Testicular atrophy is reported only in cases of strangulation. Apnea is associated with premature infants who had a history of apnea and other medical problems prior to hernia repair.[5,10–12]
Heart/breathing	There are no reports of heart or breathing complications related specifically to a hernia operation.	Other health problems increase the risk for heart and breathing anesthesia related complications. Your anesthesia provider will suggest the best anesthesia option for you.
Elderly risks	Elderly patients experience less chronic pain. Complications related to general anesthesia may be higher because of other diseases/health problems.	If general anesthesia is a concern, an open repair with local anesthesia may be recommended.
Death	No deaths are reported directly related to elective inguinal and femoral hernia repair. Death can occur after treatment of a strangulated hernia or in exceptionally high risk patients.	Stopping smoking and being at the ideal body weight before surgery reduces the risks of complications. Your surgical team is prepared for all emergency scenarios.

incarcerated, you may stay longer. Premature infants may stay overnight.

Anesthesia

Let your anesthesia provider know if you have allergies, neurologic disease (epilepsy, stroke), heart disease, stomach problems, lung disease (asthma, emphysema), endocrine disease (diabetes, thyroid conditions), loose teeth, or if you smoke, drink alcohol, use drugs, or take any herbs or vitamins.

If you have a history of nausea and vomiting with anesthesia, an antivomiting drug may be given.

About My Anesthesia

For laparoscopic hernia repair, the most frequent option is general anesthesia.

For open repair local or spinal anesthesia is an option. A mild sedation medication is often given (makes you sleepy).

The Day of Your Operation

Don't eat or drink: Not eating or drinking for at least six hours before the operation reduces your risk of complications from anesthesia.

What to Bring

- Insurance card and identification
- Advance directive
- List of medicines
- Loose-fitting comfortable clothes
- Slip-on shoes that don't require you to bend over
- Leave jewelry and valuables at home

What You Can Expect

An identification bracelet with your name and hospital/clinic number will be placed on your wrist. Your ID should be checked by health care team members before providing any procedures or giving you medication. If you have any allergies, you will also get an allergy alert bracelet.

An intravenous line (IV) will be started to give you fluids and medication.

For general anesthesia, a tube will be placed down your throat to help you breathe during the operation. For spinal anesthesia, a small needle with medication will be placed in your back alongside your spinal column.

After your operation, you will be moved to a recovery room where your heart rate, breathing rate, oxygen saturation, blood pressure, and urine output will be closely watched.

During Your Operation

Preventing pneumonia and blood clots: Movement and deep breathing after your operation can help prevent postoperative complications such as blood clots, fluid in your lungs, and pneumonia. A hernia procedure is very short and these complications are uncommon.

Preventing infection: The risk of infection is lowered if your hair is removed with clippers versus shaving around the surgical site. Be sure all visitors wash their hands.

Questions to Ask

About my home medications:

- What medications should I stop taking before my operation?
- Should I take any medicines on the day of my operation?

About my operation:

- What are the risks and side effects of anesthesia?
- What technique will be used to repair the hernia—laparoscopic or open; mesh or with sutures?
- What are the risks of this procedure?
- Will you be performing the entire procedure yourself?
- What level of pain should I expect and how will it be managed?
- How long will it be before I can return to my normal activities—work, driving, lifting?

Deep Breathing

Deep breathing can be done by taking 5–10 deep breaths and holding each breath for 3–5 seconds. Young children can do deep breathing by blowing bubbles.

Your Recovery and Discharge

High-Fiber Foods

Food high in fiber include beans, bran cereals and whole grain breads, peas, dried fruit (figs, apricots, and dates), raspberries, blackberries, strawberries, sweet corn, broccoli, baked potatoes with skin, plums, pears, apples, greens, and nuts.

Thinking Clearly

If general anesthesia is given, it may cause you to feel different for two to three days. Do not drive, drink alcohol, or make any big decisions for at least two days.

Nutrition

- When you wake up from the anesthesia, you will be able to drink small amounts of liquid. If you do not feel sick, you can begin eating regular foods.

- Continue to drink about 8 to 10 glasses of fluid per day.

- Eat a high-fiber diet.

Activity

- Slowly increase your activity. Full activity may usually be resumed in one to two weeks for laparoscopic and two to three weeks for open procedures.

- Persons sexually active before the operation reported being able to return to sexual activity in 14 days (average).

- Do not strain or lift objects over 10 pounds or participate in strenuous activity for at least 2 weeks.

Work and Return to School

You can go back to work when you feel well enough. There is a wide range of time needed for recovery. The average time to return to work is 14–21 days. Discuss the timing with your surgeon.

Wound Care

- Always wash your hands before and after touching near your incision site.

- Do not soak in a bathtub until your stitches, Steri-Strips, or staples are removed. You may take a shower after the second postoperative day unless you are told not to.

- Follow your surgeon's instructions on when to change your bandages.

- A small amount of drainage from the incision is normal. If the dressing is soaked with blood call your surgeon.

- If you have Steri-Strips in place, they will fall off in 7 to 10 days.

- If you have a glue-like covering over the incision, allow the glue to flake off on its own.

- Avoid wearing tight or rough clothing. It may rub your incisions and make it harder for them to heal.

- Protect the new skin, especially from the sun. The sun can burn and cause darker scarring.

- Your scar will heal in about four to six weeks and will become softer and continue to fade over the next year.

- For infants, the site will be covered with a waterproof dressing to protect it from urine or stool.

Bowel Movements

Avoid straining with bowel movements by increasing the fiber in your diet with high-fiber foods or over-the-counter fiber medications such as Metamucil and Fibercon.

Pain

The amount of pain is different for each person. For adults, the average time narcotics were used was three days with some patients needing no additional pain medication.[8] You can use throat lozenges if you have pain from the tube placed in your throat during your anesthesia.

Home medications—pain: The medicine you will need after your operation is for pain control.

When to Contact Your Surgeon

[Contact your surgeon] if you have:

- pain that gets worse;
- pain that will not go away;
- a fever of more than 101 degrees Fahrenheit;
- vomiting;
- swelling, redness, bleeding, or bad-smelling drainage from your wound site;
- strong or continuous abdominal pain or swelling of your abdomen;
- no bowel movements three to four days after the operation.

Pain Control

Everyone reacts to pain in a different way. A scale from 0 to 10 is used to measure pain. At a 0, you do not feel any pain. A 10 is the worst pain you have ever felt. Following a laparoscopic procedure, pain is sometimes felt in the shoulder. This is due to the gas inserted into your abdomen during the procedure. Moving and walking helps to decrease the gas and the right shoulder pain.

Extreme pain puts extra stress on your body at a time when your body needs to focus on healing. Do not wait until your pain has reached a level 10 or is unbearable before telling your doctor or nurse. It is much easier to control pain before it becomes severe.

Common Medicines to Control Pain

Hernia pain is often controlled with narcotics and often combined with acetaminophen.

Narcotics or opioids are used for severe pain. Possible side effects of narcotics are sleepiness; lowered blood pressure, heart rate, and breathing rate; skin rash and itching; constipation; nausea; and difficulty urinating. Some examples of narcotics include morphine and codeine.

Non-narcotic pain medication: Most nonopioid analgesics are classified as non-steroidal antiinflammatory drugs (NSAIDs). They are used to treat mild pain and inflammation or combined with narcotics to treat severe pain. Possible side effects of NSAIDs are stomach upset, bleeding in the digestive tract, and fluid retention. These side effects usually are not seen with short-term use. Examples of NSAIDs include ibuprofen and Aleve.

Pain Control without Medicine

Distraction helps you focus on other activities instead of your pain. Music, games, or other engaging activities are especially helpful with children.

Splinting your stomach by placing a pillow over your abdomen with firm pressure before coughing or movement can help reduce the pain.

Guided imagery helps you direct and control your emotions. Close your eyes and gently inhale and exhale. Picture yourself in the center of somewhere beautiful. Feel the beauty surrounding you and your emotions coming back to your control. You should feel calmer.

Keeping You Informed: Pain after Inguinal Hernia Repair

Pain that continued one year after inguinal hernia repair is reported as 110 of 1,000 patients, with moderate/severe pain reported in 17 of 1,000. Eighty percent of patients with severe groin pain had severe pain before the operation. The pain decreased by 50% in one year. Pain was higher when heavy versus light-weight mesh was used.[8] Most studies don't report a difference in chronic pain between open versus laparoscopic repair.

Pain in Children

Groin pain is reported occasionally in 28 of 1,000 adults who had hernia repair during infancy or childhood.[9]

For children with a simple hernia repair, 63% reported being pain free the next day. For hernia plus orchidopexy nearly 75% reported pain the next day. More pain medication was needed.

More Information

For more information on tests and procedures, please go to the American College of Surgeons Patient Education Website at www.facs.org/patienteducation.

Glossary of Terms

Advance directives: Documents signed by a competent person giving direction to health care providers about treatment choices.

Computerized tomography (CT) scan: A diagnostic test using X-ray and a computer to create a detailed, three-dimensional picture of your abdomen. A CT scan is commonly used to detect abnormalities or disease inside the abdomen. It is sometimes used to find a hernia not obvious during physical exam.

Digital exam: The examiner will place a gloved index finger gently into the scrotal sac and feel up to the inguinal ring in the groin. Then the patient is asked to strain.

Electrocardiogram (ECG): Measures the rate and regularity of heartbeats and damage to the heart.

Hematoma: A collection of blood that has leaked into the tissues under the skin or into an organ, resulting from cutting in surgery or the blood's inability to clot.

Nasogastric tube: A soft plastic tube inserted in the nose and down to the stomach used to empty the stomach of contents and gases to rest the bowel.

Seroma: A collection of serous (clear/yellow) fluid.

Ultrasound: Sound waves are used to determine the location of deep structures in the body. A hand roller is placed on top of clear gel and rolled across the abdomen. An ultrasound may be used to find a hernia that is not obvious during the physical exam.

Urinalysis: A visual and chemical examination of the urine most often used to screen for urinary tract infections and kidney disease.

References

The information provided in this report is chosen from recent articles based on relevant clinical research or trends. The following research articles do not represent all of the information available about your operation. Ask your doctor if he or she recommends that you read any additional research.

1. Fitzgibbons RJ, Jr., Giobbie-Hurder A, Gibbs JO, et al. Watchful waiting vs. repair of inguinal hernia in minimally symptomatic men: A randomized clinical trial. *JAMA.* 2006; 295:285–292.

2. Gallegos NC, Dawson J, Jarvis M, et al. Risk of strangulation in groin hernias. *British Journal of Surgery.* 1991;78:1611–1673.

3. Malangoni MA, Rosen MJ. Hernias. In: CM Townsend, RD Beauchamp, et al. *Textbook of Surgery.* Philadelphia, PA: Saunders, 2008.

4. Fitzgibbons RJ, Jr., Filipi CJ, Quinn TH. Inguinal hernias. In: FC Brunicardi, DK Anderson, et al. *Principles of Surgery (8th Edition).* New York, NY: McGraw Hill, 2005.

5. Ein SH, Njere I, Ein A. Six thousand three hundred sixty-one pediatric inguinal hernias: A 35-year review. *Journal of Pediatric Surgery.* 2006;41:980–986.

6. Zamakshary M, To T, Guan J, et al. Risk of incarceration of inguinal hernia among infants and young children awaiting elective surgery. *Canadian Medical Association Journal.* 2008;179:1001–1005.

7. Schmedt CG, Sauerland S, Bittner R. Comparison of endoscopic procedures vs. Lichtenstein and other open mesh techniques for inguinal hernia repair. A meta-analysis of randomized controlled trials. *Surgical Endoscopy.* 2005;19:188–199.

8. Schwab JR, et al. After 10 years and 1,903 inguinal hernias, what is the outcome for the laparoscopic repair? *Surgical Endoscopy.* 2002;16:1201–1206.

9. Aasvang EK, Kehleet H. Chronic pain after childhood groin hernia repair. *J Pediatr Surg.* 2007;42:1403–1408.

10. Schier F. Laparoscopic inguinal hernia repair: A prospective series of 542 children. *J Pediatric Surg.* 2006;41:1081–1084.

11. Takehara H, Yakabe S, Kameoka K. Laparoscopic percutaneous extraperitoneal closure for inguinal hernia in children: clinical outcomes of 972 repairs done in 3 pediatric surgical institutions. *J Pediatr Surg.* 2006;41:1999–2003.

12. Murphy JJ, Swanson T, Ansermino M, et al. The frequency of apnea in premature infants after inguinal hernia repair: do they need overnight monitoring in the intensive care unit? *J Pediatr Surg.* 2008;43:865–868.

Chapter 31

Weight-Loss (Bariatric) Surgery

Chapter Contents

Section 31.1

Overview of Bariatric Surgery for Severe Obesity

"Bariatric Surgery for Severe Obesity," by the National Institute of Diabetes and Digestive and Kidney Diseases (NIDDK, www.niddk.nih.gov), part of the National Institutes of Health, June 2011.

Severe obesity is a chronic condition that is hard to treat with diet and exercise alone. Bariatric surgery is an operation on the stomach and/or intestines that helps patients with extreme obesity to lose weight. This surgery is an option for people who cannot lose weight by other means or who suffer from serious health problems related to obesity. The surgery restricts food intake, which promotes weight loss and reduces the risk of type 2 diabetes. Some surgeries also interrupt how food is digested, preventing some calories and nutrients, such as vitamins, from being absorbed. Recent studies suggest that bariatric surgery may even lower death rates for patients with severe obesity. The best results occur when patients follow surgery with healthy eating patterns and regular exercise.

Bariatric Surgery for Adults

Currently, bariatric surgery may be an option for adults with severe obesity. Body mass index (BMI), a measure of height in relation to weight, is used to define levels of obesity. Clinically severe obesity is a BMI ≥ 40 or a BMI ≥ 35 with a serious health problem linked to obesity. Such health problems could be type 2 diabetes, heart disease, or severe sleep apnea (when breathing stops for short periods during sleep).

The Food and Drug Administration (FDA) has approved use of an adjustable gastric band (or AGB) for patients with BMI ≥ 30 who also have at least one condition linked to obesity, such as heart disease or diabetes.

Who is a good adult candidate for surgery?

Having surgery to produce weight loss is a serious decision. Anyone thinking about having this surgery should know what it involves.

Answers to the following questions may help patients decide whether weight-loss surgery is right for them.

Bariatric surgery may be the next step for people who remain severely obese after trying approaches other than surgery, especially if they have a disease linked to obesity.

- Is the patient unlikely to lose weight or keep it off over the long term using other methods?

- Is the patient well informed about the surgery and treatment effects?

- Is the patient aware of the risks and benefits of surgery?

- Is the patient ready to lose weight and improve his or her health?

- Is the patient aware of how life may change after the surgery? (For example, patients need to adjust to side effects, such as the need to chew food well and the loss of ability to eat large meals.)

- Is the patient aware of the limits on food choices and occasional failures?

- Is the patient committed to lifelong healthy eating and physical activity, medical follow-up, and the need to take extra vitamins and minerals?

There is no sure method, including surgery, to produce and maintain weight loss. Some patients who have bariatric surgery may have weight loss that does not meet their goals. Research also suggests that many patients regain some of the lost weight over time. The amount of weight regain may vary by extent of obesity and type of surgery.

Habits such as snacking often on foods high in calories or not exercising can affect the amount of weight loss and weight regain. Problems that may occur with the surgery, like a stretched pouch or separated stitches, may also affect the amount of weight loss.

Success is possible. Patients must commit to changing habits and having medical follow-up for the rest of their lives.

Bariatric Surgery for Youth

Rates of obesity among youth are high. Bariatric surgery is sometimes used to treat youth with extreme obesity. Although it is becoming clear that teens can lose weight after bariatric surgery, many questions still exist about the long-term effects on teens' developing bodies and minds.

Who is a good youth candidate for surgery?

Experts in childhood obesity and bariatric surgery suggest that families consider surgery only after youth have tried for at least six months to lose weight and have not had success. Candidates should meet the following criteria:

- Have extreme obesity (BMI ≥ 40)

- Be their adult height (usually at age 13 or older for girls and 15 or older for boys)

- Have serious health problems linked to weight, such as type 2 diabetes or sleep apnea, which may improve with bariatric surgery

In addition, health care providers should assess potential patients and their parents to see how emotionally prepared they are for the surgery and the lifestyle changes they will need to make. Health care providers should also refer young patients to special youth bariatric surgery centers that focus on meeting the unique needs of youth.

Mounting evidence suggests that bariatric surgery can favorably change both the weight and health of youth with extreme obesity. Over the years, gastric bypass surgery has been the main operation used to treat extreme obesity in youth. An estimated 2,700 youth bariatric surgeries were performed between 1996 and 2003. A review of short-term data from the largest inpatient database in the United States suggests that these surgeries are at least as safe for youth as adults. As yet, AGB has not been approved for use in the United States for people younger than age 18. However, favorable weight-loss outcomes after AGB for youth have been reported abroad.

The Normal Digestive Process

Normally, as food moves along the digestive tract, digestive juices and enzymes digest and absorb calories and nutrients. After we chew and swallow our food, it moves down the esophagus to the stomach, where a strong acid continues the digestive process. The stomach can hold about three pints of food at one time. When the stomach contents move to the duodenum (the first part of the small intestine), bile and pancreatic juice speed up digestion. Most of the iron and calcium in the food we eat is absorbed there. The other two parts of the nearly 20 feet of small intestine absorb nearly all of the remaining calories and nutrients. The food particles that cannot be digested in the small intestine reside in the large intestine until eliminated.

Bariatric surgery restricts food intake, which leads to weight loss. Patients who have bariatric surgery must commit to a lifetime of healthy eating and regular exercise. These healthy habits may help patients maintain weight loss after surgery.

Types of Bariatric Surgery

The type of surgery that may help an adult or youth depends on a number of factors. Patients should discuss with their health care providers what kind of surgery is suitable for them.

What is the difference between open and laparoscopic surgery?

Bariatric surgery may be performed through open approaches, which involve cutting the stomach in the standard manner, or by laparoscopy. With the latter approach, surgeons insert complex instruments through half-inch cuts and guide a small camera that sends images to a monitor. Most bariatric surgery today is laparoscopic because it requires a smaller cut, creates less tissue damage, leads to earlier hospital discharges, and has fewer problems, especially hernias occurring after surgery.

However, not all patients are suitable for laparoscopy. Patients who are considered extremely obese, who have had previous stomach surgery, or who have complex medical problems may require the open approach. Complex medical problems may include having severe heart and lung disease or weighing more than 350 pounds.

What are the surgical options?

There are four types of operations that are commonly offered in the United States: AGB, Roux-en-Y gastric bypass (RYGB), biliopancreatic diversion with a duodenal switch (BPD-DS), and vertical sleeve gastrectomy (VSG). (See Figure 31.1.) Each surgery has its own benefits and risks. The patient and provider should work together to select the best option by considering the benefits and risks of each type of surgery. Other factors to consider include the patient's BMI, eating habits, health conditions related to obesity, and previous stomach surgeries.

Adjustable gastric band: AGB works mainly by decreasing food intake. Food intake is reduced by placing a small bracelet-like band around the top of the stomach to restrict the size of the opening from the throat to the stomach. The surgeon can then control the size of the opening with a circular balloon inside the band. This balloon can be inflated or deflated with saline solution to meet the needs of the patient.

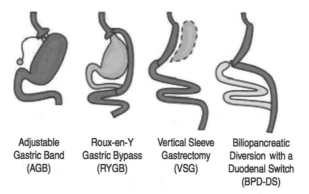

| Adjustable Gastric Band (AGB) | Roux-en-Y Gastric Bypass (RYGB) | Vertical Sleeve Gastrectomy (VSG) | Biliopancreatic Diversion with a Duodenal Switch (BPD-DS) |

Figure 31.1. Diagram of bariatric surgical options (Image credit: Walter Pories, M.D. FACS).

Roux-en-Y gastric bypass: RYGB restricts food intake. RYGB also decreases how food is absorbed. Food intake is limited by a small pouch that is similar in size to the pouch created with AGB. Also, sending food directly from the pouch into the small intestine affects how the digestive tract absorbs food. The food is absorbed differently because the stomach, duodenum, and upper intestine no longer have contact with food.

Biliopancreatic diversion with a duodenal switch: BPD-DS, usually referred to as a duodenal switch, is a complex bariatric surgery that includes three features. One feature is to remove a large part of the stomach. This step makes patients feel full sooner when eating than they did before surgery. Feeling full sooner encourages patients to eat less. Another feature is rerouting food away from much of the small intestine to limit how the body absorbs food. The third feature changes how bile and other digestive juices affect the body's ability to digest food and absorb calories. This step also helps lead to weight loss.

In removing a large part of the stomach, the surgeon creates a more tubular gastric sleeve (also known as a VSG). The smaller stomach sleeve remains linked to a very short part of the duodenum, which is then directly linked to a lower part of the small intestine. This surgery leaves a small part of the duodenum available to absorb food and some vitamins and minerals.

However, when the patient eats food, it bypasses most of the duodenum. The distance between the stomach and colon becomes much shorter after this operation, thus limiting how food is absorbed. BPD-DS produces significant weight loss. However, a decrease in the amount of food, vitamins, and minerals absorbed creates chances for long-term problems.

Some of these problems are anemia (lower than normal count for red blood cells) or osteoporosis (loss of bone mass that can make bones brittle).

Vertical sleeve gastrectomy: VSG surgery restricts food intake and decreases the amount of food used. Most of the stomach is removed during this surgery, which may decrease ghrelin, a hormone that prompts appetite. Lower amounts of ghrelin may reduce hunger more than other purely restrictive surgeries, such as AGB.

VSG has been performed in the past mainly as the first stage of BPD-DS in patients who may be at high risk for problems from more extensive types of surgery. These patients' high risk levels are due to body weight or medical issues. However, more recent research indicates that some patients who have VSG can lose a lot of weight with VSG alone and avoid a second procedure. Researchers do not yet know how many patients who have VSG alone will need a second stage procedure.

What are the side effects of these surgeries?

Some side effects may include bleeding, infection, leaks from the site where the intestines are sewn together, diarrhea, and blood clots in the legs that can move to the lungs and heart.

Examples of side effects that may occur later include nutrients being poorly absorbed, especially in patients who do not take their prescribed vitamins and minerals. In some cases, if patients do not address this problem promptly, diseases may occur along with permanent damage to the nervous system. These diseases include pellagra (caused by lack of vitamin B3—niacin), beriberi (caused by lack of vitamin B1—thiamine) and kwashiorkor (caused by lack of protein).

Other late problems include strictures (narrowing of the sites where the intestine is joined) and hernias (part of an organ bulging through a weak area of muscle).

Two kinds of hernias may occur after a patient has bariatric surgery. An incisional hernia is a weakness that sticks out from the abdominal wall's connective tissue and may cause a blockage in the bowel. An internal hernia occurs when the small bowel is displaced into pockets in the lining of the abdomen. These pockets occur when the intestines are sewn together. Internal hernias are thought to be more dangerous than incisional ones and need prompt attention to avoid serious problems.

Some patients may also require emotional support to help them through the changes in body image and personal relationships that occur after the surgery.

Medical Costs

Bariatric procedures, on average, cost from $20,000 to $25,000. Medical insurance coverage varies by state and insurance provider. In 2004, the U.S. Department of Health and Human Services reduced barriers to obtaining Medicare coverage for obesity treatments. Bariatric surgery may be covered under these conditions:

- if the patient has at least one health problem linked to obesity;

- if the procedure is suitable for the patient's medical condition;

- if approved surgeons and facilities are involved.

Patients can contact staff at their regional Medicare, Medicaid, or health insurance office to find out if the procedure is covered and to obtain facts about options.

Section 31.2

Complications and Costs for Obesity Surgery Declining

By the Agency for Healthcare Research and Quality
(AHRQ, www.ahrq.gov), April 29, 2009.

A May 2009 study by the Department of Health & Human Services' (HHS) Agency for Healthcare Research and Quality (AHRQ) found that the average rate of postsurgical and other complications in patients who have obesity surgery, also known as bariatric surgery, declined 21 percent between 2002 and 2006. They also found that payments to hospitals dropped by as much as 13 percent for bariatric surgery patients during that time period, in part because fewer complications meant fewer readmissions.

The study, "Recent Improvements in Bariatric Surgery Outcomes," published in the May 2009 *Medical Care*, found that the complication rate among patients initially hospitalized for bariatric surgery dropped from approximately 24 percent to roughly 15 percent. Much of this was driven by a reduction in the postsurgical infection rate, which plummeted 58 percent. Abdominal hernias, staple leakage, respiratory failure, and pneumonia fell by between 50 percent and 29 percent.

Rates for other complications, such as ulcers, dumping (involuntary vomiting or defecation), hemorrhage, wound reopening, deep-vein thrombosis and pulmonary embolism, heart attacks, and strokes remained relatively unchanged. With the exception of the 19 percent rate for dumping, which is especially a risk in gastric bypass surgery, rates ranged from 2.4 percent to 0.1 percent.

In addition, hospital payments for bariatric surgery patients, as a whole, fell from $29,563 to $27,905 and dropped from $41,807 to $38,175 for patients who experienced complications. Hospital payments for the most expensive patients—those who had to be readmitted because of complications—fell from $80,001 to $69,960.

"People considering an elective procedure need unbiased, science-based evidence of its benefits and risks," said AHRQ Director Carolyn M. Clancy, MD. "All surgeries involve risks, but as newer technologies emerge and surgeons and hospitals gain experience, as this study shows, risks can decrease."

Researchers led by senior economist William E. Encinosa, PhD, compared complication rates among more than 9,500 patients under age 65 who underwent obesity surgery at 652 hospitals between 2001 and 2002 and between 2005 and 2006. They found that the complication rate fell in spite of an increase in the percentage of older and sicker patients having the operations. The proportion of patients over age 50 operated on by bariatric surgeons increased from 28 percent to 44 percent during the period, and the average number of underlying illnesses in patients operated on by bariatric surgeons, such as diabetes, high blood pressure, or sleep apnea, more than doubled.

The 6-month postsurgical death rate for patients operated on between 2005 and 2006 was 0.5 percent, statistically about the same as that of patients who had bariatric surgery between 2001 and 2002. Hospital readmissions because of complications fell 31 percent, from roughly 10 percent to 7 percent, whereas complication-caused same-day hospital outpatient clinic visits declined from approximately 15 percent to 13 percent.

According to Dr. Encinosa, the improvements are largely due to a combination of three factors—increased use of laparoscopy, a technology that allows physicians to operate through small incisions; increased use of banding procedures without gastric bypass, such as vertical-banded gastroplasty and lap band; and increased surgeon experience arising from the growth in the number of bariatric surgeries performed by hospitals. For example, laparoscopy reduced the odds of having a complication by 30 percent and drove down hospital payments by 12 percent, whereas banding reduced hospital payments by 20 percent.

Section 31.3

Outpatient Bariatric Surgery May Lead to Higher Mortality and Complications

A new study of nearly 52,000 patients found that people who had gastric bypass surgery and were discharged from the hospital sooner than the national average of a two-day length of stay experienced significantly higher rates of 30-day mortality and complications. The findings were presented at the 2011 28th Annual Meeting of the American Society for Metabolic & Bariatric Surgery (ASMBS).

Stanford University researchers found patients discharged on the same day of surgery were 13 times more likely to die than patients who left after two days (risk adjusted), and were 12 times more likely to have serious complications (1.9% vs. 0.16%). Patients who spent more time in the hospital but were discharged in less than 24 hours after an overnight stay were two times more likely to die than patients who left after two days of recovery. The overall 30-day mortality rate was 0.1 percent for patients who stayed in the hospital for two or more days, and about 0.8 percent for those who were discharged on the same day of surgery.

"This study shows what a difference a day makes," said John Morton, MD, Associate Professor of Surgery and Director of Bariatric Surgery at Stanford Hospital & Clinics at Stanford University, one of the co-authors of the study. "Bariatric surgery is safer than ever, but discharging patients too soon after surgery may be pushing the envelope too far and may have serious consequences."

The data was obtained from the Bariatric Outcomes Longitudinal Database (BOLD), the world's largest and most comprehensive repository of clinical bariatric surgery patient information. Participants in the ASMBS Bariatric Surgery Center of Excellence (BSCOE) program

375

are required to enter prospective data into BOLD on all bariatric surgery patients.

"Length of stay appeared to be the leading risk factor ahead of age, gender, race, body mass index (BMI), and obesity-related conditions," added Dr. Morton.

There is an increasing focus on length of stay in bariatric surgery following an update to the Milliman Care Guidelines, which recommended shortening the length of stay for gastric bypass to cut costs and improve resource utilization. These guidelines are used by many hospitals and health plans to determine care and length of stay.

The ASMBS responded to those guidelines in October 2010 expressing concern for the shortened length of stay citing a lack of evidence demonstrating patient benefit and safety.

"A two-day length of stay appears reasonable for most people and results in a safety profile that rivals gallbladder or hip replacement surgery. To reduce it further may put patients at an increased chance of unnecessary risk," added Dr. Morton, who chairs the ASMBS Access to Care Committee. "A patient should be discharged based on his or her individual risk profile. We counsel our patients to avoid drive-thru fast food, and also advise against drive-thru gastric bypass."

Bariatric surgery has been shown to be the most effective and long lasting treatment for morbid obesity and many related conditions.[1] People with morbid obesity have BMI of 40 or more, or BMI of 35 or more with an obesity-related disease such as Type 2 diabetes, heart disease, or sleep apnea. Recently the FDA [U.S. Food and Drug Administration] approved the use of an adjustable gastric band for BMI 30 and above, recognizing that there is an increase in mortality and medical complications of obesity at even this level of obesity.

According to the ASMBS, more than 15 million Americans have morbid obesity. Studies have shown patients may lose 30 to 50 percent of their excess weight 6 months after surgery and 77 percent of their excess weight as early as one year after surgery.[2]

The federal government estimated that in 2008, annual obesity-related health spending reached $147 billion,[3] double what it was a decade ago, and projects spending to rise to $344 billion each year by 2018.[4] The Agency for Healthcare Research and Quality (AHRQ) reported significant improvements in the safety of bariatric surgery due in large part to improved laparoscopic techniques and the advent of bariatric surgical centers of excellence. The overall risk of death from bariatric surgery is about 0.1 percent[5] and the risk of major complications is about 4 percent.[6]

In addition to Dr. Morton, study co-authors include Eric DeMaria, MD, Deborah Winegar, PhD, Bintu Sherif, MS, Neil Hutcher, MD, all from Surgical Review Corporation; Robin Blackstone, MD, FACS, FASMBS, from Scottsdale Bariatric Center; and Bruce M. Wolfe, MD, FASMBS, from Oregon Health Sciences.

References

1. RA Weiner. "Indications and Principles of Metabolic Surgery." U.S. National Library of Medicine. 2010; 81(4):379–94.

2. AC Wittgrove et al. "Laparoscopic Gastric Bypass, Roux-en-Y: Technique and Results in 75 Patients With 3–30 Months Follow-up." *Obesity Surgery*. 1996. 6:500–504.

3. EA Finkelstein. "Annual Medical Spending Attributable To Obesity: Payer-And Service-Specific Estimates." *Health Affairs*. 2009. 28(5):822–831.

4. K Thorpe. America's Health Rankings. "The Future Costs of Obesity." 2009.

5. Agency for Healthcare Research and Quality (AHRQ). Statistical Brief #23. Bariatric Surgery Utilization and Outcomes in 1998 and 2004. Jan. 2007.

6. Flum et al. "Perioperative Safety in the Longitudinal Assessment of Bariatric Surgery." *New England Journal of Medicine*. 2009. 361:445–454. http://content.nejm.org/cgi/content/full/361/5/445

Chapter 32

Gynecologic and Obstetric Surgery

Chapter Contents

Section 32.1

Hysterectomy

"Hysterectomy," by the Office on Women's Health
(www.womenshealth.gov), part of the U.S. Department of
Health and Human Services, December 15, 2009.

What is a hysterectomy?

A hysterectomy is a surgery to remove a woman's uterus or womb. The uterus is where a baby grows when a woman is pregnant. The whole uterus or just part of it may be removed. After a hysterectomy, you no longer have menstrual periods and cannot become pregnant.

During the hysterectomy, your doctor also may remove your fallopian tubes and ovaries. The ovaries produce eggs and hormones. The fallopian tubes carry eggs from the ovaries to the uterus. The cervix is the lower end of the uterus that joins the vagina. These organs are located in a woman's lower abdomen.

If you have not yet reached menopause and:

- you keep your ovaries during the hysterectomy, you may enter menopause at an earlier age than most women; or

- your ovaries are removed during the hysterectomy, you will enter menopause. You can talk with your doctor about ways to manage menopausal symptoms, such as hot flashes and vaginal dryness.

The types of hysterectomy include the following:

- Partial, subtotal, or supracervical removes just the upper part of the uterus and the cervix is left in place

- Total removes the whole uterus and the cervix

- Radical removes the whole uterus, the tissue on both sides of the cervix, and the upper part of the vagina (This is done mostly when there is cancer present.)

How is a hysterectomy performed?

There are different ways that your doctor can perform a hysterectomy. It will depend on your health history and the reason for your surgery.

- Abdominal hysterectomy: This is done through a five- to seven-inch incision, or cut, in the lower part of your belly. The cut may go either up and down, or across your belly, just above your pubic hair.

- Vaginal hysterectomy: This is done through a cut in the vagina. The doctor will take your uterus out through this incision and close it with stitches.

- Laparoscopic hysterectomy: A laparoscope is an instrument with a thin, lighted tube and small camera that allows your doctor to see your pelvic organs. Your doctor will make three to four small cuts in your belly and insert the laparoscope and other instruments. He or she will cut your uterus into smaller pieces and remove them through the incisions.

- Laparoscopically assisted vaginal hysterectomy (LAVH): Your doctor will remove your uterus through the vagina. The laparoscope is used to guide the procedure.

- Robotic-assisted surgery: Your doctor uses a special machine (robot) to do the surgery through small cuts in your belly, much like a laparoscopic hysterectomy. It is most often done when a patient has cancer or is very overweight and vaginal surgery is not safe.

Why do women have hysterectomies?

Hysterectomy may be needed if you have the following:

- Cancer of the uterus, ovary, cervix, or endometrium: Hysterectomy may be the best option if you have cancer in these organs. The endometrium is the tissue that lines the uterus. If you have precancerous changes of the cervix, you might be able to have a loop electrosurgical excision procedure (LEEP) to remove the cancerous cells. Other treatment options can include chemotherapy and radiation. Your doctor will talk with you about the type of cancer you have and how advanced it is.

- Fibroids: Fibroids are non-cancerous, muscular tumors that grow in the wall of the uterus. Many women with fibroids have

381

only minor symptoms and do not need treatment. Fibroids also often shrink after menopause. In some women, fibroids can cause prolonged heavy bleeding or pain. Fibroids can be treated with medications. There are also procedures to remove the fibroids, such as uterine artery embolization, which blocks the blood supply to the tumors. Without blood, the fibroids shrink over time, which can reduce pain and heavy bleeding. Another procedure called myomectomy removes the tumors while leaving your uterus intact, but there is a risk that the tumors could come back. If medications or procedures to remove the fibroids have not helped, and a woman is either near or past menopause and does not want children, hysterectomy can cure problems from fibroids.

- Endometriosis: This health problem occurs when the tissue that lines the uterus grows outside the uterus on your ovaries, fallopian tubes, or other pelvic or abdominal organs. This can cause severe pain during menstrual periods, chronic pain in the lower back and pelvis, pain during or after sex, bleeding between periods, and other symptoms. You might need a hysterectomy when medications or less invasive surgery to remove the spots of endometriosis have not helped.

- Prolapse of the uterus: This is when the uterus slips from its usual place down into the vagina. This can lead to urinary and bowel problems and pelvic pressure. These problems might be helped for a time with an object called a vaginal pessary, which is inserted into the vagina to hold the womb in place.

- Adenomyosis: In this condition, the tissue that lines the uterus grows inside the walls of the uterus, which can cause severe pain. If other treatments have not helped, a hysterectomy is the only certain cure.

- Chronic pelvic pain: Surgery is a last resort for women who have chronic pelvic pain that clearly comes from the uterus. Many forms of pelvic pain are not cured by a hysterectomy, so it could be unnecessary and create new problems.

- Abnormal vaginal bleeding: Treatment depends on the cause. Changes in hormone levels, infection, cancer, or fibroids are some things that can cause abnormal bleeding. There are medications that can lighten heavy bleeding, correct irregular bleeding, and relieve pain. These include hormone medications, birth control pills, and nonsteroidal anti-inflammatory medications (NSAIDs).

One procedure for abnormal bleeding is dilatation and curettage (D&C), in which the lining and contents of the uterus are removed. Another procedure, endometrial ablation, also removes the lining of your uterus and can help stop heavy, prolonged bleeding. But, it should not be used if you want to become pregnant or if you have gone through menopause.

Very rarely, hysterectomy is needed to control bleeding during a cesarean delivery following rare pregnancy complications. There are other methods doctors use to control bleeding in most of these cases, but hysterectomy is still needed for some women.

Keep in mind that there may be ways to treat your health problem without having this major surgery. Talk with your doctor about all of your treatment options.

How common are hysterectomies?

A hysterectomy is the second most common surgery among women in the United States. The most common surgery in women is childbirth by cesarean section delivery.

What should I do if I am told that I need a hysterectomy?

- Ask about the possible risks of the surgery.

- Talk to your doctor about other treatment options. Ask about the risks of those treatments.

- Consider getting a second opinion from another doctor.

Keep in mind that every woman is different and every situation is different. A good treatment choice for one woman may not be good for another.

How long does it take to recover from a hysterectomy?

Recovering from a hysterectomy takes time. Most women stay in the hospital from one to two days for post-surgery care. Some women may stay longer, often when the hysterectomy is done because of cancer.

The time it takes for you to resume normal activities depends on the type of surgery.

- If you had abdominal surgery, recovery takes from four to six weeks. You will gradually be able to increase your activities.

- If you had vaginal or laparoscopic surgery, recovery takes three to four weeks.

You should get plenty of rest and not lift heavy objects for a full six weeks after surgery. About six weeks after either surgery, you should be able to take tub baths and resume sexual intercourse. Research has found that women with a good sex life before hysterectomy can maintain it after the surgery.

What are the risks of having a hysterectomy?

Most women do not have health problems during or after the surgery, but some of the risks of a hysterectomy include the following:

- Injury to nearby organs, such as the bowel, urinary tract, bladder, rectum, or blood vessels
- Pain during sexual intercourse
- Early menopause, if the ovaries are removed
- Anesthesia problems, such as breathing or heart problems
- Allergic reactions to medicines
- Blood clots in the legs or lungs. These can be fatal.
- Infection
- Heavy bleeding

Do I still need to have Pap tests after a hysterectomy?

You will still need regular Pap tests to screen for cervical cancer if you had a partial hysterectomy and did not have your cervix removed, or if your hysterectomy was for cancer. Ask your doctor what is best for you and how often you should have Pap tests.

Even if you do not need Pap tests, all women who have had a hysterectomy should have regular pelvic exams and mammograms.

Section 32.2

Dilation and Curettage

Dilation and curettage (D&C) is a minor (short) surgical procedure that removes tissue from your uterus (womb).

You may need this procedure if you have unexplained bleeding between periods or if you have delivered a baby and placental tissue remains in your womb. D&C also is performed to remove pregnancy tissue remaining from a miscarriage or an abortion.

How is the procedure done?

D&C can be done in a doctor's office or in the hospital. You may be given medications to relax you or to make you unconscious. Using special instruments, the doctor will slowly widen the opening to your uterus (cervix). Opening your cervix can cause cramping. If this procedure is performed in the doctor's office, you will receive medications that numb your cervix and make it easier to open.

After dilating (opening) the cervix (mouth of the womb), tissue from inside the uterus is removed with a scraping instrument (curette), a suction tube, or other specialized instruments. Your doctor may want to look inside your uterus by inserting a special device called a hysteroscope, which is attached to a camera. A hysteroscope will allow your doctor to see the inside of the uterus magnified on a television screen.

Is D&C safe?

Most of the time, D&C is safe. Occasionally, complications do occur during or right after surgery. Sometimes, complications will not be discovered until long after the procedure.

The possible complications include:

Uterine perforation is when a hole is accidentally made in the uterus by a surgical instrument. Though rare, this is most likely to happen if you have a D&C to control bleeding after you've delivered a baby. The doctor usually will know right away if the uterus has been perforated. Occasionally, the uterine perforation is not always obvious at the time of the D&C, and then you may need additional surgery to look inside the lower belly. The laparoscope is a small instrument attached to a camera that is placed through small incisions in your abdomen or belly to see if the organs around your uterus, such as intestines, bladder, or blood vessels, are injured. If any of these organs are injured, they must be repaired with surgery. However, if no other organs have been injured, long-term complications from a perforation are extremely rare.

Infections can occur after a D&C. If you are not pregnant at the time of your D&C, this complication is extremely rare. However, 10% of women who were pregnant before their D&C can get an infection, usually within one week of the procedure. It may be related to a sexually transmitted infection, such as chlamydia or gonorrhea, or due to normal bacteria that pass from the vagina into the uterus during or after the procedure. The symptoms can consist of vaginal discharge, uterine cramping and pain, and fever.

You must see a doctor immediately if you experience these symptoms. These infections usually do not result in long-term complications.

However, in some cases, the infection may scar the uterus, fallopian tubes, or ovaries, which may make it difficult for you to become pregnant in the future.

Scar tissue formation in the uterus is an uncommon complication in women who have had a D&C. This is referred to as Asherman's syndrome. You are at greater risk of scar tissue formation when a D&C is performed after a miscarriage, during pregnancy, or shortly after delivery of a baby. The most common symptom is very light or missed periods. If you have scar tissue in your uterus, you may have difficulty becoming pregnant or may have repeated miscarriages. To treat this condition, scar tissue is surgically removed. This type of surgery is performed with a hysteroscope, or a thin telescope attached to a small camera that is inserted through your vagina and cervix in order to view the inside of your uterus.

Other rare complications of a D&C include tears in the cervix, uterine bleeding, and reactions to anesthesia. These complications usually occur at the time of surgery.

Section 32.3

Cesarean Section

Excerpted from "Labor and Birth," by the Office on Women's Health (www.womenshealth.gov), part of the U.S. Department of Health and Human Services, September 27, 2010.

Cesarean delivery, also called C-section, is surgery to deliver a baby. The baby is taken out through the mother's abdomen. Most cesarean births result in healthy babies and mothers. But C-section is major surgery and carries risks. Healing also takes longer than with vaginal birth.

Most healthy pregnant women with no risk factors for problems during labor or delivery have their babies vaginally. Still, the cesarean birth rate in the United States has risen greatly in recent decades. Today, nearly one in three women have babies by C-section in this country. The rate was one in five in 1995.

Public health experts think that many C-sections are unnecessary. So it is important for pregnant women to get the facts about C-sections before they deliver. Women should find out what C-sections are, why they are performed, and the pros and cons of this surgery.

Reasons for C-Sections

Your doctor might recommend a C-section if she or he thinks it is safer for you or your baby than vaginal birth. Some C-sections are planned. But most C-sections are done when unexpected problems happen during delivery. Even so, there are risks of delivering by C-section. Limited studies show that the benefits of having a C-section may outweigh the risks when the following are true:

- The mother is carrying more than one baby (twins, triplets, etc.)

- The mother has health problems including HIV [human immunodeficiency virus] infection, herpes infection, and heart disease

- The mother has dangerously high blood pressure

- The mother has problems with the shape of her pelvis

- There are problems with the placenta

- There are problems with the umbilical cord
- There are problems with the position of the baby, such as breech
- The baby shows signs of distress, such as a slowed heart rate
- The mother has had a previous C-section

Patient-Requested C-Section: Can a Woman Choose?

A growing number of women are asking their doctors for C-sections when there is no medical reason. Some women want a C-section because they fear the pain of childbirth. Others like the convenience of being able to decide when and how to deliver their baby. Still others fear the risks of vaginal delivery including tearing and sexual problems.

But is it safe and ethical for doctors to allow women to choose C-section? The answer is unclear. Only more research on both types of deliveries will provide the answer. In the meantime, many obstetricians feel it is their ethical obligation to talk women out of elective C-sections. Others believe that women should be able to choose a C-section if they understand the risks and benefits.

Experts who believe C-sections should only be performed for medical reasons point to the risks. These include infection, dangerous bleeding, blood transfusions, and blood clots. Babies born by C-section have more breathing problems right after birth. Women who have C-sections stay at the hospital for longer than women who have vaginal births. Plus, recovery from this surgery takes longer and is often more painful than that after a vaginal birth. C-sections also increase the risk of problems in future pregnancies. Women who have had C-sections have a higher risk of uterine rupture. If the uterus ruptures, the life of the baby and mother is in danger.

Supporters of elective C-sections say that this surgery may protect a woman's pelvic organs, reduces the risk of bowel and bladder problems, and is as safe for the baby as vaginal delivery.

The National Institutes of Health (NIH) and American College of Obstetricians (ACOG) agree that a doctor's decision to perform a C-section at the request of a patient should be made on a case-by-case basis and be consistent with ethical principles. ACOG states that "if the physician believes that (cesarean) delivery promotes the overall health and welfare of the woman and her fetus more than vaginal birth, he or she is ethically justified in performing" a C-section. Both organizations also say that C-section should never be scheduled before a pregnancy is 39 weeks, or the lungs are mature, unless there is medical need.

The C-Section Experience

Most C-sections are unplanned. So, learning about C-sections is important for all women who are pregnant. Whether a C-section is planned or comes up during labor, it can be a positive birth experience for many women. The overview that follows will help you to know what to expect during a nonemergency C-section and what questions to ask.

Before Surgery

Cesarean delivery takes about 45 to 60 minutes. It takes place in an operating room. So if you were in a labor and delivery room, you will be moved to an operating room. Often, the mood of the operating room is unhurried and relaxed. A doctor will give you medicine through an epidural or spinal block, which will block the feeling of pain in part of your body but allow you to stay awake and alert. The spinal block works right away and completely numbs your body from the chest down. The epidural takes away pain, but you might be aware of some tugging or pushing. Medicine that makes you fall asleep and lose all awareness is usually only used in emergency situations. Your abdomen will be cleaned and prepped. You will have an IV [intravenous line] for fluids and medicines. A nurse will insert a catheter to drain urine from your bladder. This is to protect the bladder from harm during surgery. Your heart rate, blood pressure, and breathing also will be monitored. Questions to ask:

- Can I have a support person with me during the operation?

- What are my options for blocking pain?

- Can I have music played during the surgery?

- Will I be able to watch the surgery if I want?

During Surgery

The doctor will make two incisions. The first is about six inches long and goes through the skin, fat, and muscle. Most incisions are made side to side and low on the abdomen, called a bikini incision. Next, the doctor will make an incision to open the uterus. The opening is made just wide enough for the baby to fit through. One doctor will use a hand to support the baby while another doctor pushes the uterus to help push that baby out. Fluid will be suctioned out of your baby's mouth and nose. The doctor will hold up your baby for you to see. Once your baby is delivered, the umbilical cord is cut, and the placenta is

389

removed. Then, the doctor cleans and stitches up the uterus and abdomen. The repair takes up most of the surgery time. Questions to ask:

- Can my partner cut the umbilical cord?
- What happens to my baby right after delivery?
- Can I hold and touch my baby during the surgery repair?
- When is it okay for me to try to breastfeed?
- When can my partner take pictures or video?

After Surgery

You will be moved to a recovery room and monitored for a few hours. You might feel shaky, nauseated, and very sleepy. Later, you will be brought to a hospital room. When you and your baby are ready, you can hold, snuggle, and nurse your baby. Many people will be excited to see you. But don't accept too many visitors. Use your time in the hospital, usually about four days, to rest and bond with your baby. C-section is major surgery, and recovery takes about six weeks (not counting the fatigue of new motherhood). In the weeks ahead, you will need to focus on healing, getting as much rest as possible, and bonding with your baby—nothing else. Be careful about taking on too much and accept help as needed. Questions to ask:

- Can my baby be brought to me in the recovery room?
- What are the best positions for me to breastfeed?

Vaginal Birth after C-Section (VBAC)

Some women who have delivered previous babies by C-section would like to have their next baby vaginally. This is called vaginal delivery after C-section or VBAC. Women give many reasons for wanting a VBAC. Some want to avoid the risks and long recovery of surgery. Others want to experience vaginal delivery.

Today, VBAC is a reasonable and safe choice for most women with prior cesarean delivery, including some women who have had more than one cesarean delivery. Moreover, emerging evidence suggests that multiple C-sections can cause serious harm. If you are interested in trying VBAC, ask your doctor if you are a good candidate. A key factor in this decision is the type of incision made to your uterus with previous C-sections.

Your doctor can explain the risks of both repeat cesarean delivery and VBAC. With VBAC, the most serious danger is the chance that the C-section scar on the uterus will open up during labor and delivery.

This is called uterine rupture. Although very rare, uterine rupture is very dangerous for the mother and baby. Less than 1 percent of VBACs lead to uterine rupture. But doctors cannot predict if uterine rupture is likely to occur in a woman. This risk, albeit very small, is unacceptable to some women.

The percent of VBACs is dropping in the United States for many reasons. Some doctors, hospitals, and patients have concerns about the safety of VBAC. Some hospitals and doctors are unwilling to do VBACs because of fear of lawsuits and insurance or staffing expenses. Many doctors, however, question if this trend is in the best interest of women's health.

Choosing to try a VBAC is complex. If you are interested in a VBAC, talk to your doctor and read up on the subject. Only you and your doctor can decide what is best for you. VBACs and planned C-sections both have their benefits and risks. Learn the pros and cons and be aware of possible problems before you make your choice.

Section 32.4

Episiotomy

"Episiotomy," © 2006 American Pregnancy Association (www.americanpregnancy.org). Reprinted with permission. Reviewed by David A. Cooke, MD, FACP, October 10, 2012.

An episiotomy is a surgical incision used to enlarge the vaginal opening to help deliver a baby.

What are some circumstances that would require an episiotomy?

An episiotomy may be needed for any of the following reasons:

- Birth is imminent and the perineum hasn't had time to stretch slowly.
- The baby's head is too large for the vaginal opening.
- The baby is in distress.
- The mother needs a forceps or vacuum assisted delivery.

- The baby is in a breech presentation and there is a complication during delivery.
- The mother isn't able to control her pushing.

How is an episiotomy performed?

If you have already had an epidural, you will probably not need any further anesthetic. If otherwise, it will be necessary to utilize a local anesthetic called a pudendal block in your perineum.

The mediolateral cut is angled down, away from the vagina and the perineum, into the muscle. The midline cut is performed by cutting straight down into the perineum, between the vagina and anus.

How can I prevent the need to have an episiotomy?

The following measures can reduce the need for an episiotomy:

- Good nutrition (healthy skin stretches more easily!)
- Kegels (exercise for your pelvic floor muscles)
- A slowed second stage of labor where pushing is controlled
- Warm compresses and support during delivery
- Use of perineum massage techniques
- Avoiding lying on your back while pushing

Can episiotomies be harmful?

Episiotomies have the following potential side effects:

- Infection
- Bruising
- Swelling
- Bleeding
- Extended healing time
- Painful scarring that might require a period of abstinence from sexual intercourse
- Future problems with incontinence

What are some pain relief options for episiotomies and tears?

If you end up having an episiotomy or tearing you can try some of the following solutions to help ease the pain.

- Cold packs on the perineum: Ask your health care provider about special maxi pads that have built in cold packs.

- Take a sitz bath—a portable bath that you place over a toilet that allows warm water to cover the wound.

- Use medication such as Tucks Medicated Pads.

- Use a personal lubricant such as KY Jelly when you resume sexual intercourse.

- After using the bathroom, wash yourself with a squirt bottle instead of wiping. Patting dry, instead of wiping, can also help.

What if I want to avoid having an episiotomy?

Clearly state in your birth plan that you do not want an episiotomy unless absolutely necessary. Also, discuss the issue with your health care provider during routine prenatal care.

Section 32.5

Tubal Ligation

"Tubal Ligation," © 2012 A.D.A.M., Inc. Reprinted with permission.

Tubal ligation (or tying the tubes) is surgery to close a woman's fallopian tubes. These tubes connect the ovaries to the uterus. A woman who has this surgery can no longer get pregnant. This means she is sterile.

Description

Tubal ligation is done in a hospital or outpatient clinic.

- You may receive general anesthesia. You will be asleep and unable to feel pain.

- Or, you will be awake and given local or spinal anesthesia. You will likely also receive medicine to make you sleepy.

The procedure takes about 30 minutes.

- Your surgeon will make one or two small surgical cuts in your belly, usually around the belly button. Gas may be pumped into your belly to expand it. This helps your surgeon see your uterus and fallopian tubes.

- Your surgeon will insert a narrow tube with a tiny camera on the end (laparoscope) into your belly. Instruments to block off your tubes will be inserted through the laparoscope or through a separate, very small cut.

- The tubes are either burned shut (cauterized) or clamped off with a small clip or ring (band).

Tubal ligation can also be done right after you have a baby through a small cut in the navel or during a cesarean section.

Another sterilization method involves going through the cervix and placing coils or plugs in the tubes where they connect with the uterus (hysteroscopic tubal occlusion procedure). This technique does not involve cuts in the abdomen.

Why the Procedure Is Performed

Tubal ligation may be recommended for adult women who know for sure they do not want to get pregnant in the future.

Even though many women choose to have tubal ligation, some are sorry later that they did. The younger the woman is, the more likely she will regret having her tubes tied as she gets older.

Tubal ligation is considered a permanent form of birth control. It is not recommended as a short-term method or one that can be reversed. However, major surgery can sometimes restore your ability to have a baby. This is called a reversal. More than half of women who have their tubal ligation reversed are able to become pregnant.

A hysteroscopic tubal occlusion procedure is very hard to reverse.

Risks

Risks for any surgery are:

- bleeding;

- damage to other organs (bowel or urinary systems) needing more surgery for repair;

- infection.

Risks for any anesthesia are:

- allergic reactions to medicines;

- breathing problems or pneumonia;

- heart problems.

Risks for tubal ligation are:

- incomplete closing of the tubes, which could make pregnancy still possible (About 1 out of 200 women who have had tubal ligation get pregnant later.);

- increased risk of a tubal (ectopic) pregnancy if pregnancy occurs after a tubal ligation;

- injury to nearby organs or tissues from surgical instruments.

Before the Procedure

Always tell your doctor or nurse:

- if you are or could be pregnant;

- what drugs you are taking, even drugs, herbs, or supplements you bought without a prescription.

During the days before your surgery:

- You may be asked to stop taking aspirin, ibuprofen (Advil, Motrin), warfarin (Coumadin), and any other drugs that make it hard for your blood to clot.

- Ask your doctor which drugs you should still take on the day of your surgery.

- If you smoke, try to stop. Ask your doctor or nurse for help quitting.

- If you are having the tubal occlusion procedure, you will be asked to take a hormone for at least two weeks before the procedure.

On the day of your surgery:

- You will usually be asked not to drink or eat anything after midnight the night before your surgery, or eight hours before the time of your surgery.

- Take the drugs your doctor told you to take with a small sip of water.

- Your doctor or nurse will tell you when to arrive at the hospital or clinic.

After the Procedure

You will probably go home the same day you have the procedure. Some women may need to stay in the hospital overnight. You will need a ride home.

You will have some tenderness and pain. Your doctor will give you a prescription for pain medicine or tell you what over-the-counter pain medicine you can take.

After laparoscopy, many women will have shoulder pain for a few days. This is caused by the gas used in the abdomen to help the surgeon see better during the procedure. You can relieve the gas by lying down.

You should avoid heavy lifting for three weeks, but you can return to most normal activities within a few days.

If you have the hysteroscopic tubal occlusion procedure, you will need to keep using a birth control method until you have a test three months after the procedure to make sure it worked.

Outlook (Prognosis)

Most women will have no problems. Tubal ligation is an effective form of birth control for women. You will not need to have any tests to make sure you cannot get pregnant in the future if the procedure is done with laparoscopy or after delivering a baby.

Some women may need to have a test called hysterosalpingogram about three months after the procedure to make sure their tubes are blocked.

Your periods should return to whatever pattern is normal for you. If you used hormonal birth control or the Mirena IUD [intrauterine device] before, then your periods will change to whatever is normal for you after you stop using these methods.

Women who have a tubal ligation have a decreased risk of developing ovarian cancer.

Section 32.6

Uterine Fibroid Surgery

Excerpted from "Uterine Fibroids Fact Sheet," by the
Office on Women's Health (www.womenshealth.gov), part of the U.S.
Department of Health and Human Services, May 13, 2008.

Fibroids are muscular tumors that grow in the wall of the uterus (womb). Another medical term for fibroids is leiomyoma or just myoma. Fibroids are almost always benign (not cancerous). Fibroids can grow as a single tumor, or there can be many of them in the uterus. They can be as small as an apple seed or as big as a grapefruit. In unusual cases they can become very large.

About 20 percent to 80 percent of women develop fibroids by the time they reach age 50. Fibroids are most common in women in their 40s and early 50s. Not all women with fibroids have symptoms. Women who do have symptoms often find fibroids hard to live with. Some have pain and heavy menstrual bleeding. Fibroids also can put pressure on the bladder, causing frequent urination, or the rectum, causing rectal pressure. Should the fibroids get very large, they can cause the abdomen (stomach area) to enlarge, making a woman look pregnant.

Most fibroids do not cause any symptoms, but some women with fibroids can have the following:

- Heavy bleeding (which can be heavy enough to cause anemia) or painful periods

- Feeling of fullness in the pelvic area (lower stomach area)

- Enlargement of the lower abdomen

- Frequent urination

- Pain during sex

- Lower back pain

- Complications during pregnancy and labor, including a six-time greater risk of cesarean section

- Reproductive problems, such as infertility, which is very rare

397

Treatment for Uterine Fibroids

Most women with fibroids do not have any symptoms. For women who do have symptoms, there are treatments that can help. Talk with your doctor about the best way to treat your fibroids. She or he will consider many things before helping you choose a treatment. Some of these things include the following:

- Whether or not you are having symptoms from the fibroids
- If you might want to become pregnant in the future
- The size of the fibroids
- The location of the fibroids
- Your age and how close to menopause you might be

If you have fibroids but do not have any symptoms, you may not need treatment. Your doctor will check during your regular exams to see if they have grown.

If you have fibroids with moderate or severe symptoms, surgery may be the best way to treat them.

Myomectomy

A myomectomy is surgery to remove fibroids without taking out the healthy tissue of the uterus. It is best for women who wish to have children after treatment for their fibroids or who wish to keep their uterus for other reasons. You can become pregnant after myomectomy. But if your fibroids were imbedded deeply in the uterus, you might need a cesarean section to deliver. Myomectomy can be performed in many ways. It can be major surgery (involving cutting into the abdomen) or performed with laparoscopy or hysteroscopy. The type of surgery that can be done depends on the type, size, and location of the fibroids. After myomectomy new fibroids can grow and cause trouble later. All of the possible risks of surgery are true for myomectomy. The risks depend on how extensive the surgery is.

Hysterectomy

A hysterectomy is surgery to remove the uterus. This surgery is the only sure way to cure uterine fibroids. Fibroids are the most common reason that hysterectomy is performed. This surgery is used when a woman's fibroids are large, if she has heavy bleeding, is either near or past menopause, or does not want children. If the fibroids are large, a woman may need a hysterectomy that involves cutting into the abdomen to remove the uterus. If the fibroids are smaller, the doctor may be able to reach the uterus through the vagina, instead of making a cut in the abdomen. In some cases hysterectomy can be performed through the laparoscope. Removal of the ovaries and the cervix at the time of hysterectomy is usually optional. Women whose ovaries are not removed do not go into menopause at the time of hysterectomy. Hysterectomy is a major surgery. Although hysterectomy is usually quite safe, it does carry a significant risk of complications. Recovery from hysterectomy usually takes several weeks.

Endometrial Ablation

Endometrial ablation is when the lining of the uterus is removed or destroyed to control very heavy bleeding. This can be done with laser, wire loops, boiling water, electric current, microwaves, freezing, and other methods. This procedure usually is considered minor surgery. It can be done on an outpatient basis or even in a doctor's office. Complications can occur, but are uncommon with most of the methods. Most people recover quickly. About half of women who have this procedure have no more menstrual bleeding. About three in 10 women have much lighter bleeding. But, a woman cannot have children after this surgery.

Myolysis

Myolysis is when a needle is inserted into the fibroids, usually guided by laparoscopy, and electric current or freezing is used to destroy the fibroids.

Uterine Fibroid Embolization (UFE), or Uterine Artery Embolization (UAE)

UFE or UAE is when a thin tube is thread into the blood vessels that supply blood to the fibroid. Then, tiny plastic or gel particles are injected into the blood vessels. This blocks the blood supply to the fibroid, causing it to shrink. UFE can be an outpatient or inpatient procedure. Complications, including early menopause, are uncommon but can occur. Studies suggest fibroids are not likely to grow back after UFE, but more long-term research is needed. Not all fibroids can be treated with UFE. The best candidates for UFE are women who:

- have fibroids that are causing heavy bleeding;

- have fibroids that are causing pain or pressing on the bladder or rectum;
- don't want to have a hysterectomy;
- don't want to have children in the future.

Chapter 33

Urological Surgery

Chapter Contents

Section 33.1

Circumcision

Circumcision is a common procedure in which the skin covering the tip of the penis is surgically removed. It's usually performed on a newborn boy before he leaves the hospital, and often within the first two days of life. In the Jewish faith, it is performed in a special ceremony when a baby is eight days old.

Boys are born with a hood of skin, called the foreskin, covering the head (glans) of the penis. In circumcision, the foreskin is removed to expose the head of the penis. Normally the procedure causes very little bleeding and stitches aren't needed. A protective bandage may be placed over the wound, which generally heals on its own within a week to 10 days.

In the United States, many newborn males are circumcised. Circumcision is not medically required, but studies show that it lowers certain health risks. In fact, according to the American Academy of Pediatrics (AAP), the benefits of the procedure outweigh the risks. Sometimes older boys are circumcised, but the procedure can become a little more complicated as a child grows.

Most parents make the decision about circumcision based on cultural, religious, or personal reasons (such as whether other male family members have been circumcised).

Although a circumcision itself is relatively simple and takes only 10 to 20 minutes to perform, it helps to understand how it's done so you can feel confident about what is happening.

Preparing for the Circumcision

Once you decide your baby will be circumcised, discuss it with the doctor who'll perform the procedure. Many circumcisions are done by obstetricians, but pediatricians, family practitioners, urologists, neonatologists, and pediatric surgeons also can do them.

Most healthy babies can be circumcised within one to two days after birth. However, circumcision is delayed for babies with certain medical conditions. Your child's examining pediatrician or neonatologist will decide if your newborn should wait to be circumcised.

If it is OK for your child to have a circumcision, the doctor will review any risks, potential benefits, and instructions on caring for your baby after the procedure. The doctor will also ask about any family history of bleeding disorders (like hemophilia or von Willebrand's disease). Ask the doctor to explain anything you don't understand.

When you feel comfortable with the information and your questions have been fully answered, you will be asked to sign an informed consent form, which states that you understand the procedure and its risks and give your permission for your child to have the circumcision.

Circumcisions are often performed in the hospital's nursery treatment room. Some parents choose to be in the treatment room during the circumcision, while others prefer to wait for the baby to be returned to the nursery. If you'd like to be in the room, let your doctor know.

What Happens during the Procedure?

A baby is typically awake for circumcision. He is usually positioned in a molded plastic seat that helps hold him safely in place. The penis and surrounding skin are cleansed with antiseptic before the procedure begins.

Pain-Control Measures

Several safe and effective pain-control methods can lessen a baby's pain during circumcision. It's important to ask your doctor about the type of pain control your baby will have ahead of time.

Often, the first pain-control measure will be an acetaminophen suppository inserted into the baby's rectum. This helps reduce discomfort during the procedure and lasts for several hours afterward.

Next, a local anesthetic is given to numb the area of the penis where the incision will be made. A topical anesthetic, which is a numbing cream, is first applied to the skin of the penis and takes up to 30 minutes to take effect.

After the cream has numbed the area of skin, a nerve block is given. The two main types are:

1. A dorsal penile nerve block (DPNB), which is a liquid medicine injected through a tiny needle into the bottom of the penis, numbing the whole penis within minutes

2. A ring block, which is very similar to the DPNB, except that the numbing medication is injected at least three times in a ring pattern around the shaft of the penis

Often several methods of pain control are used in combination. For example, doctors may first insert the suppository, then apply the topical cream, and then give the injections where the numbing cream was applied. When the injections are given after the numbing cream, your baby will feel very little as the needle goes through the skin, although the medication may burn a little as it's being injected.

To further reduce a baby's stress and discomfort, the nurse may give the baby a sucrose pacifier (a pacifier dipped in sugar water), which has been shown to reduce newborn distress.

Circumcision Methods

In newborns, circumcision can be performed in several ways. The most common techniques protect the head of the penis with special devices while the foreskin is removed. Your doctor will determine which method is appropriate.

In newborns, the three most common circumcision techniques are [the following]:

1. The Gomco Clamp

A special instrument called a probe is used to separate the foreskin from the head of the penis (they are usually joined by a thin membrane). Next a bell-shaped device is fitted over the head of the penis and under the foreskin (an incision may be made in the foreskin to allow this). The foreskin is then pulled up and over the bell and a clamp is tightened around it to reduce blood flow to the area. A scalpel is used to cut and remove the foreskin.

2. The Mogen Clamp

Again, the foreskin is separated from the head of the penis with a probe. The foreskin is then pulled out in front of the head and inserted through a metal clamp with a slot in it. The clamp is held in place while the foreskin is cut with a scalpel and remains for a few minutes after this to make sure that bleeding has been controlled.

3. The Plastibell Technique

This method is similar to the Gomco clamp technique. After separation with a probe, the plastic bell is placed under the foreskin and over the head of the penis. A piece of suture is tied directly around the foreskin, which cuts off the blood supply to the foreskin. A scalpel may then be used to cut off the extra foreskin, but the plastic ring is left on. About three to seven days later it falls off on its own.

After the Procedure

After a circumcision, doctors will apply petroleum ointment over the wound and wrap the baby's penis in gauze to keep the wound from sticking to his diaper (unless the doctors have used the Plastibell method, which requires no dressing). The baby will usually be brought to you shortly after the procedure.

There is very little bleeding after circumcision, no matter which technique is used. Though you may see a little bit of blood oozing from the edge of the incision or on the diaper when you first take the dressing off, this will generally stop on its own.

Often, the suppository that was given before the procedure is enough pain management for the baby, but doctors or nurses may decide to give more if the baby seems uncomfortable.

It's important to talk to your doctor to learn how to care for the circumcised penis.

Because your baby's penis may be sore for a few days after the procedure, you will want to be gentle when bathing him. Cotton swabs, astringents, or any special bath products aren't necessary—most doctors recommend keeping the area clean with warm, soapy water.

If there is a bandage on the incision, for a day or two after the procedure you might need to apply a new one whenever you change his diaper. You should also put a dab of petroleum jelly on the baby's penis or on the front of the diaper to alleviate any potential discomfort caused by friction against the diaper.

It usually takes between 7 to 10 days for a circumcised penis to heal from the procedure. Until it does, the tip might be raw or yellowish. Call your doctor right away if you notice any of the following:

- Bleeding that continues
- Redness around the tip of the penis that gets worse
- Fever
- Signs of infection, such as the presence of pus-filled blisters

- Not urinating within 12 hours after the circumcision

Benefits

In the first year of life, a circumcised infant is less likely to get a urinary tract infection. It may be easier to keep a circumcised penis clean and uninfected, though boys who don't have circumcisions can be taught to properly clean beneath the foreskin once it becomes retractable (usually by age 5).

Later in life, studies show that circumcised men may also be at lower risk for developing cancer of the penis (although the disease is rare). Circumcision may lower the risk of contracting HIV [human immunodeficiency virus] from an infected female partner.

Risks and Complications

A circumcision is considered a safe procedure with minimal, if any, risks. Most of the time, there are no complications.

In rare instances, complications can include [the following]:

- Infection: Infection is rare because doctors always use sterile techniques to perform the procedure. Most circumcision-related infections are mild and easily treatable with antibiotics. Signs of infection include worsening redness, pus, pain, and swelling around the incision, or fever. If you notice any of these signs, call the doctor.

- Bleeding at the site: This is more likely when the child has a bleeding disorder, which is why it's important to let the doctor know about any family history of bleeding or clotting problems. Very rarely, a small blood vessel may be nicked during the procedure. In most cases, this bleeding will stop on its own, but occasionally stitches are required.

- Risks associated with anesthesia: Local anesthesia is very safe. But in rare cases it can cause complications in children (such as irregular heart rhythms, breathing problems, allergic reactions to medications, and, in very rare cases, death). These complications are not common, and usually involve patients who have other medical problems.

- Incomplete removal of the foreskin: Sometimes too much skin is left behind. This becomes less apparent as the child ages. Occasionally, if the excess skin is uneven, a corrective procedure may be required at a later date.

406

- Damage to the penis: In rare cases, the head of the penis can be injured during a circumcision. However, precautions doctors take almost always prevent this from happening.

When your child is having any kind of procedure or surgery, it's understandable to be a little uneasy. But it helps to know that in most cases, circumcisions are common procedures and complications are rare. A child who has a circumcision typically heals without any difficulty or health problems. If you have any questions about circumcision, talk with your doctor.

Section 33.2

Prostate Cancer Surgery

Excerpted from "Treatment Choices for Men with Early-Stage Prostate Cancer," by the National Cancer Institute (NCI, www.cancer.gov), part of the National Institutes of Health, February 11, 2011.

As a man with early-stage prostate cancer, you will be able to choose which kind of treatment is best for you. And while it is good to have choices, this fact can make the decision hard to make. Yet, each choice has benefits (how treatment can help) and risks (problems treatment may cause).

Treatment often begins a few weeks to months after diagnosis. While you are waiting for treatment, you should meet with different doctors to learn about your treatment choices.

You will want to think about what is important to you. It's also a good idea to include your spouse or partner in your decision. After all, having prostate cancer and the treatment choice you make affect both of you.

Surgery

Surgery is a treatment choice for men with early-stage prostate cancer who are in good health. Surgery to remove the prostate is called prostatectomy. There are different types of surgery for prostate cancer.

Open Prostatectomy

This surgery is also called retropubic prostatectomy. In this surgery, your doctor removes the prostate through a single long cut made in your abdomen from a point below your navel to just above the pubic bone. He or she might also check nearby lymph nodes for cancer. This type of surgery can be used for nerve-sparing surgery. Nerve-sparing surgery lessens the chances that the nerves near your prostate will be harmed. These important nerves control erections and normal bladder function.

Laparoscopic Surgery

In this type of surgery, your doctor uses a laparoscope to see and remove the prostate. A laparoscope is a long slender tube with a light and camera on the end. This surgery is done through four to six small cuts in the navel and the abdomen, instead of a single long cut in the abdomen. The laparoscope is inserted through one of the cuts, and surgery tools are inserted through the others. A robot can be used to do this type of surgery. This type of surgery can also be used for nerve-sparing surgery.

Perineal Prostatectomy

In this type of surgery, your doctor removes the prostate through an incision between your scrotum and anus. With this method, the surgeon is not able to check the lymph nodes for cancer and nerve-sparing surgery is more difficult to do. This type of surgery is not used very often.

Section 33.3

Urinary Incontinence Surgery

This section contains text from "Urinary Incontinence in Men," National Institute of Diabetes and Digestive and Kidney Disorders (NIDDK, www .niddk.nih.gov), part of the National Institutes of Health, June 29, 2012, and "Urinary Incontinence in Women," by the NIDDK, September 2, 2010.

Urinary Incontinence in Men

Surgical treatments can help men with incontinence that results from nerve-damaging events, such as spinal cord injury or radical prostatectomy.

Artificial sphincter: Some men may eliminate urine leakage with an artificial sphincter, an implanted device that keeps the urethra closed until you are ready to urinate. This device can help people who have incontinence because of weak sphincter muscles or because of nerve damage that interferes with sphincter muscle function. It does not solve incontinence caused by uncontrolled bladder contractions.

Surgery to place the artificial sphincter requires general or spinal anesthesia. The device has three parts: A cuff that fits around the urethra, a small balloon reservoir placed in the abdomen, and a pump placed in the scrotum. The cuff is filled with liquid that makes it fit tightly around the urethra to prevent urine from leaking. When it is time to urinate, you squeeze the pump with your fingers to deflate the cuff so that the liquid moves to the balloon reservoir and urine can flow through the urethra. When your bladder is empty, the cuff automatically refills in the next two to five minutes to keep the urethra tightly closed.

Male sling: Surgery can improve some types of urinary incontinence in men. In a sling procedure, the surgeon creates a support for the urethra by wrapping a strip of material around the urethra and attaching the ends of the strip to the pelvic bone. The sling keeps constant pressure on the urethra so that it does not open until the patient consciously releases the urine.

Urinary diversion: If the bladder must be removed or all bladder function is lost because of nerve damage, you may consider surgery

409

to create a urinary diversion. In this procedure, the surgeon creates a reservoir by removing a piece of the small intestine and directing the ureters to the reservoir. The surgeon also creates a stoma, an opening on the lower abdomen where the urine can be drained through a catheter or into a bag.

Urinary Incontinence in Women

Millions of women experience involuntary loss of urine called urinary incontinence (UI). Some women may lose a few drops of urine while running or coughing. Others may feel a strong, sudden urge to urinate just before losing a large amount of urine. Many women experience both symptoms. UI can be slightly bothersome or totally debilitating. For some women, the risk of public embarrassment keeps them from enjoying many activities with their family and friends. Urine loss can also occur during sexual activity and cause tremendous emotional distress.

Surgery for Stress Incontinence

In some women, the bladder can move out of its normal position, especially following childbirth. Surgeons have developed different techniques for supporting the bladder back to its normal position. The three main types of surgery are retropubic suspension and two types of sling procedures.

Retropubic suspension uses surgical threads called sutures to support the bladder neck. The most common retropubic suspension procedure is called the Burch procedure. In this operation, the surgeon makes an incision in the abdomen a few inches below the navel and then secures the threads to strong ligaments within the pelvis to support the urethral sphincter. This common procedure is often done at the time of an abdominal procedure such as a hysterectomy.

Sling procedures are performed through a vaginal incision. The traditional sling procedure uses a strip of your own tissue called fascia to cradle the bladder neck. Some slings may consist of natural tissue or man-made material. The surgeon attaches both ends of the sling to the pubic bone or ties them in front of the abdomen just above the pubic bone.

Midurethral slings are newer procedures that you can have on an outpatient basis. These procedures use synthetic mesh materials that the surgeon places midway along the urethra. The two general types of midurethral slings are retropubic slings, such as the transvaginal tapes (TVT), and transobturator slings (TOT). The surgeon makes small incisions behind the pubic bone or just by the sides of the vaginal opening as well as a small incision in the vagina. The surgeon uses specially designed needles to position a synthetic tape under the urethra. The surgeon pulls the ends of the tape through the incisions and adjusts them to provide the right amount of support to the urethra.

If you have pelvic prolapse, your surgeon may recommend an anti-incontinence procedure with a prolapse repair and possibly a hysterectomy.

Recent women's health studies performed with the Urinary Incontinence Treatment Network (UITN) compared the suspension and sling procedures and found that, two years after surgery, about two-thirds of women with a sling and about half of women with a suspension were cured of stress incontinence. Women with a sling, however, had more urinary tract infections, voiding problems, and urge incontinence than women with a suspension. Overall, 86 percent of women with a sling and 78 percent of women with a suspension said they were satisfied with their results.

Talk with your doctor about whether surgery will help your condition and what type of surgery is best for you. The procedure you choose may depend on your own preferences or on your surgeon's experience. Ask what you should expect after the procedure. You may also wish to talk with someone who has recently had the procedure. Surgeons have described more than 200 procedures for stress incontinence, so no single surgery stands out as best.

Section 33.4

Urostomy

For the thousands of people every year suffering from bladder disease, urostomy (urinary diversion) surgery can be the beginning of a new and healthier life. If you have been burdened with a chronic or even life-threatening disease, after your initial recovery period you can look forward to feeling much better, and to resuming all the activities you have enjoyed in the past.

This text has been developed to help you better understand what is happening to you. Please read the following pages carefully. Many of the words [in this text] will be used in your presence again and by doctors, your Wound Ostomy Continence Nurse (WOCN), hereinafter referred to as ostomy nurse.

Urostomy is one of a number of surgical procedures that detour, or divert, urine away from a diseased or defective bladder. This text discusses only those operations which bring the urine to the outside of the body through an opening in the abdominal wall. The bladder is either bypassed or removed, and the urine is passed from the body through a surgically created opening called a stoma. You will not have voluntary control of the urine that comes out through the stoma, therefore a collection pouch will be fitted for your individual needs.

In addition to getting you ready for abdominal surgery, your doctor or your ostomy nurse will explain the surgery and examine your abdomen to determine the best location for the stoma. You may be asked to wear a sample pouch to make sure that the site chosen is on the flattest possible surface and that you are comfortable in all positions. If you have any hobbies or habits which might be affected by the location of the pouch, talk to the doctor or the ostomy nurse.

A special source of help is an ostomy visitor. The visitor is a person who, like you, has had urostomy surgery and has successfully adapted to the changes that occur with ostomy surgery. He or she can answer many of your questions about day-to-day life. You may also benefit from taking part in an ostomy support group. A support group allows you to share your feelings and ask questions as you make progress with your recovery. You can also share your story with others that may benefit from your experience. You can find a list of UOAA Affiliated Support Groups at www.ostomy.org or by calling 800-826-0826.

Facts about Urostomies

A urinary diversion/urostomy is needed when the bladder is not functioning properly. There are four major reasons for performing a urinary diversion. The most common reason is for bladder cancer. Others include neurologic dysfunction of the bladder, birth defects, and chronic inflammation of the bladder.

The urinary tract consists of two kidneys, two ureters, the bladder, and the urethra.

Urine is made in the kidneys, transported by squeezing movements called peristalsis through the ureters to the bladder for storage, and expelled through the urethra. One can live without a bladder, but must have a minimum amount of kidney function to grow and be healthy.

Should there be a malignancy (cancerous growth) in the bladder, the entire bladder may be removed or bypassed and the urine detoured through an abdominal stoma and patients may be cured of their disease.

Some patients find a urostomy easier to manage than a defective bladder that is caused by several reasons such as birth defect, surgery, or spinal injury.

With these bladder injuries, patients cannot control the flow of urine, causing them embarrassment and annoyance with skin problems that can occur with constant wetting. Some people have requested urostomy surgery over dealing with incontinence.

If a child is born with a defect in the urinary tract, causing the urine to back up into the kidneys resulting in chronic infection, a urostomy may be lifesaving. The surgical construction of a pathway through which the urine may travel rapidly, without interference, will allow the kidneys to function at their maximum efficiency.

There are two basic options for surgery: The conventional urostomy and the continent urinary reservoir. Not every person will be a candidate for the continent urostomy as there are factors that must be considered other than the person's preference. The surgeon, upon examination of a person's diagnosis, condition, and surgical need, will present these considerations.

Normal Urinary System

- Kidneys: The kidneys are paired organs lying behind the peritoneum, against the posterior abdominal wall, one on either side of the vertebral column. The kidneys serve a number of important body functions. They process and excrete urine, and maintain the fluid, electrolyte, and acid/base balances of the body.

- Ureters: The two ureters are tubes from the kidneys approximately 10–12 inches in length. They collect the urine as it is excreted from the kidneys. Peristaltic waves force the urine down the ureters into the bladder.

- Bladder: The urinary bladder serves as a reservoir for urine. Periodically, the bladder expels urine from the body, via the urethra.

- Urethra: The urethra is a tube from the bladder to the outside of the body.

Conventional Urostomy

Indications

- Cancer of bladder
- Neurologic dysfunction
- Birth defects
- Chronic inflammation of bladder

Discharge

- Urine
- Some mucus

Management

- Skin protection
- Drainable, valve-end pouch
- Adaptable to night drainage

To create an ileal conduit, a segment of the small bowel (ileum) 6–8 inches long is excised near the entrance into the large bowel. The ileum is reconnected. The ureters are detached from the bladder and implanted into the ileal segment. The bladder may or may not be removed. The distal end of the ileal segment is brought through the abdominal wall and a stoma is formed on the abdomen, usually the right side. The proximal end of the ileal segment is sutured closed. This surgery is permanent. The urine is not controlled and will require wearing a collection pouch attached to the abdomen at all times.

The small intestine produces mucous naturally. The segment of intestine that was used to form the ileal conduit will continue to produce mucous and will collect in the pouch.

Urostomy Management

Learning to care for your urostomy may seem like a complicated procedure at first, but with practice and your own adaptations, the entire process will become second nature, just like shaving or bathing.

Pouching Systems

A successful pouching system should provide the following:

- Security with a good leak-proof seal, lasting for three to seven days

- Skin protection

- Be inconspicuous

- Easy to apply and to remove

A pouching system is used to collect urine. There are two main types of systems available: One-piece pouches with attached skin barrier and two-piece systems composed of a skin barrier and detachable pouch. The skin barrier will require a hole to be cut for the stoma or may be purchased pre-cut to size.

Each urostomy pouch has a drain valve at the bottom of the pouch, so the pouch can be emptied as needed.

Generally, it is a good idea to empty your pouch when it is about one-third full. During the day most people find it necessary to empty the pouch about as often as they did before urostomy surgery or any other bladder defects.

At nighttime a length of flexible tubing can be attached to the drain valve on your pouch. This allows the urine to flow into a bedside collector while you sleep.

Many people find a bedside drainage unit preferable to getting up during the night and emptying the pouch.

In the hospital where there are ostomy nurses, your personal needs will be evaluated and your pouching system will be selected for you. For some, this pouch is the type worn for a lifetime. For others, weight gain, a child's normal growth, and other factors may later on require a new or different type of pouching system. Do not continue using a recommended pouch if it is not satisfactory. Try different types until you find one that is both comfortable and convenient to use.

Skin Protection

The constant flow of urine from the stoma can be very irritating to a person's skin, so most urostomy pouches have protective skin barriers. Pouching systems come with either a pre-cut opening or can be cut to fit the stoma size and shape.

Immediately after surgery the stoma is swollen but will decrease in size in six to eight weeks. During this postop period the stoma should be measured about once a week.

A measuring card may be included in boxes of pouches or skin barriers or you may create your own template that matches your stoma shape. The opening should be no more than 1/8 inch larger than the stoma size to prevent urine drainage on the skin.

There are several other factors that can influence how long the pouch stays sealed. These include:

- Proper fitting, weather, skin characteristics, scars, weight changes, diet, activity, and abdominal contours near the stoma

- Perspiration during the summer months in warm, humid climates will shorten the number of days you can wear a pouch.

- Moist, oily skin may reduce adhesion time.

- Weight gain or loss will also affect the wearing time of a pouch. Weight gained or lost after urostomy surgery changes abdominal contours. You may need an entirely different pouching system.

- Physical activities will have some influence on your pouch wearing time. Very active sports or work that causes perspiration may cut down on pouch wearing time as well.

Changing the Pouching System

Applying the pouch may be accomplished with greater ease if you change it in the morning before you eat or drink anything. If this is not convenient for you, try to wait at least one to two hours after you have had fluids so that urine is not dribbling on the skin.

You will be able to decide whether sitting, standing, or lying down is the best position for putting on your pouch. This position should be the one that gives you the best view of your stoma and is the easiest when making a change. Some people stand facing the toilet so the urine, dripping from the stoma, may be caught in the toilet. When changing while sitting in a wheelchair, it is helpful to slide your buttocks toward the front of the chair and recline.

Using a mirror will help you center the pouch over the stoma. And some people find it helpful to use rolled gauze or paper towels to absorb dibbling urine from the stoma.

The first several times you change your pouch, you may find it takes 30 minutes or more. Once you gain confidence and experience, you may be able to change it in 10 minutes or less. Remember that your pouch should be changed on a schedule that fits in with your routine. In other words, do not wait for it to leak to change it.

Clean pouches will decrease the chances of introducing bacteria into the urinary system. Bacteria will multiply rapidly even in the tiniest droplet of urine. These bacteria may travel up the ureters and cause a kidney infection. Furthermore, the bacteria can cause odor by acting on the urine. Keeping all items immaculately clean will save you time and money. Always have at least two complete pouches, one on your body and one ready for your next change.

Emptying the Pouch

It is important to empty the pouch at regular intervals. During the day, you probably will find it necessary to empty the pouch every two to four hours and more often if you drink a lot of fluids. Children may have to empty more frequently because their pouch is smaller. The volume of urine could jeopardize the pouch seal.

It is recommended to empty when the pouch is one-third to one-half full. Simply open the valve and drain into an appropriate receptacle, usually directly into the toilet.

Belts

Wearing a belt is a very individual matter. Some persons who have urostomies wear an ostomy belt because it makes them feel more secure or it gives support to the pouching system. Others find an ostomy belt cumbersome. If you choose to wear an ostomy belt, adjust it so that you can get two finger widths between the belt and your waist in order to avoid a deep groove or cut in the skin around the stoma. This could result in serious damage to the stoma and cause pressure ulcers on the surrounding skin. Belts should be worn so they do not ride above or below the level of the belt tabs on the pouching system. People who are in a wheelchair may need a special belt. Manufacturers carry special belts or you can make one from belting purchased at a fabric store.

Night Drainage System

At night the bottom of the pouch is connected to a night drainage system which will carry the urine away from the stoma during the sleeping hours. This allows you to sleep undisturbed, with assurance that the urine has been transported to a bedside container by gravity. Your pouch will not get so full that it pulls away from the body.

When connecting the pouch to the bedside drainage receptacle (jar or bag) leave a small amount of urine in the pouch prior to attaching the tubing to prevent setting up a vacuum in the system. The bedside container should be vented and the tubing should be secured at the top of the bottle with no more than one inch of it extending down into a half-gallon bottle. Should urine rise above the end of the tubing, drainage ceases.

The drainage container can be hung on the side of the bed, or placed in a receptacle on the floor. A decorative waste paper basket may be used for this purpose.

To clean the tubing and beside drainage collector insert two ounces of a vinegar/water solution through the outlet valve of your emptied pouch and attach to bedside drainage collector (one part of white vinegar to three parts of water).

Ostomy Supplies

For the sake of convenience keep all your supplies together on a shelf, in a drawer, or in a small box in a cool dry area away from hot or cold temperatures.

Reorder supplies several weeks before you expect to run out, to allow enough time for delivery. It is best to avoid stockpiling of supplies due to the fact that the products have a shelf life and are influenced by changes in temperatures. Supplies do not have to be sterile. The stoma and surrounding skin are not sterile and require only cleanliness.

To order additional pouches, skin barriers, and other ostomy products, you will need the manufacturer's name and product numbers. Supplies may be ordered from a mail order company or from a medical supply or pharmacy in your town. For information and help in ordering, you may contact a local ostomy nurse, the product manufacturer, telephone directory business pages, or the internet (search word: ostomy supplies).

Helpful Hints

Protecting the Skin around the Stoma

Urostomy output can be irritating to the skin area around the stoma. This skin area should appear the same as anywhere else on the abdomen. Using the following techniques will help keep your skin healthy.

- Use the correct size and type of pouch opening and skin barrier opening.

- Change the pouch regularly to avoid leakage and skin irritation. It is recommended to change the pouch if itching and/or burning occurs.

- Remove the skin barrier gently by pushing your skin from the pouch rather than pulling the pouch from the skin.

- Keep the skin clean with water. If necessary, use a mild soap and rinse very well. This can be done in the shower or tub. Pat skin dry before applying the skin barrier or pouch.

- Watch for sensitivities and allergies to adhesive, skin barrier, tape, or pouch material. They can develop weeks, months, or years after use of a product since the body can become gradually sensitized. If you have a skin irritation that is caused by the pouch material, you might try a pouch cover. These are available from several manufacturers, or you can make your own.

Spots of Blood on the Stoma

Spots of blood are no cause for alarm. Brushing against your stoma as you are changing the pouch may cause pinpoint bleeding. The blood vessels in the tissues of the stoma are very delicate at the surface and are easily disturbed. The bleeding will usually stop as easily as it started.

Urine pH Balance

Urine pH is defined as the fluid's degree of acidity or alkalinity. When the food you eat is burned in the body, it yields a mineral residue called ash. This ash can be either acidic or basic (alkaline) depending on whether the food that is burned contains mostly acidic or basic ions.

Most fruits and vegetables actually give an alkalinized ash and tend to alkaline the urine. Meats and cereals will usually produce an acidic ash residue.

Unless otherwise indicated the urine should be maintained in an acid state. To maintain an acid urine state, increase your daily fluid intake to 8 to 10 (8 ounce) glasses of water. Drink cranberry juice in place of orange juice or other citrus juices that tend to make the urine more alkaline and take vitamin C daily (if approved by physician). Some of the acid ash foods include: Most meats, breads and cereals, cheese, corn, cranberries, eggs, macaroni, nuts, pasta, prunes, fish, and poultry.

Shaving Hair under the Pouch

Some men with excessive hair find it painful to remove their pouch because of hair pulling. Hair roots can also be injured and cause irritation. Shaving with an electric razor or trimming hairs with scissors is helpful. A straight edge or safety razor is not recommended.

Bathing

Bathe or shower with or without your pouch. Soap cannot harm the stoma. Just rinse well. Do not use an oily soap around the stoma. If you bathe with your pouch off, hold a cool wash cloth over the area to close the pores of the skin. Then pat dry and apply the pouch. Sometimes the heat from a hot bath or shower will keep the skin warm and will generate moisture under the barrier and prevent a secure seal.

Urostomy Complications

Severe Skin Problems

Large areas of skin irritation which are reddened, very sore, and weeping (always wet) will prevent a good seal around the stoma. It is therefore important to combat minor irritations when they first occur. If you have an irritation that does not go away in a few days, or encrustation around the stoma, contact your physician or ostomy nurse. The severity of a problem depends on early intervention. Remember that with a properly fitted pouching system, adequate intake of fluids and good skin care, you can expect few difficulties.

Urinary Crystals

Urinary crystals on the stoma or skin are associated with alkaline urine. The crystals appear as white, gritty particles and may lead to stomal irritation and/or bleeding of the stoma. Proper cleaning, maintaining acidic urine, and careful fitting of the opening in the pouch will help prevent urinary crystals. To help reduce urinary crystals, make a vinegar compress that can be applied to the stoma for a few minutes when the pouch is changed (mix equal parts of water and white vinegar).

Medical Emergencies

You should call the doctor or WOCN when you have:

- a deep cut in the stoma;
- excessive bleeding from the stoma opening (or a moderate amount in the pouch at several emptyings);
- continuous bleeding at the junction between stoma and skin;
- severe skin irritation or deep ulcers;
- unusual change in stoma size (prolapse or retraction) and appearance (color);
- fever and strong odor that may indicate a kidney infection.

Hospitalization

Take your ostomy supplies with you as the hospital may not have your brand in supply. You may find that you are the expert on urostomies, especially if you are in a hospital where urostomy patients are rare or if you go for a condition not related to your ostomy. If you are in doubt about any procedure, ask to talk to your doctor. Ask to have the following information listed on your chart: 1) Ileal conduit or continent diversion, 2) describe in detail your management routine and products used, 3) do not take a urine specimen from the urostomy pouch. Use a catheter inserted into the stoma.

Living with a Urostomy

After any major operation, you need time to regain your strength and to feel well again. After urostomy (ileal conduit) surgery you will wear an external collection device and learn new skills to manage it. The success of your surgery is based not only on its ability to cure or eliminate the disease or defect, but also on your ability to enjoy life and resume your work and your hobbies. Support and guidance can be found at www.ostomy.org and through local, UOAA Affiliated Support Groups.

Telling Others

You might be worried about how others will accept you and how your social role may be changed. It is natural to wonder how you will explain your surgery. Your friends and relatives may ask questions about your operation. You can tell them as much as you want them to know. You need not feel a need to explain your surgery to everyone who asks. A brief explanation would be that you had abdominal surgery or that you had your bladder removed or bypassed.

If you have children, answer their questions simply and honestly. A simple explanation will be enough for them. Once you have explained what a urostomy is they may ask questions and want to see your stoma or pouch. Discussing your surgery and showing your stoma in a natural way will dispel any misunderstandings they may have. They will accept your urostomy much the same way you do.

If you are considering marriage, discussions with your future spouse about life with a urostomy and its effect on sex, children, and family acceptance will help to alleviate misconceptions and fear on the part of the spouse. Attending UOAA support group meetings together will also be helpful. Talking to other couples, in which one partner has had ostomy surgery, will provide an experienced viewpoint.

Returning to Work

As your strength returns you may go back to your regular activities. People who have urostomies can do most jobs; however, heavy lifting may cause a stoma to herniate or prolapse and should not be resumed without physician approval. A sudden blow in the pouch area could cause the barrier or pouch to shift and cut the stoma. Still, persons who have urostomies do heavy lifting such as mechanics and truck drivers. There are athletes who have stomas. Check with your doctor about your type of work. As with all major surgery, it will take time for you to regain strength after your operation. A letter from your doctor to your employer may be helpful should the employer have doubts about your physical capabilities.

Employability and insurability are issues for some individuals. If these issues develop, seek help from healthcare professionals and/or talk with others who have found solutions to these issues. When you return to your job, you may wish to confide in your employer or a good friend. You may want to tell them you have a urostomy.

Keeping it a complete secret may cause practical difficulties.

Psychosocial Issues

There are times after surgery when you may feel discouraged. You may feel alone and isolated and unable to enjoy life again. These are common feelings. Serious illness, medication, and the surgery itself may cause feelings of insecurity, dependence, and discouragement. You may wonder if you will ever be the same and you may think that no one understands how you feel. Feeling discouraged is real and normal. Talking to a trusted friend, nurse, or another person with an ostomy about your feelings can help you work through them.

Your social life can be as active as it was before surgery. You can enjoy all activities such as travel, sporting events, eating at restaurants, or whatever you enjoyed before. The first time you go out of the house after surgery, you may feel as if everyone is staring at your pouch even though it is not visible under your clothing.

You may feel your pouch on your body, but no one can see it. Did you know what a urostomy was or where the stoma was located before you had surgery?

Intimacy and Sexuality

Sexual relationships and intimacy are important and fulfilling aspects of your life that should continue after ostomy surgery. Your attitude is a key factor in re-establishing sexual expression and intimacy. A period of adjustment after surgery is to be expected. Sexual function in women is usually not impaired, while sexual potency of men may be affected. This impairment can be temporary, but may be permanent. Consult your physician with continued issues or concerns.

Any sexuality concerns you have should be discussed openly between you and your partner. It is likely that your partner will have anxieties about sexual activities due to lack of information. An intimate relationship is one is which it matters how well two people can communicate.

The first time you become intimate after surgery things may not go perfectly. Men may have trouble getting and keeping an erection and women sometimes have pain during intercourse. These conditions can improve with time; consult your physician with continued issues or concerns. Your interest in sex will gradually return as your strength is regained and management issues are mastered. Body contact during sexual activities will usually not harm the stoma or loosen the pouch from the abdomen.

Women may consider wearing crotch-less panties, teddies, or a short slip or nightie. Men may consider wearing a cummerbund around the midsection to secure the pouch. There are several types of pouch covers that can be purchased or you can make your own.

Ostomy surgery may present more concerns for single individuals. When to tell that someone special depends upon the relationship. Brief casual dates may not need to know. If the relationship grows and leads to intimacy, the partner needs to be told about the ostomy prior to a sexual experience.

Pregnancy in women who have had urostomy surgery is not uncommon. Before pregnancy is considered, it should be discussed with your doctor. The urostomy itself is not a reason to avoid pregnancy. If you are healthy, the risk during childbirth appears to be no greater than for other mothers. Of course other health problems that you may have must be taken into consideration and discussed with your physician.

For more information, the guidebook *Intimacy, Sexuality and an Ostomy* is available from UOAA or check out the sexuality fact sheets on www.ostomy.org under Ostomy Information.

Diet and Nutrition

There are no eating restrictions as a result of urostomy surgery. If the kidneys have been severely impaired, your physician will monitor your protein and salt intake, but the functions of your kidneys are not affected by the surgery. The urinary tract and digestive tract are separate. A few foods and certain medications may cause urine odor or a change of urine color. Drink plenty of liquids each day following recommendations from your urologist or ostomy nurse.

Clothing

You need no special clothing after urostomy surgery, but some minor adjustments may be necessary for personal comfort or preference. The gentle pressure of undergarments with elastic will not harm the stoma or prevent function of the urostomy. Avoid tight fitting pants that may cause some difficulty with the urine drainage.

Cotton knit or stretch underpants may give the support and security you need.

Panty hose are also comfortable. A simple pouch cover adds comfort by absorbing perspiration and keeps the pouch from resting on the skin. Men can wear either boxer or jockey-type shorts.

Sports Activities

A urostomy should not limit your participation in sports. Many physicians because of possible injury to the stoma from a severe blow discourage contact sports, but these problems can be overcome with special equipment. Weight lifting may result in a hernia at the stoma. Check with your doctor about such sports. There are many people who have had urostomy surgery who are distance runners, skiers, swimmers, and participants in many other types of athletics.

For swimming, remember these points:

- You can protect the barrier by taping the edges with waterproof or paper tape.

- You may want to choose a swimsuit that has a lining to provide a smoother profile.

- Women may wear stretch panties designed for swimsuits.

- Men may want to wear a support garment sold in men's underwear departments on athletic wear departments.

- Men may prefer to wear a tank top and trunks, if the stoma is above the belt line.

- Empty your pouch before going into the water.

Travel

All methods of travel are open to you. Many people with urostomies travel extensively, including camping trips, cruises, and plane excursions around the world.

Since you should prepare for travel, here are some suggestions:

Take along enough supplies to last the entire trip plus some extras. Double what you think you may need, because they may not be easy to get where you are going.

Even if you don't expect to change your pouch, take along everything you need to do so. Zip-Lock bags may be used for pouch disposal. Leave home fully prepared. Find out if and where supplies are available before a long trip. A local UOAA support group may be helpful in locating ostomy supplies and local medical professionals. Contact the UOAA office or visit the www.ostomy.org to find the nearest support group.

Seat belts will not harm the stoma when adjusted comfortably. You may place a clothes pin near the retraction slot to relieve tension on the belt. When traveling by car, keep your supplies in the coolest part. Avoid the trunk or back window ledge.

When traveling by plane, checked luggage sometimes gets lost. When you travel, carry an extra pouching system and other supplies on the plane with you. Small cosmetic bags with plastic linings or shaving kits work well. These should be placed in your carry-on luggage.

To avoid problems when going through customs or luggage inspection, have a note from your doctor stating that you need to carry ostomy supplies and medication by hand—i.e., medically necessary ostomy supplies. Further problems might be avoided by having this information translated into the language or languages of the places you are visiting.

Before traveling abroad, get a copy of the current directory of English-speaking physicians in various foreign cities who charge a standard fee. The International Association for Medical Assistance to Travelers (IAMAT) publishes lists of English speaking physicians in over 2,500 cities around the world. The telephone number is 716-754-4883, www.iamat.org.

In foreign countries, traveler's diarrhea is a common illness of tourists, whether you are a person with an ostomy or not. The most common cause of diarrhea is contaminated water and/or food. It may also be caused by mere changes in water, food, or climate. It is wise to avoid unpeeled fruits and raw vegetables.

Section 33.5

Vasectomy

Vasectomy at a Glance

- Sterilization for men that prevents pregnancy

- Safe and effective

- Costs $350 to $1,000

- Meant to be permanent

- Thinking about getting a vasectomy? Find a health center

Is Vasectomy Right for Me?

All of us who need birth control want to find the method that is best for us.

Here are some of the most common questions we hear people ask about vasectomy. We hope you find the answers helpful.

What Is Vasectomy?

Vasectomy is a form of birth control for men that is meant to be permanent.

During vasectomy, a health care provider closes or blocks the tubes that carry sperm. When the tubes are closed, sperm cannot leave a man's body and cause pregnancy.

How Does Vasectomy Work?

Sperm are made in the testicles. They pass through two tubes called the vasa deferentia to other glands and mix with seminal fluids to form semen. Vasectomy blocks each vas deferens and keeps sperm out of the seminal fluid. The sperm are absorbed by the body instead of being ejaculated. Without sperm, your cum (ejaculate) cannot cause pregnancy.

How Effective Is Vasectomy?

Effectiveness is an important and common concern when choosing a birth control method. Vasectomy is the most effective birth control for men. It is nearly 100 percent effective.

However, vasectomy is not immediately effective. Sperm remains beyond the blocked tubes. You must use other birth control until the sperm are used up. It usually takes about three months. A simple test—semen analysis—shows when there are no more sperm in your ejaculate.

How Is Semen Analysis Done?

You will provide a sample of your semen by masturbating or by using a special condom during sexual intercourse. The semen will be examined under a microscope to see if there are any sperm.

Very rarely, tubes grow back together again and pregnancy may occur. This happens in about 1 out of 1,000 cases.

Keep in mind that vasectomy offers no protection against sexually transmitted infection. Sexually transmitted infections can be carried in ejaculate, whether or not it contains sperm. Latex or female condoms can reduce your risk of infection.

What Are the Types of Vasectomy?

There are different ways for men to be sterilized. One type does not require an incision—a cut. The other types of vasectomy require an incision. Incision methods take about 20 minutes. The no-incision method takes less time.

Incision methods: Usually, a local anesthetic is injected into the pelvic area. Then, the doctor makes an incision on each side of the scrotum to reach each vas deferens—the tubes that carry sperm. Sometimes a single incision is made in the center. Each tube is blocked. In most procedures, a small section of each tube is removed. Tubes may be tied off or blocked with surgical clips. Or, they may be closed using an instrument with an electrical current.

No-incision method: With the no-incision (no-scalpel) method, the skin of the scrotum is not cut. One tiny puncture is made to reach both tubes. The tubes are then tied off, cauterized, or blocked. The tiny puncture heals quickly. No stitches are needed, and no scarring takes place.

The no-scalpel method reduces bleeding and decreases the possibility of infection, bruising, and other complications.

How Safe Is Vasectomy?

Most men can have a vasectomy safely. But like any medical procedure, there are risks. Talk with your health care provider about whether vasectomy is likely to be safe for you.

What Are the Benefits of Vasectomy?

Vasectomy is safe and, because it lasts for life, it is simple and convenient. It allows women and men to enjoy sex without worrying about pregnancy.

Vasectomy does not change your hormones or masculinity. And it will not affect your ability to get and stay erect. It also will not affect your sex organs, sexuality, and sexual pleasure. No glands or organs are removed or altered. Your hormones and sperm continue being produced. Your ejaculate will look just like it always did. And there will be about the same amount as before.

Vasectomy may be right for you if:

- You want to enjoy having sex without causing pregnancy.

- You don't want to have a child biologically in the future.

- Other methods are unacceptable.

- You don't want to pass on a hereditary illness or disability.

- Your partner's health would be threatened by a future pregnancy.

- You and your partner have concerns about the side effects of other methods.

- You and your partner agree that your family is complete, and no more children are wanted.

- You want to spare your partner the surgery and expense of tubal sterilization—sterilization for women is more complicated and costly.

What Are the Disadvantages of Vasectomy?

Vasectomy may not be a good choice for you if you:

- may want to have a child biologically in the future;

- are being pressured by a partner, friends, or family;

- want to use it to solve problems that may be temporary—such as marriage or sexual problems, short-term mental or physical illnesses, financial worries, or being out of work.

Considering Other Birth Control Options

It is important to consider other methods before you choose vasectomy, like condoms, outercourse, withdrawal, and abstinence. Women have other options. IUDs [intrauterine devices] and the implant are as effective as vasectomy, simple to use, offer long-term protection, but are not permanent.

You should consider any possible life changes, such as divorce, remarriage, or death of children. You don't need your partner's permission to have a vasectomy, but it may be helpful to discuss it with your partner or anyone else who could be part of the decision-making process.

Saving Sperm in Sperm Banks

If you're thinking of getting a vasectomy and banking sperm just in case you change your mind, vasectomy may not be the best choice for you. Sperm banks collect, freeze, and thaw sperm for alternative insemination. However, some men's sperm do not survive freezing. And it is generally easier for a woman to get pregnant with fresh sperm than frozen sperm.

Can Vasectomy Be Reversed?

If you are thinking about reversal, vasectomy may not be right for you. Sometimes it is possible to reverse the operation, but there are no guarantees. Reversal involves complicated surgery and costs thousands of dollars. Success in restoring fertility is uncertain.

The success of reversal surgery depends on:

- the length of time since the vasectomy was performed;

- whether or not antibodies to sperm have developed;

- the method used for vasectomy and the length and location of the segments of vas deferens that were removed or blocked.

Possible Risks of Vasectomy

There are risks with any medical procedure, including vasectomy. Major complications with vasectomy are rare and are usually caused by infection.

Complication rates for vasectomy are generally lower for the no-incision method than for methods that include cutting the skin.

After you've had a vasectomy, look for signs of infection:

- A fever over 100 degrees Fahrenheit

- Blood or pus oozing from the site of the incision

- Excessive pain or swelling

See a health care provider if you have signs of infection. You may need an antibiotic.

Other potential problems include:

- Bruising, which usually clears up on its own

- Hematomas—swellings that contain blood: They usually clear up by themselves, or with bed rest or ice packs. In rare cases, they need to be drained by a health care provider.

- Hydroceles—swellings that contain fluid and tenderness near the testicles: They usually clear up in about a week. Applying heat and wearing an athletic supporter can help. In rare cases, they need to be drained with by a health care provider.

430

- Granuloma—sperm that leaks from the tubes and causes a small lump under the skin near the site of the surgery: This usually clears up by itself. Surgical treatment is sometimes required.

- Pain or discomfort in the testicles: This is usually temporary, but in about 2 out of 100 cases the pain may be chronic and severe. Most of the time, pain is relieved by taking anti-inflammatory drugs or other medications. Very rarely, an injection called a spermatic cord block can be used to deaden the pain temporarily. Vasectomy reversal is very rarely needed to relieve pain permanently.

Very rarely, the cut ends of a tube grow back together. This most often happens within four months of the operation and may allow pregnancy to happen.

Decreased sexual desire or an inability to have an erection occurs in 4 out of 1,000 cases. The most likely cause is emotional—there is no physical cause for sexual dysfunction associated with vasectomy.

Does Vasectomy Hurt?

Your health care provider will give you medicine to make it as comfortable as possible. Numbing medication and/or sedatives will be used. The choice depends on your health and the method of sterilization being used. Conscious sedation allows you to be awake but deeply relaxed. Local anesthesia blocks the feeling of pain in a certain area of your body. It is much safer than general anesthesia.

General anesthesia is entirely painless. It allows you to sleep through the procedure.

When you get local anesthesia, you may feel brief discomfort. You may also feel some pain when the tubes are brought out through the incision.

How Will I Feel after Vasectomy?

As with any surgery, there's some discomfort after the operation. It will be different for each man. However, most men say the pain is slight or moderate and not excessive. An athletic supporter, ice bag, and non-aspirin pain reliever may help ease the pain. Avoid strenuous physical work or exercise for about a week. There seems to be less pain associated with no-incision procedures.

How Long Does Recovery Take after Vasectomy?

That depends on your general health and lifestyle. Most men lose little or no time from work. A few need a day or two to rest. You will have to avoid strenuous work or exercise for about a week.

Rare complications may require more days at home. However, prompt medical attention usually clears up any problems.

For most men, sexual activity can begin again within a week. Others have sex sooner. Some wait longer. But remember, after the procedure, it takes about three months to clear sperm out of your system. Use another form of birth control for vaginal intercourse until a semen analysis shows there are no longer any sperm in your seminal fluid.

How Do I Get a Vasectomy? How Much Does a Vasectomy Cost?

If you are interested in getting a vasectomy, talk with a health care provider. Contact your local Planned Parenthood health center, your family doctor, a local hospital, a local public health department, or a urologist. A vasectomy can be performed in a medical office, hospital, or clinic.

Nationwide, the cost of a vasectomy ranges from $350–$1,000, including the follow-up sperm count. (Sterilization for women costs up to six times as much.) Some clinics and doctors use a sliding scale according to income.

There may be state or federal requirements for sterilization, such as age restrictions or waiting periods. Ask if there are any restrictions when you make an appointment.

Planned Parenthood works to make health care accessible and affordable. Some health centers are able to charge according to income. Most accept health insurance. If you qualify, Medicaid or other state programs may lower your health care costs.

Call your local Planned Parenthood health center to get specific information on costs.

Chapter 34

Cosmetic and Reconstructive Surgery

Chapter Contents

Section 34.1

Abdominoplasty

What Is a Tummy Tuck?

Also known as abdominoplasty, a tummy tuck removes excess fat and skin, and in most cases restores weakened or separated muscles creating an abdominal profile that is smoother and firmer.

A flat and well-toned abdomen is something many of us strive for through exercise and weight control. Sometimes these methods cannot achieve our goals.

Even individuals of otherwise normal body weight and proportion can develop an abdomen that protrudes or is loose and sagging. The most common causes of this include:

- pregnancy;
- aging;
- significant fluctuations in weight;
- heredity;
- prior surgery.

Tummy tuck surgery is a highly individualized procedure and you should do it for yourself, not to fulfill someone else's desires or to try to fit any sort of ideal image.

Abdominoplasty is a good option for you if:

- you are physically healthy and at a stable weight;
- you have realistic expectations;
- you do not smoke.

Although the results of an abdominoplasty procedure are technically permanent, the positive outcome can be greatly diminished by significant fluctuations in your weight. For this reason, individuals who are planning substantial weight loss or women who may be considering future pregnancies may be advised to postpone abdominoplasty surgery.

What a tummy tuck won't do: Tummy tucks are not a substitute for weight loss or an appropriate exercise program. Also, tummy tuck operations cannot correct stretch marks, although these may be removed or somewhat improved if they are located on the areas of excess skin that will be excised, generally the treated areas below the belly button.

Tummy Tuck Risks and Safety Information

The decision to have tummy tuck surgery is extremely personal and you'll have to decide if the benefits will achieve your goals and if the risks and potential abdominoplasty complications are acceptable.

Your plastic surgeon and/or staff will explain in detail potential tummy tuck complications. You will be asked to sign consent forms to ensure that you fully understand the procedure you will undergo and any risks or potential complications.

Possible abdominoplasty risks include:

- unfavorable scarring;
- bleeding (hematoma);
- infection;
- fluid accumulation;
- poor wound healing;
- skin loss;
- blood clots;
- numbness or other changes in skin sensation;
- anesthesia risks;
- skin discoloration and/or prolonged swelling;
- fatty tissue found deep in the skin might die (fat necrosis);
- major wound separation;
- asymmetry;
- recurrent looseness of skin;
- pain, which may persist;
- deep vein thrombosis, cardiac and pulmonary complications;

- persistent swelling in the legs;

- nerve damage;

- possibility of revisional surgery;

- suboptimal aesthetic result.

You'll need help: If your abdominoplasty is performed on an outpatient basis, be sure to arrange for someone to drive you to and from surgery and to stay with you for at least the first night following surgery.

What Happens during Tummy Tuck Surgery?

Step 1—Anesthesia: Medications are administered for your comfort during abdominoplasty surgery. The choices include intravenous sedation and general anesthesia. Your doctor will recommend the best choice for you.

Step 2—The incision: A full tummy tuck procedure requires a horizontally-oriented incision in the area between the pubic hairline and navel. The shape and length of the incision will be determined by the degree of correction necessary.

Through this incision, weakened abdominal muscles are repaired and sutured while excess fat, tissue, and skin is removed.

A second incision around the navel may be necessary to remove excess skin in the upper abdomen.

Step 3—Closing the incisions: Sutures, skin adhesives, tapes, or clips close the skin incisions.

Step 4—See the results: Your abdominoplasty procedure will result in a flatter, firmer abdominal contour that is more proportionate with your body type and weight.

The final results may be initially obscured by swelling and your inability to stand fully upright until internal healing is complete.

Within a week or two, you should be standing tall and confident about your new slimmer profile.

Tummy Tuck Recovery

Following your surgery, dressings or bandages may be applied to your incisions, and you may be wrapped in an elastic bandage or a compression garment to minimize swelling and to support your abdomen as it heals.

A small, thin tube may be temporarily placed under the skin to drain any excess blood or fluid that may collect to minimize swelling after tummy tuck surgery.

You will be given specific instructions to aid your recovery from tummy tuck surgery: How to care for the surgical site and drains, medications to apply or take orally to aid healing and reduce the potential for infection, specific concerns to look for at the surgical site or in your general health, and when to follow-up with your plastic surgeon.

Be sure to ask your plastic surgeon specific questions about what you can expect during your individual abdominoplasty recovery period.

- Where will I be taken after my surgery is complete?

- What medication will I be given or prescribed after surgery?

- Will I have dressings/bandages after surgery? When will they be removed?

- Are stitches removed? When?

- When can I resume normal activity and exercise?

- When do I return for follow-up care?

Previous abdominal surgery may limit the potential results of a tummy tuck. In women who have undergone cesarean section, the existing scars may often be incorporated into the new scar.

Section 34.2

Blepharoplasty

What Is Cosmetic Eyelid Surgery?

Also known as blepharoplasty, eyelid surgery improves the appearance of the upper eyelids, lower eyelids, or both. It gives a rejuvenated appearance to the surrounding area of your eyes, making you look more rested and alert.

Treatable conditions:

- Upper eyelid surgery can remove excess fatty deposits that appear as puffiness in the upper eyelids.

- Loose or sagging skin that creates folds or disturbs the natural contour of the upper eyelid, sometimes impairing vision, can be treated by eyelid lift surgery.

- Lower eyelid blepharoplasty can remove excess skin and fine wrinkles of the lower eyelid.

- Bags under the eyes can be corrected by blepharoplasty.

- Lower eyelid surgery can correct droopiness of the lower eyelids, showing white below the iris (colored portion of the eye).

Is It Right for Me?

A blepharoplasty procedure is usually performed on adult men and women who have healthy facial tissue and muscles and have realistic goals for improvement of the upper and/or lower eyelids and surrounding area.

You should undergo blepharoplasty surgery for yourself, not to fulfill someone else's desires or to try to fit any sort of ideal image.

Good candidates for cosmetic eyelid surgery are:

- healthy individuals who do not have a life-threatening illness or medical conditions that can impair healing;

- non-smokers;
- individuals with a positive outlook and specific goals in mind for blepharoplasty;
- individuals without serious eye conditions.

You must tell your doctor if you have any of these medical conditions:

- Eye disease such as glaucoma, dry eye, or a detached retina
- Thyroid disorders such as Graves' disease and under or overactive thyroid
- Cardiovascular disease, high blood pressure, or other circulatory disorders or diabetes

Preparing for Eyelid Surgery

Before blepharoplasty surgery, you may be asked to:

- get lab testing or a medical evaluation;
- take certain medications or adjust your current medications;
- stop smoking well in advance of surgery;
- avoid taking aspirin, anti-inflammatory drugs, and herbal supplements as they can increase bleeding.

Special instructions you receive will cover:

- what to do on the night before and the morning of surgery;
- the use of anesthesia during your procedure;
- post-operative care and follow-up.

Your plastic surgeon will also discuss where your procedure will be performed. Blepharoplasty may be performed in an accredited office-based surgical center, outpatient or ambulatory surgical center, or a hospital.

You'll Need Help

If your eyelid surgery is performed on an outpatient basis, be sure to arrange for someone to drive you to and from surgery and to stay with you for at least the first night following surgery.

Blepharoplasty Surgery Steps

What happens during an eyelid surgery?

Step 1—Anesthesia

Medications are administered for your comfort during the eyelid surgery procedure. The choices include intravenous sedation or general anesthesia. Your doctor will recommend the best choice for you.

Step 2—The Incision

The incision lines for eyelid surgery are designed for scars to be well concealed within the natural structures of the eyelid region.

Droopy conditions of the upper eyelid can be corrected through an incision within the natural crease of the upper eyelid allowing repositioning of fat deposits, tightening of muscles and tissue, and/or removal of excess skin.

Conditions of the lower eyelid may be corrected with an incision just below the lower lash line. Through this incision, excess skin in the lower eyelids is removed.

A transconjunctival incision, one hidden inside the lower eyelid, is an alternate technique to correct lower eyelid conditions and redistribute or remove excess fat.

Step 3—Closing the Incisions

Eyelid incisions typically are closed with:

• removable or absorbable sutures;

• skin adhesives;

• surgical tape.

Your surgeon may use a laser chemical peel to erase dark discoloration of the lower eyelids.

Step 4—See the Results

The results of eyelid surgery will appear gradually as swelling and bruising subside to reveal a smooth, better-defined eyelid and surrounding region, and an alert and rejuvenated appearance.

Eyelid Surgery Risks and Safety Information

The decision to have cosmetic surgery is extremely personal and you'll have to decide if the benefits will achieve your goals and if the risks and potential blepharoplasty complications are acceptable.

Your plastic surgeon and/or staff will explain potential eyelid surgery complications in detail. You will be asked to sign consent forms to ensure that you fully understand the procedure you will undergo and any risks or potential complications.

- Unfavorable scarring
- Temporarily blurred or impaired vision
- Dry eyes
- Difficulty closing your eyes
- Lid lag, a pulling down of the lower eyelid may occur and is often temporary
- Ectropion, rolling of the eyelid outwards
- Bleeding (hematoma)
- Poor wound healing
- Infection
- Fluid accumulation
- Blood clots
- Numbness and other changes in skin sensation
- Anesthesia risks
- Eyelid disorders that involve abnormal position of the upper eyelids (eyelid ptosis), loose eyelid skin, or abnormal laxness of the lower eyelid (ectropion) can coexist with sagging forehead and eyebrow structures; brow lift surgery will not correct these disorders; additional surgery may be required
- Pain, which may persist
- Skin discoloration and swelling
- Sutures may spontaneously surface through the skin, become visible, or produce irritation that require removal
- Deep vein thrombosis, cardiac and pulmonary complications
- Possibility of revisional surgery
- Loss of eyesight

Be sure to ask questions: It's very important to ask your plastic surgeon questions about your eyelid procedure. It's natural to feel some anxiety, whether it's excitement for your anticipated new look or a bit of preoperative stress. Don't be shy about discussing these feelings with your plastic surgeon.

A Special Note about the Use of Fibrin Sealants (Tissue Glue)

Fibrin sealants (made from heat-treated human blood components to inactivate virus transmission) are used to hold tissue layers together at surgery and to diminish post-operative bruising following surgery.

This product has been carefully produced from screened donor blood plasma for hepatitis, syphilis, and human immunodeficiency virus (HIV). These products have been used safely for many years as sealants in cardiovascular and general surgery. This product is thought to be of help in diminishing surgical bleeding and by adhering layers of tissue together.

When You Go Home

If you experience shortness of breath, chest pains, or unusual heart beats, seek medical attention immediately. Should any of these complications occur, you may require hospitalization and additional treatment.

The practice of medicine and surgery is not an exact science. Although good results are expected, there is no guarantee. In some situations, it may not be possible to achieve optimal results with a single surgical procedure. Another surgery may be necessary.

Be Careful

Following your physician's instructions is key to the success of your surgery. It is important that the surgical incisions are not subjected to excessive force, abrasion, or motion during the time of healing. Your doctor will give you specific instructions on how to care for yourself.

Section 34.3

Body Contouring Surgery after Weight Loss Surgery

What Is Body Contouring after Major Weight Loss?

Body contouring after major weight loss improves the shape and tone of your underlying tissue that supports fat and skin and removes excess sagging fat and skin.

Beauty for Life: Enhancing Your Appearance with Body Contouring Surgery

Following weight reduction surgery, or any substantial amount of weight loss, the skin and tissues often lack elasticity and cannot conform to the reduced body size. As a result, skin that has been severely stretched now is unsupported:

- Upper arms may sag and appear loose and full.

- Breasts may flatten and hang with nipples pointed downward.

- Abdominal area may extend around the sides and into the lower back area, resulting in an apron-like overhang.

- Buttocks, groin, and thighs can sag and cause hanging pockets of skin.

Surgical body contouring following major weight loss improves the shape and tone of your underlying tissue that supports fat and skin, and removes excess sagging fat and skin.

The result is a more normal appearance to the body, with smoother contours. This is, in essence, the final phase of your total weight loss experience.

Is It Right for Me?

Before you decide to undergo body contouring following major weight loss, your weight loss must be stabilized.

- If you continue to lose weight, sagging pockets will redevelop.
- If you rapidly regain the weight, you will traumatically stress your already weakened and thinned skin, causing further stress to the skin, visible stretch marks, and wide scars.

If you had weight reduction surgery, your plastic surgeon will work closely with your physician to determine when it is appropriate for you to begin body contouring.

Good candidates for body contouring are:

- adults of any age whose weight loss has stabilized;
- healthy individuals who do not have medical conditions that can impair healing or increase risk of surgery;
- non-smokers;
- individuals with a positive outlook and realistic goals for what body contouring can accomplish;
- individuals committed to leading a healthy lifestyle including proper nutrition and fitness.

Preparing for Body Contouring Surgery

Prior to surgery, you may be asked to:

- get lab testing or a medical evaluation;
- take certain medications or adjust your current medications;
- stop smoking well in advance of surgery;
- avoid taking aspirin, anti-inflammatory drugs, and herbal supplements as they can increase bleeding.

Special instructions you receive will cover:

- what to do on the day of surgery;
- the use of anesthesia during your body contouring surgery;
- post-operative care and follow-up.

Your plastic surgeon will also discuss where your procedure will be performed. Body contouring surgery may be performed in an accredited office-based surgical center, outpatient or ambulatory surgical center, or a hospital.

You'll Need Help

If a component of your body contouring surgery is performed on an outpatient basis, be sure to arrange for someone to drive you to and from surgery and to stay with you for at least the first night following surgery.

Body Contouring Risks and Safety Information

The decision to have body contouring surgery is extremely personal and you'll have to decide if the benefits will achieve your goals and if the risks and potential complications are acceptable.

Your plastic surgeon and/or staff will explain in detail the risks associated with surgery. You will be asked to sign consent forms to ensure that you fully understand the procedure you will undergo and any risks and potential complications.

Possible risks of body contouring following major weight loss include:

- unfavorable scarring;
- bleeding (hematoma);
- infection;
- fluid accumulation;
- poor wound healing;
- skin loss;
- blood clots;
- numbness or other changes in skin sensation;
- anesthesia risks;
- skin discoloration and/or prolonged swelling;
- fatty tissue found deep in the skin might die (fat necrosis);
- major wound separation;
- asymmetry;
- recurrent looseness of skin;
- pain, which may persist;
- deep vein thrombosis, cardiac and pulmonary complications;

- persistent swelling in the legs;

- possibility of revisional surgery.

Be sure to ask questions: It's very important to ask your plastic surgeon questions about your body contouring procedure. It's natural to feel some anxiety, whether it's excitement for your anticipated new look or a bit of preoperative stress. Don't be shy about discussing these feelings with your plastic surgeon.

Body Contouring Procedure Steps

What happens during body contouring surgery?

The procedures necessary to achieve your goals will be defined along with a plan for the timing of these procedures. Plastic surgery procedures that may be recommended by your physician include [the following]:

- Lower body lift: To correct sagging of the abdomen, buttocks, groin, and outer thighs

- Breast lift: To correct sagging, flattened breasts

- Arm lift: To correct sagging of the upper arms

- Thigh lift: To correct sagging of the inner, outer, and mid-thigh

Step 1—Anesthesia

Medications are administered for your comfort during the surgical procedures. The choices include intravenous sedation and general anesthesia. Your doctor will recommend the best choice for you.

Step 2—The Incision

All body contouring procedures require incisions to remove excess skin. In many cases, these incisions may be extensive.

Incision length and pattern depend on the amount and location of excess skin to be removed, as well as personal preference and your doctor's surgical judgment.

Advanced techniques usually allow incisions to be placed in strategic locations where they can be hidden by most types of clothing, but this is not always the case.

Body contouring is often performed in stages. Your particular condition and goals, as well as your plastic surgeon's best judgment, will all influence how your doctor defines a surgical plan. While it may have taken you two years or more to lose all the excess weight, it may take equally as long for the results of your body contouring to be complete.

Body Lift

A complete lower body lift treats sagging buttocks, abdomen, waist, hips, and outer thighs in one procedure or in staged procedures. Incision patterns vary, and may include a circumferential incision around the body to remove the belt of excess skin and fat.

Breast Lift

The incision patterns for lifting a woman's sagging breasts will be determined based on the amount of excess skin to be removed.

These may include one or a combination of incisions in a circular pattern around the areola, in a line extending from the areola to the breast crease, and horizontally along the breast crease.

A breast implant also may be recommended to enhance breast shape and size.

Arm Lift

Sagging skin in the upper arms is treated with an incision from the underarm area extending along the inside or back of the upper arm. Additional incisions on the arms may be necessary anywhere excess skin has formed sagging pockets.

The smoother, tighter contours that result from upper arm contouring are apparent almost immediately, although initially obscured by swelling and bruising. In addition, skin quality is dramatically improved in both appearance and texture.

Thigh Lift

Reshaping of the thighs is achieved through incisions in the groin that can extend downward to the knee along the inner portion of the thigh.

Improving contours of the outer thigh may require an incision extending from the groin around the hip. Through these incisions your plastic surgeon will tighten tissues for a smoother, better toned thigh.

Body Contouring Recovery

After your body contouring procedure is completed, dressings or bandages will be applied to the incisions. A small, thin tube may be temporarily placed under the skin to drain any excess blood or fluid that may collect.

You will be given specific instructions that may include: How to care for your surgical site(s) following surgery, medications to apply or take orally to aid healing and reduce the risk of infection, specific concerns to look for at the surgical site or in your general health, and when to follow-up with your plastic surgeon.

Be sure to ask your plastic surgeon specific questions about what you can expect during your individual recovery period.

- Where will I be taken after my surgery is complete?
- What medication will I be given or prescribed after surgery?
- Will I have dressings/bandages after surgery? When will they be removed?
- Are stitches removed? When?
- When can I resume normal activity and exercise?
- When do I return for follow-up care?

When You Go Home

If you experience shortness of breath, chest pains, or unusual heart beats, seek medical attention immediately. Should any of these complications occur, you may require hospitalization and additional treatment.

The practice of medicine and surgery is not an exact science. Although good results are expected, there is no guarantee. In some situations, it may not be possible to achieve optimal results with a single surgical procedure and another surgery may be necessary.

Be Careful

Following your physician's instructions is key to the success of your surgery. It is important that the surgical incisions are not subjected to excessive force, abrasion, or motion during the time of healing. Your doctor will give you specific instructions on how to care for yourself.

Section 34.4

Liposuction

"Liposuction Information," by the U.S. Food and
Drug Administration (FDA, www.fda.gov), February 2, 2012.

Liposuction is a surgical procedure intended to remove fat deposits and shape the body. Fat is removed from under the skin with the use of a vacuum-suction canula (a hollow pen-like instrument) or using an ultrasonic probe that emulsifies (breaks up into small pieces) the fat and then removes it with suction.

Persons with localized fat may decide to have liposuction to remove fat from that area. Liposuction is a procedure for shaping the body and is not recommended for weight loss.

Liposuction may be performed on the abdomen, hips, thighs, calves, arms, buttocks, back, neck, or face. A liposuction procedure may include more than one site, for instance, the abdomen, back, and thighs all on the same day.

Liposuction is also used to reduce breast size in men with large breasts (gynecomastia) or to remove fat tumors (lipomas) but it is most commonly used for cosmetic body shaping.

Who performs liposuction and where is liposuction performed?

Many liposuction surgeries are performed by plastic surgeons or by dermatologists. Any licensed physician may perform liposuction. While some physicians' professional societies may recommend training before performing liposuction surgery, no standardized training is required. As a result, there will be differences in experience and training in physicians performing liposuction. You can ask your physician to tell you whether he or she has had specialized training to do liposuction and whether he or she has successfully done liposuction before. But remember, even the best screened patients under the care of the best trained and experienced physicians may experience complications as a result of liposuction.

Liposuction may be performed in a:

- doctor's office;

- surgical center;

- hospital.

Because liposuction is a surgical procedure, it is important that it be performed in a clean environment. Emergencies may arise during any surgery and access to emergency medical equipment and/or a nearby hospital emergency room is important. These are things that you should ask your physician before the liposuction.

How can I find the right doctor for me?

The FDA cannot recommend physicians to you. However, there are some things that you may consider:

Ask questions: If you decide to take the step to talk to a doctor about liposuction, be sure that you ask questions and understand what happens during the liposuction procedure and what you can expect. Your physician should also answer any and all questions you have about potential problems with liposuction. Remember that you are purchasing a service when you pay a physician to do a liposuction procedure and you shouldn't feel embarrassed to ask hard questions about the procedure or about the physician's experience in performing liposuction.

Beware advertising: Be wary of advertisements that say or imply that you will have a perfect appearance after liposuction. Remember that advertisements are meant to sell you a product or service, not to inform you of all the potential problems with that service.

Don't base your decision simply on cost and remember that you don't have to settle for the first doctor or procedure you investigate: The decision you make about liposuction surgery is an important one but not one that you must make right away.

Read: You should learn as much as you can about liposuction. It is important for you to read the patient information that your doctor provides.

Don't be pressured: Do not feel that because you speak to a physician about this procedure that you must go through with it. Take your time to decide whether liposuction is right for you and whether you are willing to take the risks of undergoing liposuction for its benefits.

Section 34.5

Rhinoplasty

What Is Rhinoplasty Surgery?

Rhinoplasty or nose surgery, sometimes referred to as nose reshaping or a nose job, improves the appearance and proportion of your nose, enhancing facial harmony and self-confidence. Surgery of the nose may also correct impaired breathing caused by structural abnormalities in the nose.

Enhancing Your Appearance with Nose Plastic Surgery

While the shape of your nose is usually the result of heredity, the appearance may have been altered in an injury or during prior surgery.

What Can Surgery of the Nose Accomplish?

Rhinoplasty surgery can change:

- nose size, in relation to the other facial structures;
- nose width, at the bridge;
- nose profile, with visible humps or depressions on the bridge;
- nasal tip, that is large or bulbous, drooping, or too upturned;
- nostrils that are large, wide, or upturned;
- nasal asymmetry and deviation.

Is It Right for Me?

Nose cosmetic surgery is a highly individualized procedure and you should do it for yourself, not to fulfill someone else's desires or to try to fit any sort of ideal image.

A rhinoplasty procedure is a good option for you if:

- your facial growth is complete and you are 13 years of age or older;

- you are physically healthy;

- you do not smoke;

- you have specific, but realistic goals in mind for the improvement of your appearance.

Rhinoplasty Risks and Safety Information

The decision to have nose surgery is extremely personal and you'll have to decide if the benefits will fulfill your goals and if the risks and potential rhinoplasty complications are acceptable.

Your plastic surgeon and/or staff will explain in detail the risks associated with surgery. You will be asked to sign consent forms to ensure that you fully understand the procedure you will undergo and any risks or potential complications.

The risks of rhinoplasty include:

- rupture of small surface vessels of the nose;

- infection;

- poor wound healing;

- anesthesia risks;

- bleeding (hematoma);

- nose asymmetry;

- cardiac and pulmonary complications can occur in longer surgical procedures and may be associated with the formation of, or increase in, blood clots in the venous system;

- change in skin sensation (numbness);

- nasal airway alterations may occur after a rhinoplasty or septoplasty that may interfere with normal passage of air through the nose;

- nasal septal perforation (a hole in the nasal septum) may develop but is rare; additional surgical treatment may be necessary to repair the nasal septum but in some cases, it may be impossible to correct this complication;

- pain, which may persist;

- unfavorable rhinoplasty scarring;

- skin contour irregularities;

- skin discoloration and post rhinoplasty swelling;
- sutures may spontaneously surface through the skin, become visible, or produce irritation that requires removal;
- possibility of revisional surgery.

Be sure to ask questions: It's very important to ask your plastic surgeon questions about your nose procedure. It's natural to feel some anxiety, whether it's excitement for your anticipated new look or a bit of preoperative stress. Don't be shy about discussing these feelings with your plastic surgeon.

When You Go Home

If you experience shortness of breath, chest pains, or unusual heart beats, seek medical attention immediately. Should any of these complications occur, you may require hospitalization and additional treatment.

The practice of medicine and surgery is not an exact science. Although good results are expected, there is no guarantee. In some situations, it may not be possible to achieve optimal results with a single surgical procedure. Another minor surgery may be necessary to reach the intended aesthetic goal.

Be Careful

Following your physician's instructions is key to the success of your surgery. It is important that the surgical incisions are not subjected to excessive force, abrasion, or motion during your recovery from rhinoplasty. Your doctor will give you specific instructions on how to care for yourself.

Rhinoplasty Surgery Steps

Step 1—Anesthesia

Medications are administered for your comfort during rhinoplasty surgery. The choices include intravenous sedation or general anesthesia. Your doctor will recommend the best choice for you.

Step 2—The Incision

Surgery of the nose is performed either using a closed procedure, where incisions are hidden inside the nose, or an open procedure, where an incision is made across the columella, the narrow strip of tissue that separates the nostrils.

Through these incisions, the soft tissues that cover the nose are gently raised, allowing access to reshape the structure of the nose.

Step 3—Reshaping the Nose Structure

Surgery of the nose can reduce or augment nasal structures with the use of cartilage grafted from other areas of your body.

Most commonly, pieces of cartilage from the septum, the partition in the middle of the nose, is used for this purpose.

Occasionally a piece of cartilage from the ear and rarely a section of rib cartilage can be used.

Step 4—Correcting a Deviated Septum

If the septum is deviated, it is now straightened and the projections inside the nose are reduced to improve breathing.

Step 5—Closing the Incision

Once the underlying structure of the nose is sculpted to the desired shape, nasal skin and tissue is redraped and incisions are closed. Additional incisions may be placed in the natural creases of the nostrils to alter their size.

Step 6—See the Results

Splints and internal tubes will likely support the nose as it begins to heal for approximately one week.

While initial swelling subsides within a few weeks, it may take up to a year for your new nasal contour to fully refine.

During this time you may notice gradual changes in the appearance of your nose as it refines to a more permanent outcome. Swelling may come and go and worsen in the morning during the first year following your nose surgery.

A nose surgery procedure to improve an obstructed airway requires careful evaluation of the nasal structure as it relates to airflow and breathing. Correction of a deviated septum, one of the most common causes of breathing impairment, is achieved by adjusting the nasal structure to produce better alignment.

My Nose Surgery Recovery

After your procedure is completed, a splint, internal tubes, or packing will likely be placed inside your nose and a splint or bandages placed on the outside to support and protect the new structures during initial healing.

You will be given specific instructions to follow during your recovery from rhinoplasty: How to care for the surgical site, medications to apply or take orally to aid healing and reduce the potential for infection, specific concerns to look for at the surgical site or in your general health, and when to follow up with your plastic surgeon.

Be sure to ask your plastic surgeon specific questions about what you can expect during your individual recovery period.

- Where will I be taken after my surgery is complete?

- What medication will I be given or prescribed after surgery?

- Will I have dressings/bandages after surgery? When will they be removed?

- Are stitches removed? When?

- When can I resume normal activity and exercise?

- When do I return for follow-up care?

- How long will swelling after rhinoplasty surgery persist?

Section 34.6

Scar Revision Surgery after Injury or Previous Surgery

Enhancing Your Appearance with Scar Revision Surgery

Scars are visible signs that remain after a wound has healed. They are unavoidable results of injury or surgery, and their development can be unpredictable. Poor healing may contribute to scars that are obvious, unsightly, or disfiguring. Even a wound that heals well can result in a scar that affects your appearance. Scars may be raised or recessed, different in color or texture from surrounding healthy tissue, or particularly noticeable due to their size, shape, or location.

Your treatment options may vary based on the type and degree of scarring and can include:

- simple topical treatments;

- minimally invasive procedures;

- surgical revision with advanced techniques in wound closure.

Scar revision surgery is meant to minimize the scar so that it is more consistent with your surrounding skin tone and texture.

Although scar revision can provide a more pleasing cosmetic result or improve a scar that has healed poorly, a scar cannot be completely erased.

Is It Right for Me?

Scar revision is a highly individualized procedure and you should do it for yourself, not to fulfill someone else's desires or to try to fit any sort of ideal image. Scar revision can be performed on people of any age and is a good option for you if:

- you are bothered by a scar anywhere on your body;

- you are physically healthy;

- you do not smoke;

- you have a positive outlook and realistic goals for your scar revision surgery;

- you do not have active acne or other skin diseases in the area to be treated.

Scar Revision Surgery Risks and Safety Information

The decision to have scar revision surgery is extremely personal and you'll have to decide if the benefits will achieve your goals and if the risks and potential complications are acceptable. Your plastic surgeon and/or staff will explain in detail the risks associated with surgery.

You will be asked to sign consent forms to ensure that you fully understand the procedure you will undergo, the alternatives, and the most likely risks and potential complications.

Some of the risks include:

- bleeding (hematoma);

- infection;

- delayed healing;

- anesthesia risks;

- change in skin sensation;

- damage to deeper structures including nerves, blood vessels, muscles, and lungs can occur and may be temporary or permanent;

- allergies to tape, suture materials and glues, blood products, topical preparations, or injected agents;

- skin contour irregularities;

- skin discoloration and swelling;

- skin sensitivity;

- deep vein thrombosis, cardiac and pulmonary complications;

- pain, which may persist;

- possibility of revisional surgery or staged procedures.

Be sure to ask questions: It's very important to ask your plastic surgeon questions about your procedure. It's natural to feel some anxiety, whether it's excitement for your anticipated new look or a bit of preoperative stress. Don't be shy about discussing these feelings with your plastic surgeon.

Where Will My Surgery Be Performed?

Scar revision surgery may be performed in your plastic surgeon's office, accredited office-based surgical facility, an ambulatory surgical facility, or a hospital. Your plastic surgeon and the assisting staff will fully attend to your comfort and safety.

When your procedure is finished, bandages or dressings may be applied to keep the surgical site clean.

You will be given specific instructions that may include: How to care for yourself following surgery, medications to apply or take orally to aid healing and reduce the risk of infection, and when to follow-up with your plastic surgeon.

When You Go Home

If you experience shortness of breath, chest pains, or unusual heart beats, seek medical attention immediately. Should any of these complications occur, you may require hospitalization and additional treatment.

Be Careful

Following your physician's instructions is key to the success of your surgery. It is important that the surgical incisions are not subjected to excessive force, abrasion, or motion during the time of healing. Your doctor will give you specific instructions on how to care for yourself.

Follow all postoperative instructions carefully, including cleansing and at-home treatment regimens, and avoid sun exposure. Your cooperation will influence the outcome of your surgery.

What Happens during Scar Revision Surgery?

Step 1—Anesthesia

Medications are administered for your comfort during the surgical procedures. The choices include local anesthesia, intravenous sedation, and general anesthesia. Your doctor will recommend the best choice for you.

Step 2—The Treatment

The degree of improvement that can be achieved with scar revision will depend on the severity of your scarring, and the type, size, and location of the scar. In some cases, a single technique may provide significant improvement. However, your plastic surgeon may recommend a combination of scar revision techniques to achieve the best results.

Topical treatments, such as gels, tapes, or external compression, can help in wound closure and healing, or to reduce the ability of skin to produce irregular pigment. These products may be used to treat existing surface scars and discoloration, and to aid in healing of scar revision procedures.

Injectable treatments are often used to fill depressed or concave scars. Depending on the injectable substance used and your particular scar conditions, results may last from three months to several years. Therapy must be repeated to maintain results. One form of injection therapy uses steroidal-based compounds to reduce collagen formation and can alter the appearance, size, and texture of raised scar tissue.

Surface treatments are most often used for cosmetic improvement of scars. These methods can soften surface irregularities and reduce uneven pigmentation. Surface treatments are a controlled means of either mechanically removing the top layers of skin or changing the nature of tissue. These treatment options include:

- Dermabrasion is a mechanical polishing of the skin.

- Laser or light therapy causes changes to the surface of the skin that allow new, healthy skin to form at the scar site.

- Chemical peel solutions penetrate the skin's surface to soften irregularities in texture and color.

- Skin bleaching agents are medications applied topically to lighten the skin.

Step 3—Remove the Old Scar

Sometimes for deeper scars an incision is needed to surgically remove the old scar.

Step 4—Closing the Incisions

Some scars require layered closure. Layered closure is often used where excision extends to tissue below the skin surface or in areas with a high degree of movement. The first step, or layer, requires sub-dermal closure (below the skin surface) with absorbable or non-removable sutures. Layers of closure continue to build, concluding with closure of the remaining surface wound.

Advanced techniques in scar revision include complex flap closure to reposition a scar so that it is less conspicuous, or improve flexibility where contracture has restricted mobility.

Pharmaceutical tissue substitutes may be used if ample healthy tissue is not present for closure of a scar excision. This is more likely with revision of severe burn scars.

Tissue expansion can be a substitute for skin grafts. In this procedure, an inflatable balloon called a tissue expander is placed under the skin near the scar site. Over time, the balloon is slowly filled with sterile solution to expand the area of healthy skin. Once the skin has been stretched sufficiently, the expander and the scar is removed and the stretched skin is moved to replace the scar tissue. This process can involve multiple surgical stages or procedures in order to achieve the final results.

Scar Revision Recovery

Progress and Healing

The initial healing phase of a surgical scar revision may include localized swelling, discoloration, or discomfort and may take one to two weeks. Healing will continue for several weeks and as the new scar heals it will slowly refine and fade. With dermabrasion, chemical peel, or laser resurfacing, you will experience similar conditions at the treated area, in addition to overall sensitivity.

The Results Will Be Long-Lasting

The final results of your scar revision surgery will be long-lasting, however it may take several months for your final results to become apparent and in some cases it may take a year for the new scar to fully heal and fade.

The practice of medicine and surgery is not an exact science. Although good results are expected, there is no guarantee, in some situations, it may not be possible to achieve optimal results with a single surgical procedure and another surgery may be necessary.

Section 34.7

Skin Graft Surgery

"Skin graft," © 2012 A.D.A.M., Inc. Reprinted with permission.

A skin graft is a patch of skin that is removed by surgery from one area of the body and transplanted, or attached, to another area.

Description

Your surgery will probably be done while you are under general anesthesia (you will be unconscious and will not feel pain).

Healthy skin is taken from a place on your body called the donor site. Most people who are having a skin graft have a split-thickness skin graft. This takes the two top layers of skin from the donor site (the epidermis) and the layer under the epidermis (the dermis).

The donor site can be any area of the body. Most times, it is an area that is hidden by clothes, such as the buttock or inner thigh.

The graft is carefully spread on the bare area where it is being transplanted. It is held in place either by gentle pressure from a well-padded dressing that covers it, or by staples or a few small stitches. The donor-site area is covered with a sterile dressing for three to five days.

People with deeper tissue loss may need a full-thickness skin graft. This requires an entire thickness of skin from the donor site, not just the top two layers.

A full-thickness skin graft is a more complicated procedure. The flap of skin from the donor site includes the muscles and blood supply. It is transplanted to the area of the graft. Common donor sites for full-thickness skin grafts include the chest wall, back, or abdominal wall.

Why the Procedure Is Performed

Skin grafts may be recommended for:

- areas where there has been infection that caused a large amount of skin loss;

- burns;

461

- cosmetic reasons or reconstructive surgeries where there has been skin damage or skin loss;
- skin cancer surgery;
- surgeries that need skin grafts to heal;
- venous ulcers, pressure ulcers, or diabetic ulcers that do not heal;
- very large wounds;
- when the surgeon is unable to close a wound properly.

Full-thickness grafts are done when a lot of tissue is lost. This can happen with open fractures of the lower leg, or after severe infections.

Risks

Risks for any anesthesia are:

- reactions to medicines;
- problems with breathing.

Risks for this surgery are:

- bleeding;
- chronic pain (rarely);
- infection;
- loss of grafted skin (the graft not healing, or the graft healing slowly);
- reduced or lost skin sensation, or increased sensitivity;
- scarring;
- skin discoloration;
- uneven skin surface.

Before the Procedure

Always tell your doctor or nurse:

- what drugs you are taking, even drugs or herbs you bought without a prescription;
- if you have been drinking a lot of alcohol.

During the days before your surgery:

- You may be asked to stop taking aspirin, ibuprofen, warfarin (Coumadin), and any other drugs that make it hard for your blood to clot.
- Ask your doctor which drugs you should still take on the day of your surgery.
- If you smoke, try to stop.

If you have diabetes, follow your diet and take your medicines as usual.

On the day of the surgery:

- Usually you will be asked not to drink or eat anything for 8 to 12 hours before the surgery.
- Take the drugs your doctor told you to take with a small sip of water.

Prepare your home. Plan to have the help you will need from your spouse, a friend, or a neighbor.

Make sure the bathroom and the rest of the house are set up safely so that you do not trip or fall. Make sure you can get in and out of your house easily.

After the Procedure

You should recover quickly after split-thickness skin grafting, except in cases of major burns. The skin graft must be protected from trauma, such as being hit, or heavy stretching for at least two to three weeks.

Depending on the location of the graft, you may need to wear a dressing for one to two weeks. Avoid exercise that might stretch or injure the graft for three to four weeks. Some people need physical therapy after their skin graft.

Full-thickness grafts need a longer recovery period. Most people with these grafts need to stay in the hospital for one to two weeks.

Outlook (Prognosis)

New blood vessels begin growing within 36 hours. Most skin grafts are successful, but some do not heal well. You may need a second graft.

Section 34.8

Surgery for Facial Injuries

"Facial trauma," © 2012 A.D.A.M., Inc. Reprinted with permission.

Facial trauma is any injury of the face and upper jaw bone (maxilla).

Causes

Blunt or penetrating trauma can cause injury to the area of the face that includes the upper jaw, lower jaw, cheek, nose, or forehead. Common causes of injury to the face include:

- automobile accidents;
- penetrating injuries;
- violence.

Symptoms

- Changes in sensation and feeling over the face
- Deformed or uneven face or facial bones
- Difficulty breathing through the nose due to swelling and bleeding
- Double vision
- Missing teeth
- Swelling around the eyes that may cause vision problems

Exams and Tests

The doctor will perform a physical exam, which may show:

- bleeding from the nose, eyes, or mouth, or nasal blockage;
- breaks in the skin (lacerations);
- bruising around the eyes or widening of the distance between the eyes, which may mean injury to the bones between the eye sockets.

The following may suggest bone fractures:

- Abnormal sensations on the cheek and irregularities that can be felt

- An upper jaw that moves when the head is still

A CT scan of the head may be done.

Treatment

Patients who cannot function normally or who have significant deformity will need surgery.

The goal of treatment is to:

- control bleeding;

- create a clear airway;

- fix broken bone segments with titanium plates and screws;

- leave the fewest scars possible;

- rule out other injuries;

- treat the fracture.

Treatment should be immediate, as long as the person is stable and there are no neck fractures or life-threatening injuries.

Outlook (Prognosis)

Patients generally do very well with proper treatment. You will probably look different than you did before your injury. You may need to have more surgery 6–12 months later.

Possible Complications

General complications include, but are not limited to:

- bleeding;

- uneven face;

- infection;

- brain and nervous system problems;

- numbness or weakness;

- loss of vision or double vision;

When to Contact a Medical Professional

Go to the emergency room or call the local emergency number (such as 911) if you have a severe injury to your face.

Prevention

Wear seat belts and use protective head gear when appropriate. Avoid violent confrontations with other people.

Section 34.9

Surgery for Skin Cancer

Hearing a diagnosis of cancer is very difficult to accept. Understanding that treating your skin cancer may result in scars or disfigurement can also be troubling. Your plastic surgeon understands your concerns and will guide you through treatment and explain the resulting effect on your health and appearance.

Quick facts about skin cancer treatment:

- Treatment of skin cancer, much like any form of cancer, may require surgery to remove cancerous growths.

- Your plastic surgeon can surgically remove cancerous and other skin lesions using specialized techniques to preserve your health and your appearance.

- Although no surgery is without scars, your plastic surgeon will make every effort to treat your skin cancer without dramatically changing your appearance.

- For some people, reconstruction may require more than one procedure to achieve the best results.

Skin Cancer Surgery Risks and Safety Information

The decision to have skin cancer surgery is extremely personal. Your physician will explain all of the potential risks. Your plastic surgeon and/or staff will explain in detail the risks associated with surgery. You will be asked to sign consent forms to ensure that you fully understand the procedure you will undergo, the alternatives, and the most likely risks and potential complications.

Possible risks include:

- bleeding (hematoma);

- infection;

- poor healing of incisions;

- anesthesia risks;

- unfavorable scarring;

- frozen-section inaccuracy;

- recurrence of skin cancer;

- systemic spread of skin cancer;

- change in skin sensation;

- skin contour irregularities;

- skin discoloration/swelling;

- allergies to tape, suture materials and glues, blood products, topical preparations, or injected agents;

- damage to deeper structures— such as nerves, blood vessels, muscles, and lungs—can occur and may be temporary or permanent;

- pain, which may persist;

- possibility of revisional surgery.

Be sure to ask questions: It's very important to ask your plastic surgeon questions about your procedure. It's natural to feel some anxiety; don't be shy about discussing these feelings with your plastic surgeon.

Other important considerations: Skin grafts have an added risk that the graft will not take and therefore additional surgery may be necessary to close the wound.

Preserve your health: Once you have been diagnosed with skin cancer, you are at a higher risk to develop another skin cancer than the general population. Skin cancer also can reoccur. So, it's important to discuss the signs of skin cancer with your physician, regularly perform self-examinations for suspicious lesions, and schedule an annual skin cancer screening.

Be careful: Following your physician's instructions is key to the success of your surgery. It is important that the surgical incisions are not subjected to excessive force, abrasion, or motion during the time of healing. Your doctor will give you specific instructions on how to care for yourself.

Preparing for Surgery

Prior to surgery, you may be asked to:

- get lab testing or a medical evaluation;
- take certain medications or adjust your current medications;
- stop smoking well in advance of surgery;
- avoid taking aspirin, anti-inflammatory drugs, and herbal supplements as they can increase bleeding.

Special instructions you receive will cover:

- what to do on the day of surgery;
- the use of anesthesia during your skin cancer surgery;
- postoperative care and follow-up.

Your plastic surgeon will also discuss where your procedure will be performed. Skin cancer surgery may be performed in an accredited outpatient or ambulatory surgical center, or a hospital.

You'll need help: If your procedure is performed on an outpatient basis, be sure to arrange for someone to drive you home after surgery and to stay with you for at least the first night following surgery.

What Happens during Skin Cancer Surgery?

Depending on the size, type, and location of the lesion, there are many ways to remove skin cancer and reconstruct your appearance if necessary.

Step 1: Anesthesia

Medications are administered for your comfort during the surgical procedures. The choices include local, intravenous sedation and general anesthesia. Your doctor will recommend the best choice for you.

Step 2: Removal

A small or contained lesion may be removed with excision—a simple surgical process to remove the lesion from the skin. Closure is most often performed in conjunction with excision.

Skin cancer can be like an iceberg. What is visible on the skin surface sometimes is only a small portion of the growth. Beneath the skin, the cancerous cells cover a much larger region and there are no defined borders. In these cases, a specialized technique called Mohs surgery may be recommended.

Your plastic surgeon may order a frozen section. In this procedure, the cancerous lesion is removed and microscopically examined by a pathologist prior to wound closure to ensure all cancerous cells have been removed.

The goal is to look for a clear margin—an area where the skin cancer has not spread. If clear margins are found, the resulting wound would be reconstructed. If clear margins are not present, your plastic surgeon will remove more tissues until the entire region has a clear margin.

Step 3: Reconstruction

A large lesion or one that has been removed with frozen sections can be reconstructed with a local flap. A flap may also be necessary where excision may result in a disfiguring appearance. A local flap repositions healthy, adjacent tissue over the wound. A suture line is positioned to follow the natural creases and curves of the face if possible, to minimize the appearance of the resulting scar.

A skin graft, healthy skin removed from one area of the body and relocated to the wound site, may also be applied.

Step 4: See the Results

After your skin cancer has been removed and any primary reconstruction is completed, a dressing or bandages will be applied to your incisions.

Skin Cancer Surgery Recovery

Following your skin cancer surgery, incision sites may be sore, red, or drain small amounts of fluid.

- It is important to follow all wound care instructions such as cleansing and applying topical medications exactly as directed.

- You may be able to return to light activity the day of your surgery.

- Make certain to keep your incision sites clean and well protected from potential injury.

- Try to limit movement that may stress your wound and your sutures.

Be sure to ask your plastic surgeon specific questions about what you can expect during your individual recovery period.

- Where will I be taken after my surgery is complete?

- What medication will I be given or prescribed after surgery?

- Will I have dressings/bandages after surgery? When will they be removed?

- Are stitches removed? When?

- When can I resume normal activity and exercise?

- When do I return for follow-up care?

Healing will continue for many weeks or months as incision lines continue to improve. It may take a year or more following a given procedure for incision lines to refine and fade to some degree. In some cases, secondary procedures may be required to complete or refine your reconstruction.

Practice diligent sun protection every day of your life and quit smoking to ensure continued healing and good health. Sun exposure on healing wounds may result in irregular pigmentation and scars that can become raised, red, or dark. Sun exposure may result in a recurrence of your skin cancer, or the development of skin cancer in another region of your body.

Chapter 35

Organ Transplant Surgery

Preparing for Your Transplant

Each person's journey to transplant is unique. Some people wait for extended periods of time, hoping for the day when they will be called for a transplant. Others come to transplant with compatible living donor candidates and move quickly to surgery and life with their new organ.

No matter the circumstances, nearly everyone finds it difficult to completely absorb that they have an end-stage disease that can best be treated with a transplant.

The fear and anxiety that nearly every transplant candidate feels are further compounded by the complex system for transplant evaluation and organ matching. To make the process easier to understand, here's what you can expect when your doctor recommends that you be evaluated for a transplant and refers you to a transplant center.

The Transplant Process

1. You are evaluated for a transplant by the medical team at a transplant center.

Excerpted from "Talking about Transplantation: What Every Patient Needs to Know," © 2011 United Network for Organ Sharing (www.unos.org). These materials were originally developed by United Network for Organ Sharing (UNOS), under contract with the Health Resource Services Administration and originally published using a grant from Astellas. These materials are reprinted with permission of UNOS.

471

2. If accepted as a transplant candidate, you are registered on the national organ transplant waiting list. A living donor may also be identified and evaluated for living donation.

3. You begin organizing your support system.

4. You begin developing your financial strategy.

5. Your waiting period begins.

6. Your transplant takes place.

7. Your medical team manages your posttransplant care.

In the following text is presented step-by-step instructions to get you started, based on experiences of transplant recipients and their donors.

Transplant Centers

A transplant center is a hospital that has staff that specializes in transplant medicine.

Your primary doctor or organ specialist can refer you to a transplant center that:

• is near your home;

• specializes in your medical situation;

• accepts your insurance.

Choosing a Transplant Center

One of the biggest decisions you will make as a transplant candidate is choosing a transplant center. There are nearly 250 transplant centers in the United States and all of them must meet strict professional standards. Go to http://optn.transplant.hrsa.gov (click on Members>Member Directory) to access transplant center listings and links. Many patients simply choose the facility closest to them, but there are several questions to ask when choosing a transplant center:

• Can you easily reach the transplant center for all appointments before and after the transplant?

• Can you easily reach the transplant center when called to receive an organ?

• If the center is a distance from your home, can your caregivers stay near the transplant center without causing an undue burden?

- Is the center within the network of your health insurance?

- Do you feel comfortable with the transplant team?

For more information, call UNOS patient services at 888-894-6361 or go to www.transplantliving.org.

For More Information

When choosing a transplant center, you may want to compare the number of transplants performed, waiting list size, and survival rates at the centers you are considering. There is more data available to patients about transplants than for other procedures.

- Go to http://optn.transplant.hrsa.gov (click on Data>View Data Reports>Center Data) for the number of transplants and waiting list size by center.

- Visit www.srtr.org for median wait time and survival rates by center.

The Transplant Evaluation

The transplant evaluation process involves long days of tests and clinic visits and can be stressful.

The transplant team will test every major system in your body. Tests could find other medical conditions that could complicate your transplant or make it less likely to succeed.

It's perfectly normal to feel anxious or vulnerable, like your life is in the hands of the medical team.

They understand and can help. These are some questions to ask as you go through the process.

Questions for the Transplant Center and Team

- Do I have choices other than transplantation?

- What are the benefits and risks of transplantation?

- What are your criteria for accepting organs for transplant?

- Who are the members of the transplant team, and what do they do?

- How many surgeons are available here to do my type of transplant?

- How do I find out about the transplant process?

- Is there a special hospital unit for transplant patients?

- May I tour the transplant center's units?

- Will I be asked to take part in research studies?

- What are the organ and patient survival rates for my type of transplant at this hospital?

- How many of my type of transplant do you perform each year? How long have you been doing them?

Questions about Your Evaluation

- What should I bring with me?

- What should I do to prepare for the appointment?

- Does your center offer parking permits or overnight accommodations?

- What does the evaluation and testing process include? How does it affect whether I am put on the list?

Financial Questions

- What part of the transplant cost is covered by my insurance?

- What if my insurance does not pay for medications?

- What financial coverage is accepted by this hospital?

- What happens if my financial coverage runs out?

- How much will I have to pay in the end?

Questions about Living Donation

- What types of living donor transplants does the center do? Is a living donor transplant a choice in my case? If so, where can the living donor evaluation occur?

- What are the costs if I have a living donor?

Write your questions down and bring them to the appointment. You might also want to bring a trusted friend or family member with you and ask them to take notes.

The Standard Transplant Evaluation

The standard transplant evaluation usually includes the following tests:

- blood typing;
- tissue typing;
- dental exam;
- chest X-ray;
- cardiac work-up;
- pulmonary work-up;
- infectious disease testing;
- gender-specific testing;
- psychological evaluation to determine emotional preparedness;
- evaluation of social and financial supports and ability to care for yourself and your new organ after transplant.

Other testing may be required depending on the organ you need and your health history.

After the Evaluation

You will likely receive a huge amount of information during your evaluation. Afterward, spend some time alone to let it all sink in. It may also be helpful to talk with others who have had a transplant. This is a good way to spend your time as you wait for insurance approval and test results.

It is normal to feel unsure if you want a transplant, even though you may need one. You may doubt your ability to get through the process. Or you may be frozen with fear. Your transplant team is there for you. It is okay if you decide that a transplant is not for you—it is your decision to make.

The Waiting List

The waiting list is a computer database that contains medical information on every person who is waiting for any type of organ transplant in the United States and Puerto Rico. You will not have a number ranking for transplant based on all the other persons who are waiting for your organ.

You also will not move up or down each time someone receives a transplant.

Each organ has different criteria for allocation, but wealth, social status, and citizenship are never factors. To learn more about OPTN/

UNOS policies, visit http://optn.transplant.hrsa.gov (click on Policy Management>Policies).

- Livers: Medical test results and geography determine priority for transplant.

- Hearts, lungs, intestines: Priority is based on clinical or medical status and geography.

- Kidneys and pancreata: Waiting time is a factor, but others such as tissue type matching are also considered.

You're on the List

Congratulations. The evaluation is over and you're on the organ transplant waiting list. Your transplant center will confirm your waiting list status in writing, and they will do so any time there is a change in status. It is normal to feel relief and hope, and also fear and regret.

Now the waiting begins. Waiting for a donor organ can be stressful, since you don't know how long that wait will be. Now is the time to mobilize your resources so you're ready when the call comes.

While you wait, others may get their transplants quickly. Transplant is not a first-come, first served process. Organ allocation is based on many criteria. Often a sicker patient will get an organ in a very short time. Each patient is unique and is handled as such.

Being on the waiting list simply means that your transplant team found you to be a good candidate for transplant and you're being considered for organs.

Multiple Listing

After talking with staff and other patients and doing your own research, you may decide to be on the waiting list at more than one center. Listing at centers in different geographic regions can provide advantages:

- You will have access to multiple donor pools.

- There may be different rules in other regions (pilot projects or other agreements).

- Average wait times for your organ may be shorter in another region.

Each center decides who it accepts as a candidate and a center can refuse patients who are listed elsewhere. Every center can require that tests be redone at their own center. Insurance may not pay for duplicate tests so confirm your health plan's stance on coverage before going forward.

Inform both your primary center and any others you contact of your plans. There is no advantage to listing at more than one transplant center in the same OPO's local service area. Waiting time starts after a center evaluates you and adds you to the list.

Transferring Waiting Time

If you would like to change transplant centers, you can transfer your primary waiting time to the new center when you list there. Notify your original center that you want to transfer to a new one, so they can remove you from that center's list.

What If I Am Not Accepted?

Ask your transplant team about your options. You may need to manage other medical conditions first. You may be too healthy for a transplant now but might need one in the future. You may still be a candidate at another transplant center. If a transplant is not an option, you should commend yourself on putting forth your best effort to survive. This may now be a time for personal, spiritual, and emotional reflection.

What If I Have a Living Donor?

If your transplant center identifies you as a good candidate and you also have a compatible living donor, the center will work with you and your donor to coordinate surgery. The timing of your transplant depends on your and your donor's health, the schedules of all involved, and administrative factors like the availability of operating rooms.

For more information on living donation, go to www.transplant living.org.

Preparing for Your Transplant

Wait times for transplants vary. Not everyone who needs a transplant will get one. Because of the shortage of organs that are suitable for donation, only slightly more than 50% of people on the waiting list will receive an organ within five years.

After your evaluation, it's important to prepare for your transplant while you are waiting. Work closely with your transplant team. Keep all scheduled appointments. Build a solid support system of family, friends, clergy, and medical professionals. Let people know what's going on in your life. They can be a tremendous source of support and information. Taking these steps puts you in control.

To help yourself prepare, address the following areas:

- Medical

- Practical

- Emotional

- Educational

- Financial

- Spiritual

Preparing Yourself Medically

While you are on the waiting list, your transplant team will monitor you continuously to make sure you remain suitable for transplant. If your condition improves or complications arise, you may be taken off the transplant list. Always discuss any concerns with your transplant team. If you need to make lifestyle changes before getting a transplant, you should continue with them after your transplant to ensure the best outcome.

Remaining healthy and active before the transplant will make recovery easier.

- Take care of your health. Take your prescribed medicines. Notify your transplant coordinator about all of your health issues and any other prescriptions.

- Keep your scheduled appointments with your physicians. Until your transplant, you will need to meet with the transplant team so that they can evaluate your overall health.

- Follow diet and exercise guidelines. Weight management is important while waiting for your transplant. A dietician and physical therapist can help you develop a program that will give you the best results. Ask about ways to reduce the use of painkillers and how to manage issues with alcohol, tobacco, or drugs.

- Make sure you are available. Your transplant team needs to know how to reach you at all times. Cell phones, pagers, or answering machines may be required by your transplant center. Your transplant coordinator may ask you to stay within a certain geographic range.

- Complete medical tests and procedures. Ask your transplant team about other elective or required surgeries (not related to your organ failure) before your transplant.

- Women of childbearing age: Ask your medical team about birth control and pregnancy and what precautions you should take before and after your transplant.

- Stay organized. Keep a binder of your records to help you manage your medical information.

- Stay in contact with your transplant team to learn about your waiting list status.

Preparing Yourself Practically

- Select your primary support person. Choose someone you feel close to who has the time, health, and flexibility to be your caregiver. You need to know you are a not a burden to this person.

- Prepare a phone/email tree. This will make it easier for your caregiver to update friends and family and cut down on phone or email volume.

- Organize your personal affairs. Consider filling out an advanced directive, writing a will, and sharing access to bank accounts, email, or blogs. You may also need to fill out Family Medical Leave Act, insurance, or loan deferment paperwork.

- Consider dependent care. Find someone you trust and set up a plan to take care of your children and/or pets. Ask your doctor when you can expect to see your children and pets after your transplant.

- Arrange transportation. When you are on the organ waiting list, your first responsibility is to plan how to get to the transplant center quickly when you get the call that an organ is available. Make arrangements well in advance.

- Plan the driving route and think about traffic conditions. If you are relocating, make housing arrangements in advance.

- Pack your bags. You'll need to be ready to leave as soon as you get the call that an organ is available. Include insurance information, a list of medications, an extra 24-hour supply of medication, and other necessities.

Preparing Yourself Emotionally

Many portrayals of the transplant process in the media are inaccurate or sensationalized. In the real world you get sick, you wait, and hopefully, you get a transplant. Your transplant team should be the main source of information about your care. You'll find a wealth of information on www.transplantliving.org, a UNOS website designed for transplant candidates, patients, and loved ones.

Preparing Yourself Educationally

Transplantation is a whole new world with a whole new language to learn—one filled with medical terms, abbreviations, and acronyms. The best way to navigate this world is to choose to become a lifelong learner. Carefully review any educational materials provided by your transplant center. Many organ- or disease-specific organizations provide patient education. This text is just one example of the patient-focused resources that are available through UNOS. Join a transplant support group, either in person or online, for information and support. As you learn about the transplant and what to expect, you will gain control of your transplant experience and your life. Education leads to empowerment.

For more information go to www.transplantliving.org or www.unos.org (click on Donation & Transplantation>Patient Education), or to request printed materials call 888-894-6361.

Preparing Yourself Financially

Major health problems can impact your finances. Success in transplant includes having a realistic financial plan. It can be scary to face concerns about loss of income, employment, or insurance; high medical bills; and the need to apply for financial help. Yet facing these possibilities helps you gain a degree of control over the unimaginable.

A good financial plan begins by talking with your loved ones about your situation. Also inform your transplant team about financial issues of your transplant.

Preparing Yourself Spiritually

Spiritual growth and challenges await many transplant candidates and recipients. Some find that life-threatening illness makes them question their faith; others find their faith strengthened through the transplant process. Your second chance at a healthy life may come with the knowledge that another life was lost. Receiving a donor organ may create a sense of spiritual rebirth. This may create a profound change in your beliefs, and spiritual guidance and counseling can help you deal with these issues. Just as every patient has different medical issues, spiritual needs vary as well. Talking to your pastor, your rabbi, or the hospital chaplain may help.

Preparing for Your Loved One's Transplant

A caregiver may be a family member or friend. Some caregivers have been supporting a medically fragile loved one for years. The transplant team social worker may be able to suggest resources for caregivers, but here are some basic tips:

- Physical health: Ask the transplant team and your own doctor what you need to do to stay healthy in your care-giving role, such as using medications or vaccinations. Make sure you are in good physical condition.

- Mental health: Spending time with one person can be the best of times and the worst of times. Make sure you arrange some respite time to take a walk, call friends, or do something for yourself. This can keep you from feeling burned out.

- Living arrangements: Where will you stay while the patient is in the hospital? If you are away from home, be sure your mail and phone calls are forwarded and you've packed necessities.

- Support network: Caregivers need support too. Find people to help you with respite care, errands, or meals. The best resource for caregivers may be other caregivers who have survived a transplant. Ask your social worker if your transplant center offers these types of support groups.

- Financial arrangements: Make financial and insurance plans or take leave from work or other duties.

- Manage expectations: To avoid questions and stress later, find out the hospital's visiting hours, limits on visitation, storage, parking, hygiene requirements, and cafeteria hours.

- Saying no: Being a caregiver is a great reason to cut back on other responsibilities and de-stress your life. You have enough on your plate.

A transplant is a life-saving gift for both the recipient and the caregiver. It is what you have hoped for during the long wait and time of illness. Transplant is not only life-saving; it is life-altering.

A transplant will help the patient become more independent so he can return to work and other activities. For the caregiver, transplant may mean a big change in roles. This can bring on feelings of sadness, resentment, and stress. All of this is perfectly normal and can be resolved with open communication and a little adjustment time.

If more is required, talk to your transplant social worker about counseling and support groups.

Receiving the Call

Answer your phone at all times of day and night, especially if it's from the hospital. If they call to tell you that an organ is available, you will likely have to stop eating and drinking to get ready for surgery. You may wish to shower or bathe. You may be asked whether you have a cold, cough, fever, or other infection. Your doctor will explain which medications and treatments to stop or continue.

You will be asked to go to the hospital within a certain window of time. Plan ahead and have directions to the hospital handy, and find out where to park. Ask where your caregiver will stay during the surgery. Bring the bag you packed and your insurance card. Your caregiver should also bring his or her packed bag. When you arrive at the hospital, be ready for medical tests and possibly a long wait for surgery.

You may feel a surge of adrenalin, excitement, eagerness, a peaceful state of readiness, or a sense of dread, shock, and disbelief. You may also feel sadness for the family who lost someone at the same moment you are thrilled to receive the gift of life. All of these feelings are normal.

After receiving the call, contact your support person to make sure he or she can be with you.

Your support person can help you contact other close family or friends and take care of children, pets, and other matters such as paying bills.

A Dry Run

Sometimes an organ may be evaluated more closely after you've arrived at the hospital, and it is found to be in poor condition for transplant.

You could be told that you will not receive a transplant and must go home. This can be very disappointing after a long wait. Your transplant team is looking out for your best interests and outcome, and maybe this organ just wasn't right for you. Be patient.

One patient suggested thinking of this waiting time as a sort of sabbatical during which you get to consider your plans and goals for the potentially "very long and reasonably healthy life" you will have after transplant.

The Surgery

Transplant surgery can last from four to nine hours, but each transplant is unique. Most patients are placed on a breathing machine.

You will likely spend some time in intensive care or intermediate care. It is normal to go through some challenges, which your medical team will manage. Everyone adjusts to surgery and medications differently. Ask your transplant team when you can expect to eat, walk, use the bathroom, and go home after transplant.

Going Home

Going home after a transplant is something to celebrate. You made it through the hardest part, and now you can start to recover and live again.

Make sure you and your caregiver know your medication routine, clinic visit schedule, and diet and exercise restrictions. Ask your medical team what your caregiver needs to do to prepare your home for your arrival for your health and safety.

Most patients feel more like themselves within six months of transplant, although this varies by age, health, and the organ they receive.

Life after Transplant

Every transplant candidate has a dream of what life will be like on the day after transplant surgery. Those dreams can be both thrilling and frightening, so it helps to know what you might expect.

Transplant recipients will tell you two truths: No two transplants are alike, and a transplant is not a cure. Even after your transplant, you may still have a serious chronic illness that must be closely managed.

Immediately after Transplant

After dealing with the effects of long-term illness (lack of energy, shortness of breath), you may feel euphoric when you awake after surgery to find those symptoms gone. Anesthesia often protects you from post-surgical pain for a short time. Follow your team's pain management instructions to make the overall experience as comfortable as possible.

Transplant is major surgery. It may take time to get back to eating normally, moving around, and managing your own care. Don't be discouraged.

Most recipients report feeling much better just after transplant. Others take longer to feel better, move around, and manage their care. Remember that you now have a functioning organ, which gives you a new lease on life.

Going Home

There is no set time when people go home after transplant. These factors can affect how soon you will be able to go home:

- The organ that you received; recovery for each organ is different
- Your overall health status and ability to take care of yourself
- Your lab results
- Other chronic health problems
- Availability of support at home

After you are discharged from the hospital, here are a few things to expect.

Medications

Immunosuppressants, or anti-rejection medications, "hide" your new transplanted organ from your body's immune system to protect it from being attacked and destroyed. Take these and other medications just as your doctor prescribes.

Talk to your transplant team before making any changes. You will take immunosuppressants for the lifetime of your transplanted organ. Visit www.transplantliving.org (click on After the Transplant> Medications) for more information.

You also will take other medications to help the immunosuppressants to do their job, or to control side effects. You may need medications for other chronic health problems. In the beginning it seems like you are taking lots and lots of medications, but this likely will change as you recover.

Doctor Visits and Wellness Appointments

In the first few months after transplant, you will visit with your transplant team frequently to be sure that your new organ is functioning well and to help you develop good health habits. A big part of keeping your new organ healthy means keeping your body as healthy as possible. Keeping all wellness appointments will help you meet this goal.

- Keep up with other check-ups—dental, gender specific, eye exams.

- Monitor your blood pressure, weight, and cholesterol.

- Get all recommended health screenings on schedule.

Get Moving

Every person is different. The amount and type of activity you can handle after your transplant depends on your age and health. The goal is still to get moving. For one person, moving may mean sitting up in a chair. For another, it might mean walking several times a day. If moving is challenging, your transplant team may prescribe physical rehabilitation to get you started in the safest manner possible. Rehabilitation may be done at home or at an outpatient facility.

Sometimes a stay in a rehab facility is necessary. Don't be alarmed if you need rehab. It is one resource your transplant team uses to get you back to a more normal life. Once you have found your new normal, keep exercising so that you stay as fit as possible.

Lifestyle Changes

You may be able to return to activities that you gave up because of your illness. Many people return to playing sports, gardening, or hiking.

Remember, don't start or resume any activity without getting approval from your transplant doctor first.

After transplant you may need to change your diet. You may need to drink more water. You'll need to get laboratory tests done frequently. If you are a kidney recipient, you won't go to dialysis anymore. This is a good time to curb cigarette or alcohol use.

Back to Work or School

Many people go back to their jobs or classes, or even start new careers based on insights gained during their transplant journey. Vocational rehabilitation helps people who have been out of the workforce because of a disability get assistance that allows them to go back to work.

Ask your transplant social worker about vocational rehabilitation services in your state.

Physical Changes and Challenges

It is common to have at least one episode of rejection, when your body attacks the newly transplanted organ. Rejection is a very scary word, but it doesn't always mean you are losing your transplanted organ. Your transplant team knows how to manage rejection with medication.

After treatment, most people live normally with their transplanted organ. Other complications may require re-hospitalization.

Going back into the hospital allows you to be properly monitored and treated so that you can get healthy quickly.

Many transplant patients experience annoying short-term side effects from the anti-rejection medications—hair growth, acne, mood swings, and weight gain, to name a few. Symptoms diminish as the initial high dose of medications is tapered down in the early months after transplant. Talk with your transplant team about your concerns.

Relationship Changes

While you were ill, family members and friends may have managed many things for you or helped you with your care. After your transplant, you may be able to handle more of these issues on your own. As you change and feel better, everyone will have to adapt their thoughts and behaviors to a new you.

Before your transplant, sexual activity may have been out of the question. Now that you feel better, you may be ready to reconsider. Talk to your transplant team before resuming sexual activity. Open communication will be important to maintaining good relationships.

Take It All In

It may be difficult to absorb all that has happened. If you received an organ from a deceased donor, you may feel sad or guilty because someone else died so that you could have a chance at a healthier life. Take advantage of emotional and spiritual supports to help you understand how you feel about your transplant.

Communicate with Your Donor or Donor Family

When you are ready, you may want to express your feelings to or about your donor. If you received your organ from an unknown deceased donor, you could write a letter to the donor family.

Your transplant team can help get your letter or other communication to a living donor or donor family.

Pay It Forward

Your transplant is an awesome gift. You can never truly repay your donor, but you can honor the sacrifice that was made:

- Take good care of yourself and your new organ.

    - Take your medications.

    - Exercise.

    - Keep up with wellness checks.

- Get involved in promoting organ and tissue donation in your community so that someone else can receive the same wonderful gift.

Chapter 36

Emergency, Critical Care, or Traumatic Surgery

Chapter Contents

Section 36.1

Amputation Surgery

Traumatic amputation is the loss of a body part—usually a finger, toe, arm, or leg—that occurs as the result of an accident or injury.

Considerations

If an accident or trauma results in complete amputation (the body part is totally severed), the part sometimes can be reattached, especially when proper care is taken of the severed part and stump.

In a partial amputation, some soft-tissue connection remains. Depending on the severity of the injury, the partially severed extremity may or may not be able to be reattached.

There are various complications associated with amputation of a body part. The most important of these are bleeding, shock, and infection.

The long-term outcome for amputees has improved due to better understanding of the management of traumatic amputation, early emergency and critical care management, new surgical techniques, early rehabilitation, and new prosthetic designs. New limb replantation techniques have been moderately successful, but incomplete nerve regeneration remains a major limiting factor.

Often, the patient will have a better outcome from having a well-fitting, functional prosthesis than a nonfunctional replanted limb.

Causes

Traumatic amputations usually result directly from factory, farm, or power tool accidents or from motor vehicle accidents. Natural disasters, war, and terrorist attacks can also cause traumatic amputations.

Symptoms

- A body part that has been completely or partially cut off

- Bleeding (may be minimal or severe, depending on the location and nature of the injury)

- Pain (the degree of pain is not always related to the severity of the injury or the amount of bleeding)

- Crushed body tissue (badly mangled, but still partially attached by muscle, bone, tendon, or skin)

First Aid

1. Check the person's airway (open if necessary); check breathing and circulation. If necessary, begin rescue breathing, CPR [cardiopulmonary resuscitation], or bleeding control.

2. Try to calm and reassure the person as much as possible. Amputation is painful and extremely frightening.

3. Control bleeding by applying direct pressure to the wound. Raise the injured area. If the bleeding continues, recheck the source of the bleeding and reapply direct pressure, with help from someone who is not tired. If the person has life-threatening bleeding, a tight bandage or tourniquet will be easier to use than direct pressure on the wound. However, using a tight bandage for a long time may do more harm than good.

4. Save any severed body parts and make sure they stay with the patient. Remove any dirty material that can contaminate the wound, if possible. Gently rinse the body part if the cut end is dirty.

5. Wrap the severed part in a clean, damp cloth, place it in a sealed plastic bag and place the bag in ice cold water.

6. Do not directly put the body part in water without using a plastic bag.

7. Do not put the severed part directly on ice. Do not use dry ice as this will cause frostbite and injury to the part.

8. If cold water is not available, keep the part away from heat as much as possible. Save it for the medical team, or take it to the hospital. Cooling the severed part will keep it useable for about 18 hours. Without cooling, it will only remain useable for about four to six hours.

9. Keep the patient warm.

10. Take steps to prevent shock. Lay the person flat, raise the feet about 12 inches, and cover the person with a coat or blanket. Do not place the person in this position if a head, neck, back, or leg injury is suspected or if it makes the victim uncomfortable.

11. Once the bleeding is under control, check the person for other signs of injury that require emergency treatment. Treat fractures, additional cuts, and other injuries appropriately.

12. Stay with the person until medical help arrives.

Do Not

- Do not forget that saving the person's life is more important than saving a body part.

- Do not overlook other, less obvious, injuries.

- Do not attempt to push any part back into place.

- Do not decide that a body part is too small to save.

- Do not place a tourniquet, unless the bleeding is life threatening, as the entire limb may be harmed.

- Do not raise false hopes of reattachment.

When to Contact a Medical Professional

If someone severs a limb, finger, toe, or other body part, you should call immediately for emergency medical help.

Prevention

Use safety equipment when using factory, farm, or power tools. Wear seat belts when driving a motor vehicle. Always use good judgment and observe appropriate safety precautions.

Section 36.2

Chest Tube Thoracostomy

Chest tube thoracostomy, commonly referred to as "putting in a chest tube," is a procedure that is done to drain fluid, blood, or air from the space around the lungs. This procedure may be done when a patient has a disease, such as pneumonia or cancer, that causes extra fluid to build up in the space around the lungs (called a pleural effusion). A chest tube may also be needed when a patient has had a severe injury to the chest wall that causes bleeding around the lungs (called a hemothorax). Sometimes, a patient's lung can be accidentally punctured, allowing air to gather outside the lung, causing its collapse (called a pneumothorax).

Chest tube thoracostomy involves placing a hollow plastic tube between the ribs and into the chest to drain fluid or air from around the lungs. The tube is often hooked up to a suction machine to help with drainage. The tube remains in the chest until all or most of the air or fluid has drained out, usually a few days. Occasionally special medicines are given through a chest tube.

Why Do I Need a Chest Tube?

Common reasons why a chest tube is needed include:

- **Collapsed lung (pneumothorax):** This occurs when air has built up in the area around the lungs (the pleural space) from a leak in the lung. This leak may be the result of lung disease. It can also occur as a complication of certain medical procedures. Chest tubes are frequently needed to remove air from around the lung. Failure to remove such air can be life-threatening. Removing the air allows the lung to re-expand and seal the leak.

- **Infection:** If the fluid building up around the lung is infected, it may be necessary to insert a chest tube to remove the fluid.

Getting the fluid out sometimes helps clear the infection faster. A culture can also be done on the fluid to try to figure out what type of infection is present.

- **Cancer:** Some cancers spread to the lung or pleura (lining of the lung). This can cause large amounts of fluid to build up around the lung. Doctors usually drain the fluid with a needle. If the fluid keeps coming back, however, it may be necessary to insert a chest tube to first drain the fluid, and then deliver special medicines into the chest that reduce the likelihood of the fluid building up again.

- **Comfort:** A large buildup of fluid or air in the chest can make it difficult to breathe. Removing some of the fluid or air may decrease discomfort and make it easier for the patient to breathe.

- **Chest surgery:** Sometimes a chest tube is left in place after surgery. The surgeon can usually tell you if it will be needed and how long it may need to stay in.

Risks of Chest Tube Insertion

Below are listed some risks of chest tube thoracostomy. It should be noted that the risk of serious complications (bleeding and infection) is uncommon (usually less than 5% of cases). Your doctor will explain the risks and how likely they may be for you when you give consent for the procedure.

- **Pain during placement:** Discomfort often occurs as the chest tube is inserted. Doctors try to lessen any pain or discomfort by giving a local numbing medicine. The discomfort usually decreases once the tube is in place.

- **Bleeding:** During insertion of the tube, a blood vessel in the skin or chest wall may be accidentally nicked. Bleeding is usually minor and stops on its own. Rarely, bleeding can occur into or around the lung and may require surgery. Usually bleeding can just be watched with the chest tube in place.

- **Infection:** Bacteria can enter around the tube and cause an infection around the lung. The longer the chest tube stays in the chest, the greater the risk for infection. The risk of infection is decreased by special care in bandaging the skin at the point where the tube goes into the chest.

Preparation for Chest Tube Insertion

Fluid or air in the chest that needs to be drained is identified using a chest radiograph (X-ray). Sometimes other tests, such as a chest ultrasound or chest CT are also done to evaluate pleural fluid. If the X-ray shows a need for a chest tube to drain fluid or air, the procedure is likely to be done by a surgeon, a pulmonary/critical care physician or an interventional radiologist.

Often an adult or older child remains awake when a chest tube is inserted, except when it is placed in the operating room during an open chest procedure. Sometimes a person, particularly a younger child, is given a small amount of medicine (a sedative) that causes sleepiness before a chest tube is inserted. The skin will be thoroughly cleaned and a local anesthetic medication will be injected into the skin. This numbing medicine will also be injected deeper in the tissue along the path through the ribs that the tube will follow. The doctor will use a scalpel to make a cut, from three quarters of an inch to one and a half inches long, between the ribs (the exact location depends on what is being drained and its location in the lungs). Then the doctor will guide the tube into the chest. The tube is usually a little thinner than a pinky finger, although there are different sizes that can be used. It will be stitched into place to prevent it from slipping out. A sterile dressing bandage is placed over the insertion site.

What Happens When the Chest Tube Is in?

Most patients will need to stay in the hospital the entire time the chest tube is in. You will be checked often for possible air leaks, plugging of the tube, and any breathing problems you may be having. Usually, you will be able to breathe more comfortably with the tube in place. Sometimes pain around the area where the tube enters the chest may cause you to take more shallow breaths. The nurse or doctor will tell you how much you can move around with the chest tube in place. Sometimes the tube is clamped and left in place to make sure no fluid or air comes back before it is pulled out.

Will There Be Any Pain or Possible Complications When the Chest Tube Is Removed?

When the doctor determines that you no longer need the chest tube, it will be removed. Usually it can be taken out right at your bedside. There rarely is a need for sedation medication. You will be told how to breathe as the tube is being pulled. A secure bandage will be put in place. You will be told when the bandage can be removed. Often, a follow-up chest X-ray will be done to make sure that fluid or air haven't come back. Generally there are no complications from the chest tube once it has been removed. You will only have a small scar.

Source: Manthous, CA, Tobin, MJ, A Primer on Critical Care for Patients and Their Families, ATS Website: http://www.thoracic.org/clinical/critical-care/patient-information/index.php

Reviewed and revised August 2012 by Kevin Wilson, MD and Colin Cooke, MD. Revised version available at: http://patients.thoracic.org/information-series/index.php

Additional Information

- American Thoracic Society: www.thoracic.org

- ATS Patient Advisory Roundtable: www.thoracic.org/aboutats/par/par.asp

- National Heart, Lung, and Blood Institute: www.nhlbi.nih.gov/index.htm

- Centers for Disease Control and Prevention: www.cdc.gov

Action Steps

You/your loved one has or is scheduled to have a chest tube inserted to remove excess fluid, blood, or air from the area around their lungs.

- Talk with the doctor about the use of numbing medicine or medicine that causes sleepiness (sedation) before the procedure.

- Talk to your doctor or nurse about any pain or shortness of breath you may have after the chest tube is in place.

- Have your nurse show you how the chest tube site is watched to monitor any potential problems.

Section 36.3

Tracheostomy

A tracheostomy is a surgical procedure to create an opening through the neck into the trachea (windpipe). A tube is usually placed through this opening to provide an airway and to remove secretions from the lungs. This tube is called a tracheostomy tube or trach tube.

Description

General anesthesia is used, unless the situation is critical. In that case, local anesthesia is injected into the area to reduce the discomfort caused by the procedure.

The neck is cleaned and draped. Surgical cuts are made to expose the tough cartilage rings that make up the outer wall of the trachea. The surgeon then creates an opening into the trachea and inserts a tracheostomy tube.

Why the Procedure Is Performed

A tracheostomy may be done if you have:

- a large object blocking the airway;
- an inability to breathe on your own;
- an inherited abnormality of the larynx or trachea;
- breathed in harmful material such as smoke, steam, or other toxic gases that swell and block the airway;
- cancer of the neck, which can affect breathing by pressing on the airway;
- paralysis of the muscles that affect swallowing;
- severe neck or mouth injuries;
- surgery around the voice box (larynx) that prevents normal breathing and swallowing.

497

Risks

The risks for any anesthesia are:

- problems breathing;
- reactions to medications, including heart attack and stroke.

The risks for any surgery are:

- bleeding;
- infection;
- nerve injury, including paralysis.

Other risks include:

- damage to the thyroid gland;
- erosion of the trachea (rare);
- puncture of the lung and lung collapse;
- scar tissue in the trachea that causes pain or trouble breathing.

After the Procedure

If the tracheostomy is temporary, the tube will eventually be removed. Healing will occur quickly, leaving a minimal scar. Sometimes, a surgical procedure may be needed to close the site (stoma).

Occasionally a stricture, or tightening of the trachea may develop, which may affect breathing.

If the tracheostomy tube is permanent, the hole remains open.

Outlook (Prognosis)

Most patients need one to three days to adapt to breathing through a tracheostomy tube. It will take some time to learn how to communicate with others. At first, it may be impossible for the patient to talk or make sounds.

After training and practice, most patients can learn to talk with a tracheostomy tube. Patients or family members learn how to take care of the tracheostomy during the hospital stay. Home-care service may also be available.

You should be able to go back to your normal lifestyle. When you are outside, you can wear a loose covering (a scarf or other protection) over the tracheostomy stoma (hole). Use safety precautions when you are exposed to water, aerosols, powder, or food particles.

Part Four

Managing Pain and Surgical Complications

Chapter 37

Pain Control and Surgery

Pain control following surgery is a major priority for both you and your doctors. While you should expect to have some pain after your surgery, your doctor will make every effort to safely minimize your pain.

We provide the following information to help you understand your options for pain treatment, to describe how you can help your doctors and nurses control your pain, and to empower you to take an active role in making choices about pain treatment. Be sure to tell your doctor about all medications (prescribed and over-the-counter), vitamins and herbal supplements you are taking. This may affect which drugs are prescribed for your pain control.

Why Is Pain Control So Important?

In addition to keeping you comfortable, pain control can help you recover faster and may reduce your risk of developing certain complications after surgery, such as pneumonia and blood clots. If your pain is well controlled, you will be better able to complete important tasks such as walking and deep breathing exercises.

What Kinds of Pain Will I Feel after Surgery?

You may be surprised at where you experience pain after surgery. Often times the incision itself is not the only area of discomfort. You may or may not feel the following:

- Muscle pain: You may feel muscle pain in the neck, shoulders, back, or chest from lying on the operating table.

- Throat pain: Your throat may feel sore or scratchy.

- Movement pain: Sitting up, walking, and coughing are all important activities after surgery, but they may cause increased pain at or around the incision site.

What Can I Do to Help Keep My Pain under Control?

Important: Your doctors and nurses want and need to know about pain that is not adequately controlled. If you are having pain, please tell someone. Don't worry about being a bother.

You can help the doctors and nurses measure your pain. While you are recovering, your doctors and nurses will frequently ask you to rate your pain on a scale of 0 to 10, with 0 being "no pain" and 10 being "the worst pain you can imagine." Reporting your pain as a number helps the doctors and nurses know how well your treatment is working and whether to make any changes. Keep in mind that your comfort level (i.e., ability to breathe deeply or cough) is more important than absolute numbers (i.e., pain score).

Pain Score

- 0: I'm not in pain and I do not feel uncomfortable.

- 1–2: I'm not pain-free, but would be okay if no pain medication or treatment was available.

- 3–4: I'm a bit uncomfortable. It's not awful, but if Tylenol, aspirin, or ibuprofen were available, I would take it.

- 5–6: I can only concentrate on an activity for a short period of time due to my pain. I need more than Tylenol. I could wait an hour or so if I had to but I need some relief.

- 7–8: My pain is dominating my thoughts. I don't feel like doing anything until I get some relief. Please get me something strong as soon as possible. I don't think I can wait. I need some relief.

- 9–10: I barely feel like talking. I don't want to do anything. I can't enjoy any activity at all—maybe not even eating. All I can think about is getting rid of this pain. Please give me something strong—even sooner than right now.

Who Is Going to Help Manage My Pain?

You and your surgeon will decide what type of pain control would be most acceptable for you after surgery. Your surgeon may choose to consult the Acute Pain Management Service to help manage your pain following surgery. Doctors with this service are specifically trained in the types of pain control options described in the following text.

You are the one who ultimately decides which pain control option is most acceptable. The manager of your post-surgical pain—your surgeon or the Acute Pain Management Service doctor—will review your medical and surgical history, check the results from your laboratory tests and physical exam, and then advise you about which pain management option may be best suited to safely minimize your discomfort.

After surgery, you will be assessed frequently to ensure that you are comfortable and safe. When necessary, adjustments or changes to your pain management regimen will be made.

Types of Pain-Control Treatments

You may receive more than one type of pain treatment, depending on your needs and the type of surgery you are having. All of these treatments are relatively safe, but like any therapy, they are not completely free of risk. Dangerous side effects are rare. Nausea, vomiting, itching, and drowsiness can occur. These side effects are usually easily treated in most cases.

Intravenous Patient-Controlled Analgesia (PCA)

Patient-controlled analgesia (PCA) uses a computerized pump that safely permits you to push a button and deliver small amounts of pain medicine into your intravenous (IV) line, usually in your arm. No needles are injected into your muscle. PCA provides stable pain relief in most situations. Many patients like the sense of control they have over their pain management.

The PCA pump is programmed to give a certain amount of medication when you press the button. It will only allow you to have so much medication, no matter how often you press the button, so there is little worry that you will give yourself too much.

One way that you may get too much medication from the PCA pump is if a family member presses the PCA button for you. This removes the patient control aspect of the therapy, which is a major safety feature. Do not allow family members or friends to push your PCA pump button for you. You need to be awake enough to know that you need pain medication.

Patient-Controlled Epidural Analgesia

Many people are familiar with epidural anesthesia because it is frequently used to control pain during childbirth. Patient-controlled epidural analgesia uses a PCA pump to deliver pain-control medicine into an epidural catheter (a very thin plastic tube) that is placed into your back.

Placing the epidural catheter (to which the PCA pump is attached) usually causes no more discomfort than having an IV started. A sedating medication, given through your IV, will help you relax. The skin of your back will be cleaned with a sterile solution and numbed with a local anesthetic. Next, a thin needle will be carefully inserted into an area called the epidural space. A thin catheter will be inserted through this needle into the epidural space, and the needle will then be removed. During and after your surgery, pain medications will be infused through this epidural catheter with the goal of providing you with excellent pain control when you awaken. If additional pain medication is required, you can press the PCA button.

Epidural analgesia is usually more effective in relieving pain than intravenous medication. Patients who receive epidural analgesia typically have less pain when they take deep breaths, cough, and walk, and they may recover more quickly. For patients with medical problems such as heart or lung disease, epidural analgesia may reduce the risk of serious complications, such as heart attack or pneumonia.

Epidural analgesia is safe, but like any procedure or therapy, is not risk-free. Sometimes the epidural does not adequately control pain. In this situation, you will be given alternative treatments or be offered replacement of the epidural. Nausea, vomiting, itching, and drowsiness can occur. Occasionally, numbness and weakness of the legs can occur, which disappear after the medication is reduced or stopped. Headache can occur, but this is rare. Severe complications, such as nerve damage and infection, are extremely rare.

Nerve Blocks

You may be offered a nerve block to control your pain after surgery. Whereas an epidural controls pain over a broad area of your body, a nerve block is used when pain from surgery affects a smaller region of your body, such as an arm or leg. Sometimes a catheter similar to an epidural catheter is placed for prolonged pain control. There are several potential advantages of a nerve block. It may allow for a significant reduction in the amount of opioid (narcotic) medication, which may result in fewer side effects, such as nausea, vomiting, itching, and drowsiness.

In some cases, a nerve block can be used as the main anesthetic for your surgery. In this case, you will be given medications during your surgery to keep you sleepy, relaxed, and comfortable. This type of anesthesia provides the added benefit of pain relief both during and after your surgery. It may reduce your risk of nausea and vomiting after surgery. You, your anesthesiologist, and your surgeon will decide before surgery if a nerve block is a suitable pain management or anesthetic option for you.

Pain Medications Taken by Mouth

At some point during your recovery from surgery, your doctor will order pain medications to be taken by mouth (oral pain medications). These may be ordered to come at a specified time, or you may need to ask your nurse to bring them to you. Make sure you know if you need to ask for the medication. Most oral pain medications can be taken every four hours.

Important: Do not wait until your pain is severe before you ask for pain medications. Also, if the pain medication has not significantly helped within 30 minutes, notify your nurse. Extra pain medication is available for you to take. You do not have to wait four hours to receive more medication.

What Are Some of the Risks and Benefits Associated with Pain Medication?

Opioids (Narcotics) after Surgery: Medications Such as Morphine, Fentanyl, Hydromorphone

- Benefits: Strong pain relievers. Many options are available if one is causing significant side effects.

- Risks: May cause nausea, vomiting, itching, drowsiness, and/or constipation. The risk of becoming addicted is extremely rare.

Opioid (Narcotics) at Home (Percocet or Vicodin, Tylenol #3)

- Benefits: Effective for moderate to severe pain. Many options are available.

- Risks: Nausea, vomiting, itching, drowsiness, and/or constipation. Stomach upset can be lessened if the drug is taken with food. You should not drive or operate machinery while taking these medications. Note: These medications often contain acetaminophen (Tylenol). Make sure that other medications that you are taking do not contain acetaminophen, because too much of it may damage your liver.

Non-Opioid (Non-Narcotic) Analgesic Medications (Tylenol FeverAll)

- Benefits: Effective for mild to moderate pain. They have very few side effects and are safe for most patients. They often decrease the requirement for stronger medications, which may reduce the incidence of side effects.

- Risks: Liver damage may result if more than the recommended daily dose is used. Patients with pre-existing liver disease or those who drink significant quantities of alcohol may be at increased risk.

Nonsteroidal Anti-Inflammatory Drugs (NSAIDs), Ibuprofen (Advil), Naproxen Sodium (Aleve), Celecoxib (Celebrex)

- Benefits: These drugs reduce swelling and inflammation and relieve mild to moderate pain. Ibuprofen and naproxen sodium are available without a prescription, but you should ask your doctor about taking them. They may reduce the amount of opioid analgesic you need, possibly reducing side effects such as nausea, vomiting, and drowsiness. If taken alone, there are no restrictions on driving or operating machinery.

- Risks: The most common side effects of nonsteroidal anti-inflammatory medications (NSAIDs) are stomach upset and dizziness. You should not take these drugs without your doctor's approval if you have kidney problems, a history of stomach ulcers, heart failure, or are on blood thinner medications such as (warfarin) Coumadin, Lovenox injections, or Plavix.

Are There Ways I Can Relieve Pain without Medication?

Yes, there are other ways to relieve pain, and it is important to keep an open mind about these techniques. When used along with medication, these techniques can dramatically reduce pain.

Relaxation music or guided imagery is a proven form of focused relaxation that coaches you in creating calm, peaceful images in your mind, providing a mental escape. For the best results, practice using your listening device before your surgery, and then use it twice daily during your recovery.

At home, heat or cold therapy may be an option that your surgeon may choose to help reduce swelling and control your pain. Specific instructions for the use of these therapies will be discussed with you by your surgical team.

If you have an abdominal or chest incision, you will want to splint the area with a pillow when you are coughing or breathing deeply to decrease motion near your incision. You will be given a pillow in the hospital. Continue to use it at home as well.

Lastly, make sure you are comfortable with your treatment plan. Talk to your doctor and nurses about your concerns and needs. This will help avoid miscommunication, stress, anxiety, and disappointment, which may make pain worse. Keep asking questions until you have satisfactory answers. You are the one who will benefit.

How Can I Control Pain at Home?

You may be given prescriptions for pain medication to take at home. These may or may not be the same pain medications you took in the hospital. Talk with your doctor about which pain medications will be prescribed at discharge.

Note: Make sure your doctor knows about pain medications that have caused you problems in the past. This will prevent possible delays in your discharge from the hospital.

Preparation for Your Discharge

Your doctors may have already given you your prescription for pain medication prior to your surgery date. If this is the case, it is best to be prepared and have your medication filled and ready for you when you come home from the hospital. You may want to have your pain pills with you on your ride home if you are traveling a long distance. Check with your insurance company regarding your prescription plan and coverage for your medication. Occasionally, a pain medication prescribed by your doctor is not covered by your insurance company.

If you do not receive your prescription for pain medication until after the surgery, make sure a family member takes your prescription and gets it filled as soon as possible. It is important that you are prepared in case you have pain.

Make sure you wear comfortable clothes, and keep your coughing and deep breathing pillow with you.

You may want to have your relaxation music available for your travels.

If you are traveling by plane, make sure you have your pain pills in your carry-on luggage in case the airline misplaces your checked luggage.

While at home:

- Remember to take your pain medication before activity and at bedtime. Your doctor may advise you to take your pain medication at regular intervals (such as every four to six hours).

- Be sure to get enough rest. If you are having trouble sleeping, talk to your doctor.

- Use pillows to support you when you sleep and when you do your coughing and deep breathing exercises.

- Try using the alternative methods discussed earlier. Heating pads or cold therapy, guided imagery tapes, listening to soft music, changing your position in bed, and massage can help relieve your pain.

Note: If you need to have stitches or staples removed and you are still taking pain medications, be sure to have a friend or family member drive you to your appointment. Commonly, you should not drive or operate equipment if you are taking opioid (narcotic)-containing pain medications. Check the label of your prescription for any warnings, or ask your doctor, nurse, or pharmacist.

Frequently Asked Questions

I am nervous about getting hooked on pain pills. How do I avoid this?

The risk of becoming addicted to pain medication after surgery is very small. The bigger risk is a possible prolonged recovery if you avoid your pain medications and cannot effectively do your required activities. If you are concerned about addiction, or have a history of substance abuse (alcohol or any drug), talk with your doctors. They will monitor you closely during your recovery. If issues arise following surgery, they will consult the appropriate specialists.

I am a small person who is easily affected by medicine. I am nervous that a normal dose of pain medication will be too much for me. What should I do?

During recovery, your healthcare team will observe how you respond to pain medication and make changes as needed. Be sure to communicate with your doctors any concerns you have prior to surgery. The relatively small doses of pain medication given after surgery are highly unlikely to have an exaggerated effect based on your body size.

I don't have a high tolerance for pain. I am afraid that the pain will be too much for me to handle. What can I do?

Concern about pain from surgery is very normal. The most important thing you can do is to talk with your surgeon and anesthesiologist about your particular situation. Setting pain control goals with your doctors before surgery will help them better tailor your pain treatment plan. Treating pain early is easier than treating it after it has set in. If you have had prior experiences with surgery and pain control, let your doctor know what worked or what did not work. Remember, there are usually many options available to you for pain control after surgery.

I normally take Tylenol if I get a headache. Can I still take Tylenol for a headache if I am on other pain medication?

As discussed earlier, before taking any other medication, be sure to talk to your doctor. Some of the medications prescribed for use at home contain acetaminophen (Tylenol) and if too much is taken, you may become ill. In order to avoid getting too much of any medication, discuss this issue with your doctor before you leave the hospital.

Play an Active Role in Your Pain Control

Ask your doctors and nurses about:

- Pain and pain control treatments and what you can expect from them. You have a right to the best level of pain relief that can be safely provided.
- Your schedule for pain medicines in the hospital
- How you can participate in a pain-control plan

Inform your doctors and nurses about:

- any surgical pain you have had in the past;

- how you relieved your pain before you came to the hospital;
- pain you have had recently or currently;
- pain medications you have taken in the past and cannot tolerate;
- pain medications you have been taking prior to surgery;
- any pain that is not controlled with your current pain medications.

You should:

- help the doctors and nurses measure your pain and expect staff to ask about pain relief often and to respond quickly when you do report pain;
- ask for pain medicines as soon as pain begins;
- tell us how well your pain is relieved and your pain relief expectations;
- use other comfort measures for pain control—listening to relaxation or soft music, repositioning in bed, etc.

Your doctors are committed to providing you with the safest and most effective pain management strategy that is most acceptable to you.

Chapter 38

Assisted Breathing and Surgery

A ventilator is a machine that supports breathing. These machines mainly are used in hospitals. Ventilators:

- get oxygen into the lungs;
- remove carbon dioxide from the body;
- help people breathe easier;
- breathe for people who have lost all ability to breathe on their own.

A ventilator often is used for short periods, such as during surgery when you're under general anesthesia. The term anesthesia refers to a loss of feeling and awareness. General anesthesia temporarily puts you to sleep.

The medicines used to induce anesthesia can disrupt normal breathing. A ventilator helps make sure that you continue breathing during surgery.

A ventilator also may be used during treatment for a serious lung disease or other condition that affects normal breathing.

Some people may need to use ventilators long term or for the rest of their lives. In these cases, the machines can be used outside of the hospital—in long-term care facilities or at home.

Excerpted from "What Is a Ventilator?" by the National Heart, Lung, and Blood Institute (NHLBI, www.nhlbi.nih.gov), part of the National Institutes of Health, February 1, 2011.

A ventilator doesn't treat a disease or condition. It's used only for life support.

During Surgery

If you have general anesthesia during surgery, you'll likely be connected to a ventilator. The medicines used to induce anesthesia can disrupt normal breathing. A ventilator helps make sure that you continue breathing during surgery.

After surgery, you may not even know you were connected to a ventilator. The only sign may be a slight sore throat for a short time. The sore throat is caused by the tube that connects the ventilator to your airway.

Once the anesthesia wears off and you begin breathing on your own, the ventilator is disconnected. The tube in your throat also is taken out. This usually happens before you completely wake up from surgery.

However, depending on the type of surgery you have, you could stay on a ventilator for a few hours to several days after your surgery. Most people who have anesthesia during surgery only need a ventilator for a short time, though.

How Does a Ventilator Work?

Ventilators blow air—or air with extra oxygen—into the airways and then the lungs. The airways are pipes that carry oxygen-rich air to your lungs. They also carry carbon dioxide, a waste gas, out of your lungs.

The airways include your:

- nose and linked air passages, called nasal cavities;
- mouth;
- larynx, or voice box;
- trachea, or windpipe;
- tubes called bronchial tubes or bronchi, and their branches.

What to Expect While on a Ventilator

Ventilators normally don't cause pain. The breathing tube in your airway may cause some discomfort. It also affects your ability to talk and eat.

If your breathing tube is a trach tube, you may be able to talk. (A trach tube is put directly into your windpipe through a hole in the front of your neck.)

Instead of food, your health care team may give you nutrients through a tube inserted into a vein. If you're on a ventilator for a long time, you'll likely get food through a nasogastric, or feeding, tube. The tube goes through your nose or mouth or directly into your stomach or small intestine through a surgically made hole.

A ventilator greatly restricts your activity and also limits your movement. You may be able to sit up in bed or in a chair, but you usually can't move around much.

If you need to use a ventilator long term, you may be given a portable machine. This machine allows you to move around and even go outside, although you need to bring your ventilator with you.

Sometimes the ventilator is set so that you can trigger the machine to blow air into your lungs. But, if you fail to trigger it within a certain amount of time, the machine automatically blows air to keep you breathing.

What to Expect When You're Taken off of a Ventilator

Weaning is the process of taking you off of a ventilator so that you can start to breathe on your own. People usually are weaned after they've recovered enough from the problem that caused them to need the ventilator.

Weaning usually begins with a short trial. You stay connected to the ventilator, but you're given a chance to breathe on your own. Most people are able to breathe on their own the first time weaning is tried. Once you can successfully breathe on your own, the ventilator is stopped.

If you can't breathe on your own during the short trial, weaning will be tried at a later time. If repeated weaning attempts over a long time don't work, you may need to use the ventilator long term.

After you're weaned, the breathing tube is removed. You may cough while this is happening. Your voice may be hoarse for a short time after the tube is removed.

Chapter 39

Managing Blood Loss with Blood Transfusions

A blood transfusion is a safe, common procedure in which you receive blood through an intravenous (IV) line inserted into one of your blood vessels.

Blood transfusions are used to replace blood lost during surgery or a serious injury. A transfusion also might be done if your body can't make blood properly because of an illness.

During a blood transfusion, a small needle is used to insert an IV line into one of your blood vessels. Through this line, you receive healthy blood. The procedure usually takes one to four hours, depending on how much blood you need.

Who Needs a Blood Transfusion?

Blood transfusions are very common. Each year, almost 5 million Americans need blood transfusions. The procedure is used for people of all ages.

Some people who have surgery need blood transfusions because they lose blood during their operations. People who have serious injuries—for example, from car crashes, war, or natural disasters—also may need blood transfusions to replace blood lost during the injury.

Some people need blood or blood parts because of illnesses. For example, blood transfusions might be used to treat the following:

Excerpted from "What Is a Blood Transfusion?" by the National Heart, Lung, and Blood Institute (NHLBI, www.nhlbi.nih.gov), part of the National Institutes of Health, January 30, 2012.

- A severe infection or liver disease that stops your body from properly making blood or some blood parts

- An illness that causes anemia, such as kidney disease or cancer

- A bleeding disorder, such as hemophilia or thrombocytopenia

What to Expect before a Blood Transfusion

Before a blood transfusion, a technician tests your blood to find out your blood type (A, B, AB, or O) and whether you're Rh-positive or Rh-negative. He or she pricks your finger with a needle to get a few drops of blood or draws blood from one of your veins.

The blood type used for your transfusion must work with your blood type. If it doesn't, antibodies (proteins) in your blood attack the new blood and make you sick.

Some people have allergic reactions even when the donated blood does work with their own blood type. To prevent this, your doctor may prescribe a medicine to stop allergic reactions.

If you have allergies or have had an allergic reaction during a past transfusion, your doctor will make every effort to make sure you're safe.

Most people don't need to change their diets or activities before or after a blood transfusion. Your doctor will let you know whether you need to make any lifestyle changes prior to the procedure.

What to Expect during a Blood Transfusion

Blood transfusions take place in either a doctor's office or a hospital. Sometimes they're done at a person's home, but this is less common. Blood transfusions also are done during surgery and in emergency rooms.

A needle is used to insert an intravenous (IV) line into one of your blood vessels. Through this line, you receive healthy blood. The procedure usually takes one to four hours. The time depends on how much blood you need and what part of the blood you receive.

During the blood transfusion, a nurse carefully watches you, especially for the first 15 minutes. This is when allergic reactions are most likely to occur. The nurse continues to watch you during the rest of the procedure as well.

What to Expect after a Blood Transfusion

After a blood transfusion, your vital signs are checked (such as your temperature, blood pressure, and heart rate). The intravenous (IV) line is removed from your blood vessel. You may have some bruising or soreness for a few days at the site where the IV was inserted.

You may need blood tests to show how your body is reacting to the transfusion. Your doctor will let you know about signs and symptoms to watch for and report.

Chapter 40

Infection and Surgery

Chapter Contents

Section 40.1

Frequently Asked Questions about Surgical Site Infections

By the Centers for Disease Control and Prevention
(CDC, www.cdc.gov), November 24, 2010.

What is a surgical site infection (SSI)?

A surgical site infection is an infection that occurs after surgery in the part of the body where the surgery took place. Surgical site infections can sometimes be superficial infections involving the skin only. Other surgical site infections are more serious and can involve tissues under the skin, organs, or implanted material. CDC provides guidelines and tools to the healthcare community to help end surgical site infections and resources to help the public understand these infections and take measures to safeguard their own health when possible.

Symptoms include the following:

• Redness and pain around the area where you had surgery

• Drainage of cloudy fluid from your surgical wound

• Fever

Can SSIs be treated?

Yes. Most SSIs can be treated with antibiotics. The antibiotic given to you depends on the bacteria (germs) causing the infection. Sometimes patients with SSIs also need another surgery to treat the infection.

What are some of the things that hospitals are doing to prevent SSIs?

To prevent SSIs, doctors, nurses, and other healthcare providers should follow infection prevention guidelines including the following:

• Clean their hands and arms up to their elbows with an antiseptic agent just before the surgery

- Clean their hands with soap and water or an alcohol-based hand rub before and after caring for each patient

- If indicated, remove some of your hair immediately before your surgery using electric clippers if the hair is in the same area where the procedure will occur

- Wear special hair covers, masks, gowns, and gloves during surgery to keep the surgery area clean

- When indicated, give you antibiotics before your surgery starts (In most cases, you should get antibiotics within 60 minutes before the surgery starts and the antibiotics should be stopped within 24 hours after surgery.)

- Clean the skin at the site of your surgery with a special soap that kills germs

What can I do to help prevent SSIs?

Before surgery:

- Tell your doctor about other medical problems you may have. Health problems such as allergies, diabetes, and obesity could affect your surgery and your treatment.

- Quit smoking. Patients who smoke get more infections. Talk to your doctor about how you can quit before your surgery.

- Do not shave near where you will have surgery. Shaving with a razor can irritate your skin and make it easier to develop an infection.

At the time of surgery:

- Speak up if someone tries to shave you with a razor before surgery. Ask why you need to be shaved and talk with your surgeon if you have any concerns.

After surgery:

- If you do not see your providers clean their hands, please ask them to do so.

- Family and friends who visit you should not touch the surgical wound or dressings.

- Family and friends should clean their hands with soap and water or an alcohol-based hand rub before and after visiting you. If you do not see them clean their hands, ask them to clean their hands.

- Make sure you understand how to care for your wound before you leave the hospital.

- Always clean your hands before and after caring for your wound.

- Make sure you know who to contact if you have questions or problems after you get home.

- If you have any symptoms of an infection, such as redness and pain at the surgery site, drainage, or fever, call your doctor immediately.

Section 40.2

Simple Steps Can Reduce Health Care-Associated Infections

Excerpted from the document by the Agency for Healthcare Research and Quality (AHRQ, www.ahrq.gov), July 1, 2008.

Did you know that there is a problem in health care that causes nearly 90,000 deaths and costs billions of dollars to treat each year? It's called a health care-associated infection (HAI)—and it's preventable. That's why it's getting more attention every day.

An HAI often happens in the hospital, where patients tend to be very ill or are recovering from surgery. But this kind of infection can also occur in a doctor's office, clinic, emergency room, or ambulatory setting. Patients who are elderly, very young, or who have chronic diseases, such as diabetes, also are at a high risk for getting HAIs.

Different types of bacteria cause HAIs. Some of the infections are hard to get rid of once they get into a patient's bloodstream, even with powerful medicines. That's why preventing HAIs in the first place is so important.

Hospitals in Michigan have made great progress toward reducing the risk of these infections. Doctors and nurses at 103 intensive care units used a simple checklist that reminded them of what to do to lower the risk of infections for patients who had central venous catheters, which are tubes inserted into the body to give drugs or drain fluids.

Steps on the checklist included the following:

- Washing their hands

- Cleaning patients' skin with a bacteria-killing soap

- Removing catheters when they weren't needed

Doctors and nurses stopped and reminded each other when these practices weren't being followed in nonemergency situations. Medical staff talked about catheter infections at daily and monthly meetings.

These simple steps had a dramatic effect. Infection rates dropped to nearly zero shortly after these practices were put in place.

If you or a loved one is having surgery, there are steps you can take to lower the risk of getting an HAI. Make sure you wash your hands. Ask the hospital staff to do the same before and after they provide care, such as changing bandages. Tell the nurse if you notice that bandages are not clean, dry, or attached around wounds. And tell your friends and family members to avoid hospital visits if they have a cold or aren't feeling well. Don't be afraid to speak up.

Like many diseases, HAIs are deadly and add billions of dollars in health care spending.

Section 40.3

Catheter-Associated Urinary Tract Infections

By the Centers for Disease Control and Prevention
(CDC, www.cdc.gov), November 24, 2010.

What is a urinary catheter?

An indwelling urinary catheter is a drainage tube that is inserted into the urinary bladder through the urethra, is left in place, and is connected to a closed collection system. Alternative methods of urinary drainage may be employed in some patients. Intermittent (in-and-out) catheterization involves brief insertion of a catheter into the bladder through the urethra to drain urine at intervals. An external catheter is a urine containment device that fits over or adheres to the genitalia and is attached to a urinary drainage bag. The most commonly used external catheter is a soft flexible sheath that fits over the penis (condom catheter). A suprapubic catheter is surgically inserted into the bladder through an incision above the pubis.

What is a urinary tract infection?

A urinary tract infection (UTI) is an infection that involves any of the organs or structures of the urinary tract, including the kidneys, ureters, bladder, and urethra. Some of the common symptoms of a urinary tract infection are burning or pain in the lower abdomen (that is, below the stomach), fever, burning during urination, or an increase in the frequency of urination. UTIs are the most common type of healthcare-associated infection (HAI) and are most often caused by the placement or presence of a catheter in the urinary tract.

What is a catheter-associated urinary tract infection (CAUTI)?

A catheter-associated urinary tract infection (CAUTI) occurs when germs (usually bacteria) enter the urinary tract through the urinary catheter and cause infection. CAUTIs have been associated with increased morbidity, mortality, healthcare costs, and length of stay. The risk of CAUTI can be reduced by ensuring that catheters are used only when needed and removed as soon as possible; that catheters are placed using proper aseptic technique; and that the closed sterile drainage system is maintained.

Can CAUTIs be treated?

Yes, most CAUTIs can be treated with antibiotics and/or removal or change of the catheter. The healthcare provider will determine the best treatment for each patient.

What can patients do to help prevent CAUTI?

Patients with a urinary catheter can take the following precautions to prevent CAUTI:

- Understand why the catheter is needed and ask the healthcare provider frequently if the catheter is still needed.

- If the patient has a long-term catheter, they must clean their hands before and after touching the catheter.

- Check the position of the urine bag; it should always be below the level of the bladder.

- Do not tug or pull on the tubing.

- Do not twist or kink the catheter tubing.

Section 40.4

Central Line-Associated Bloodstream Infection

Excerpted from "Central Line-associated Bloodstream Infections:
Resources for Patients and Healthcare Providers," by the Centers for
Disease Control and Prevention (CDC, www.cdc.gov), February 7, 2011.

Central line-associated bloodstream infections (CLABSIs) result
in thousands of deaths each year and billions of dollars in added costs
to the U.S. healthcare system, yet these infections are preventable.

What is a central line?

A central line (also known as a central venous catheter) is a catheter
(tube) that doctors often place in a large vein in the neck, chest, or groin
to give medication or fluids or to collect blood for medical tests. You may
be familiar with intravenous catheters (also known as IVs) that are
used frequently to give medicine or fluids into a vein near the skin's
surface (usually on the arm or hand), for short periods of time. Central
lines are different from IVs because central lines access a major vein
that is close to the heart and can remain in place for weeks or months
and be much more likely to cause serious infection. Central lines are
commonly used in intensive care units.

What is a central line-associated bloodstream infection?

A central line-associated bloodstream infection (CLABSI) is a serious infection that occurs when germs (usually bacteria or viruses)
enter the bloodstream through the central line. Healthcare providers
must follow a strict protocol when inserting the line to make sure the
line remains sterile and a CLABSI does not occur. In addition to inserting the central line properly, healthcare providers must use stringent
infection control practices each time they check the line or change the
dressing. Patients who get a CLABSI have a fever, and might also have
red skin and soreness around the central line. If this happens, healthcare providers can do tests to learn if there is an infection present.

What can patients do to help prevent CLABSI?

Here are some ways patients can protect themselves from CLABSI:

- Research the hospital, if possible, to learn about its CLABSI rate.

- Speak up about any concerns so that healthcare personnel are reminded to follow the best infection prevention practices.

- Ask a healthcare provider if the central line is absolutely necessary. If so, ask them to help you understand the need for it and how long it will be in place.

- Pay attention to the bandage and the area around it. If the bandage comes off or if the bandage or area around it is wet or dirty, tell a healthcare worker right away.

- Don't get the central line or the central line insertion site wet.

- Tell a healthcare worker if the area around the catheter is sore or red or if the patient has a fever or chills.

- Do not let any visitors touch the catheter or tubing.

- The patient should avoid touching the tubing as much as possible.

- In addition, everyone visiting the patient must wash their hands—before and after they visit.

Section 40.5

Clostridium Difficile *Infections*

Excerpted from "Making Health Care Safer: Stopping *C. difficile* Infections," by the Centers for Disease Control and Prevention (CDC, www.cdc.gov), March 2012.

People getting medical care can catch serious infections called health care-associated infections (HAIs). While most types of HAIs are declining, one—caused by the germ *Clostridium difficile* (*C. difficile*)—remains at historically high levels. *C. difficile* causes diarrhea linked to 14,000 American deaths each year. Those most at risk are people, especially older adults, who take antibiotics and also get medical care. When a person takes antibiotics, good germs that protect against infection are destroyed for several months. During this time, patients can get sick from *C. difficile* picked up from contaminated surfaces or spread from a health care provider's hands. About 25% of *C. difficile* infections first show symptoms in hospital patients; 75% first show in nursing home patients or in people recently cared for in doctors' offices and clinics. *C. difficile* infections cost at least $1 billion in extra health care costs annually.

C. Difficile Infections Are at an All-Time High

C. difficile causes many Americans to become sick or die:

- *C. difficile* infections are linked to 14,000 deaths in the United States each year.

- Deaths related to *C. difficile* increased 400% between 2000 and 2007, due in part to a stronger germ strain.

- Most *C. difficile* infections are connected with receiving medical care.

- Almost half of infections occur in people younger than 65, but more than 90% of deaths occur in people 65 and older.

- Infection risk generally increases with age; children are at lower risk.

- About 25% of *C. difficile* infections first show symptoms in hospital patients; 75% first show in nursing home patients or in people recently cared for in doctors' offices and clinics.

C. Difficile Germs Infect Other Patients

- Half of all hospital patients with *C. difficile* infections have the infection when admitted and may spread it within the facility.

- The most dangerous source of spread to others is patients with diarrhea.

- Unnecessary antibiotic use in patients at one facility may increase the spread of *C. difficile* in another facility when patients transfer.

- When a patient transfers, health care providers are not always told that the patient has or recently had a *C. difficile* infection, so they may not take the right actions to prevent spread.

C. Difficile Infections Can Be Prevented

- Early results from hospital prevention projects show 20% fewer *C. difficile* infections in less than two years with infection prevention and control measures.

- England decreased *C. difficile* infection rates in hospitals by more than half in three years by using infection control recommendations and more careful antibiotic use.

What Patients Can Do

- Take antibiotics only as prescribed by your doctor. Antibiotics can be lifesaving medicines.

- Tell your doctor if you have been on antibiotics and get diarrhea within a few months.

- Wash your hands after using the bathroom.

- Try to use a separate bathroom if you have diarrhea, or be sure the bathroom is cleaned well if someone with diarrhea has used it.

Section 40.6

Methicillin-Resistant Staphylococcus Aureus *Infections*

"Frequently Asked Questions about MRSA (Methicillin-Resistant *Staphylococcus aureus*)," by the Centers for Disease Control and Prevention (CDC, www.cdc.gov), 2011.

Staphylococcus aureus, or staph, is a very common germ that about one out of every three people have on their skin or in their nose. This germ does not cause any problems for most people who have it on their skin. But sometimes it can cause serious infections such as skin or wound infections, pneumonia, or infections of the blood.

Antibiotics are given to kill staph germs when they cause infections. Some staph are resistant, meaning they cannot be killed by some antibiotics. Methicillin-resistant *Staphylococcus aureus* or MRSA is a type of staph that is resistant to some of the antibiotics that are often used to treat staph infections.

Who is most likely to get an MRSA infection?

In the hospital, people who are more likely to get an MRSA infection are people who:

- have other health conditions making them sick;
- have been in the hospital or a nursing home;
- have been treated with antibiotics.

People who are healthy and who have not been in the hospital or a nursing home can also get MRSA infections. These infections usually involve the skin.

How do I get infected with MRSA?

People who have MRSA germs on their skin or who are infected with MRSA may be able to spread the germ to other people. MRSA can be passed on to bed linens, bed rails, bathroom fixtures, and medical equipment. It can spread to other people on contaminated equipment and on the hands of doctors, nurses, other healthcare providers and visitors.

Can MRSA infections be treated?

Yes, there are antibiotics that can kill MRSA germs. Some patients with MRSA abscesses may need surgery to drain the infection. Your healthcare provider will determine which treatments are best for you.

What are some of the things that hospitals are doing to prevent MRSA infections?

To prevent MRSA infections, doctors, nurses, and other healthcare providers should do the following:

- Clean their hands with soap and water or an alcohol-based hand rub before and after caring for every patient.
- Carefully clean hospital rooms and medical equipment.
- Use Contact Precautions when caring for patients with MRSA. Contact Precautions mean the following:
  - Whenever possible, patients with MRSA will have a single room or will share a room only with someone else who also has MRSA.
  - Healthcare providers will put on gloves and wear a gown over their clothing while taking care of patients with MRSA.
  - Visitors may also be asked to wear a gown and gloves.
  - When leaving the room, hospital providers and visitors remove their gown and gloves and clean their hands.
  - Patients on Contact Precautions are asked to stay in their hospital rooms as much as possible. They should not go to common areas, such as the gift shop or cafeteria. They may go to other areas of the hospital for treatments and tests.

Health care professionals may test some patients to see if they have MRSA on their skin. This test involves rubbing a cotton-tipped swab in the patient's nostrils or on the skin.

What can I do to help prevent MRSA infections?

In the hospital:

- Make sure that all doctors, nurses, and other healthcare providers clean their hands with soap and water or an alcohol-based hand rub before and after caring for you.

- If you do not see your providers clean their hands, please ask them to do so.

When you go home:

- If you have wounds or an intravascular device (such as a catheter or dialysis port) make sure that you know how to take care of them.

Can my friends and family get MRSA when they visit me?

The chance of getting MRSA while visiting a person who has MRSA is very low. To decrease the chance of getting MRSA your family and friends should do the following:

- Clean their hands before they enter your room and when they leave.

- Ask a healthcare provider if they need to wear protective gowns and gloves when they visit you.

What do I need to do when I go home from the hospital?

To prevent another MRSA infection and to prevent spreading MRSA to others, do the following:

- Keep taking any antibiotics prescribed by your doctor. Don't take half-doses or stop before you complete your prescribed course.

- Clean your hands often, especially before and after changing your wound dressing or bandage.

- People who live with you should clean their hands often as well.

- Keep any wounds clean and change bandages as instructed until healed.

- Avoid sharing personal items such as towels or razors.

- Wash and dry your clothes and bed linens in the warmest temperatures recommended on the labels.

- Tell your healthcare providers that you have MRSA. This includes home health nurses and aides, therapists, and personnel in doctors' offices.

Your doctor may have more instructions for you. If you have questions, please ask your doctor or nurse.

Section 40.7

Pneumonia

Excerpted from "What Is Pneumonia?" by the National Heart,
Lung, and Blood Institute (NHLBI, www.nhlbi.nih.gov), part of the
National Institutes of Health, March 1, 2011.

Pneumonia is an infection in one or both of the lungs. Many germs—
such as bacteria, viruses, and fungi—can cause pneumonia.

The infection inflames your lungs' air sacs, which are called alveoli.
The air sacs may fill up with fluid or pus, causing symptoms such as
a cough with phlegm (a slimy substance), fever, chills, and trouble
breathing.

Outlook

Pneumonia is common in the United States. Treatment for pneumonia depends on its cause, how severe your symptoms are, and your
age and overall health. Many people can be treated at home, often
with oral antibiotics.

Children usually start to feel better in one to two days. For adults, it
usually takes two to three days. Anyone who has worsening symptoms
should see a doctor.

People who have severe symptoms or underlying health problems
may need treatment in a hospital. It may take three weeks or more
before they can go back to their normal routines.

Fatigue (tiredness) from pneumonia can last for a month or more.

What Are the Signs and Symptoms of Pneumonia?

The signs and symptoms of pneumonia vary from mild to severe.
Many factors affect how serious pneumonia is, including the type of
germ causing the infection and your age and overall health.

See your doctor promptly if you experience the following:

- High fever
- Shaking chills

533

- Cough with phlegm (a slimy substance), which doesn't improve or worsens

- Shortness of breath with normal daily activities

- Chest pain when you breathe or cough

- Feel suddenly worse after a cold or the flu

People who have pneumonia may have other symptoms, including nausea (feeling sick to the stomach), vomiting, and diarrhea.

Symptoms may vary in certain populations. Newborns and infants may not show any signs of the infection. Or, they may vomit, have a fever and cough, or appear restless, sick, or tired and without energy.

Older adults and people who have serious illnesses or weak immune systems may have fewer and milder symptoms. They may even have a lower than normal temperature. If they already have a lung disease, it may get worse. Older adults who have pneumonia sometimes have sudden changes in mental awareness.

How Is Pneumonia Treated?

Treatment for pneumonia depends on the type of pneumonia you have and how severe it is. Most people who have community-acquired pneumonia—the most common type of pneumonia—are treated at home.

The goals of treatment are to cure the infection and prevent complications.

General Treatment

If you have pneumonia, follow your treatment plan, take all medicines as prescribed, and get ongoing medical care. Ask your doctor when you should schedule followup care. Your doctor may want you to have a chest X-ray to make sure the pneumonia is gone.

Although you may start feeling better after a few days or weeks, fatigue (tiredness) can persist for up to a month or more. People who are treated in the hospital may need at least three weeks before they can go back to their normal routines.

Bacterial Pneumonia

Bacterial pneumonia is treated with medicines called antibiotics. You should take antibiotics as your doctor prescribes. You may start to feel better before you finish the medicine, but you should continue taking it as prescribed. If you stop too soon, the pneumonia may come back.

Most people begin to improve after one to three days of antibiotic treatment. This means that they should feel better and have fewer symptoms, such as cough and fever.

Viral Pneumonia

Antibiotics don't work when the cause of pneumonia is a virus. If you have viral pneumonia, your doctor may prescribe an antiviral medicine to treat it.

Viral pneumonia usually improves in one to three weeks.

Treating Severe Symptoms

You may need to be treated in a hospital if the following are true:

• Your symptoms are severe.

• You're at risk for complications because of other health problems.

If the level of oxygen in your bloodstream is low, you may receive oxygen therapy. If you have bacterial pneumonia, your doctor may give you antibiotics through an intravenous (IV) line inserted into a vein.

Section 40.8

Sepsis (Bloodstream Infection)

Excerpted from "Inpatient Care for Septicemia or Sepsis: A Challenge for Patients and Hospitals," a National Center for Health Statistics Data Brief, No. 62, by the Centers for Disease Control and Prevention (CDC, www.cdc.gov), June 2011.

Septicemia and sepsis are serious bloodstream infections that can rapidly become life-threatening. They arise from various infections, including those of the skin, lungs, abdomen, and urinary tract. Patients with these conditions are often treated in a hospital's intensive care unit. Early aggressive treatment increases the chance of survival. In 2008, an estimated $14.6 billion was spent on hospitalizations for septicemia, and from 1997 through 2008, the inflation-adjusted aggregate costs for treating patients hospitalized for this condition increased on average annually by 11.9%.

Despite high treatment expenditures, septicemia and sepsis are often fatal. Those who survive severe sepsis are more likely to have permanent organ damage, cognitive impairment, and physical disability. Septicemia is a leading cause of death.

Recent Trends in Care for Hospital Inpatients with These Diagnoses

The hospitalization rate of those with a principal diagnosis of septicemia or sepsis more than doubled from 2000 through 2008, increasing from 11.6 to 24.0 per 10,000 population. During the same period, the hospitalization rate for those with septicemia or sepsis as a principal or as a secondary diagnosis increased by 70% from 22.1 to 37.7 per 10,000 population. Reasons for these increases may include an aging population with more chronic illnesses; greater use of invasive procedures, immunosuppressive drugs, chemotherapy, and transplantation; and increasing microbial resistance to antibiotics. Greater clinical awareness of septicemia or sepsis may also have occurred during the period studied.

Septicemia or sepsis treatment involves caring for sicker patients who have longer inpatient stays than those with other diagnoses. Total nationwide inpatient annual costs of treating those hospitalized for septicemia have been rising and were estimated to be $14.6 billion in 2008. Even with this expenditure, the death rate was high. Patients who do survive severe cases are more likely to have negative long-term effects on health and on cognitive and physical functioning.

The "Surviving Sepsis Campaign" was an international effort organized by physicians that developed and promoted widespread adoption of practice improvement programs grounded in evidence-based guidelines. The goal was to improve diagnosis and treatment of sepsis. Included among the guidelines were sepsis screening for high-risk patients; taking bacterial cultures soon after the patient arrived at the hospital; starting patients on broad-spectrum intravenous antibiotic therapy before the results of the cultures are obtained; identifying the source of infection and taking steps to control it (e.g., abscess drainage); administering intravenous fluids to correct a loss or decrease in blood volume; and maintaining glycemic (blood sugar) control. These and similar guidelines have been tested by a number of hospitals and have shown potential for decreasing hospital mortality due to sepsis.

Chapter 41

Other Surgical Complications

Chapter Contents

Section 41.1

Abdominal Adhesions

Excerpted from "Abdominal Adhesions," by the National Institute of Diabetes and Digestive and Kidney Diseases (NIDDK, www.niddk.nih.gov), part of the National Institutes of Health, March 20, 2012.

What are abdominal adhesions?

Abdominal adhesions are bands of tissue that form between abdominal tissues and organs. Normally, internal tissues and organs have slippery surfaces, which allow them to shift easily as the body moves. Adhesions cause tissues and organs to stick together.

The intestines are part of the digestive system. Abdominal adhesions can cause an intestinal obstruction.

Although most adhesions cause no symptoms or problems, others cause chronic abdominal or pelvic pain. Adhesions are also a major cause of intestinal obstruction and female infertility.

What causes abdominal adhesions?

Abdominal surgery is the most frequent cause of abdominal adhesions. Almost everyone who undergoes abdominal surgery develops adhesions; however, the risk is greater after operations on the lower abdomen and pelvis, including bowel and gynecological surgeries. Adhesions can become larger and tighter as time passes, causing problems years after surgery.

Surgery-induced causes of abdominal adhesions include the following:

- Tissue incisions, especially those involving internal organs

- The handling of internal organs

- The drying out of internal organs and tissues

- Contact of internal tissues with foreign materials, such as gauze, surgical gloves, and stitches

- Blood or blood clots that were not rinsed out during surgery

A less common cause of abdominal adhesions is inflammation from sources not related to surgery, including the following:

- Appendicitis—in particular, appendix rupture
- Radiation treatment for cancer
- Gynecological infections
- Abdominal infections

Rarely, abdominal adhesions form without apparent cause.

How can abdominal adhesions cause intestinal obstruction?

Abdominal adhesions can kink, twist, or pull the intestines out of place, causing an intestinal obstruction. An intestinal obstruction partially or completely restricts the movement of food or stool through the intestines. A complete intestinal obstruction is life threatening and requires immediate medical attention and often surgery.

How are abdominal adhesions and intestinal obstructions treated?

Treatment for abdominal adhesions is usually not necessary, as most do not cause problems. Surgery is currently the only way to break adhesions that cause pain, intestinal obstruction, or fertility problems. More surgery, however, carries the risk of additional adhesions and is avoided when possible.

A complete intestinal obstruction usually requires immediate surgery. A partial obstruction can sometimes be relieved with a liquid or low-residue diet. A low-residue diet is high in dairy products, low in fiber, and more easily broken down into smaller particles by the digestive system.

Can abdominal adhesions be prevented?

Abdominal adhesions are difficult to prevent; however, surgical technique can minimize adhesions.

Laparoscopic surgery avoids opening up the abdomen with a large incision. Instead, the abdomen is inflated with gas while special surgical tools and a video camera are threaded through a few, small abdominal incisions. Inflating the abdomen gives the surgeon room to operate.

If a large abdominal incision is required, a special film-like material (Seprafilm) can be inserted between organs or between the organs and the abdominal incision at the end of surgery. The film-like material, which looks similar to wax paper, is absorbed by the body in about a week.

Other steps during surgery to reduce adhesion formation include using starch- and latex-free gloves, handling tissues and organs gently, shortening surgery time, and not allowing tissues to dry out.

Section 41.2

Deep Vein Thrombosis

Excerpted from "What Is Deep Vein Thrombosis?" by the National Heart, Lung, and Blood Institute (NHLBI, www.nhlbi.nih.gov), part of the National Institutes of Health, October 28, 2011.

Deep vein thrombosis, or DVT, is a blood clot that forms in a vein deep in the body. Blood clots occur when blood thickens and clumps together.

Most deep vein blood clots occur in the lower leg or thigh. They also can occur in other parts of the body.

A blood clot in a deep vein can break off and travel through the bloodstream. The loose clot is called an embolus. It can travel to an artery in the lungs and block blood flow. This condition is called pulmonary embolism, or PE.

PE is a very serious condition. It can damage the lungs and other organs in the body and cause death.

Blood clots in the thighs are more likely to break off and cause PE than blood clots in the lower legs or other parts of the body. Blood clots also can form in veins closer to the skin's surface. However, these clots won't break off and cause PE.

Causes of DVT

Blood clots can form in your body's deep veins if the following situations occur:

- A vein's inner lining is damaged. Injuries caused by physical, chemical, or biological factors can damage the veins. Such factors include surgery, serious injuries, inflammation, and immune responses.

- Blood flow is sluggish or slow. Lack of motion can cause sluggish or slow blood flow. This may occur after surgery, if you're ill and in bed for a long time, or if you're traveling for a long time.

- Your blood is thicker or more likely to clot than normal. Some inherited conditions (such as factor V Leiden) increase the risk of blood clotting. Hormone therapy or birth control pills also can increase the risk of clotting.

DVT Treatment

Doctors treat deep vein thrombosis (DVT) with medicines and other devices and therapies. The main goals of treating DVT are to:

- stop the blood clot from getting bigger;

- prevent the blood clot from breaking off and moving to your lungs;

- reduce your chance of having another blood clot.

Your doctor may prescribe medicines to prevent or treat DVT.

Anticoagulants

Anticoagulants are the most common medicines for treating DVT. They're also known as blood thinners.

These medicines decrease your blood's ability to clot. They also stop existing blood clots from getting bigger. However, blood thinners can't break up blood clots that have already formed. (The body dissolves most blood clots with time.)

Blood thinners can be taken as a pill, an injection under the skin, or through a needle or tube inserted into a vein (called intravenous, or IV, injection).

Warfarin and heparin are two blood thinners used to treat DVT. Warfarin is given in pill form. (Coumadin is a common brand name for warfarin.) Heparin is given as an injection or through an IV tube. There are different types of heparin. Your doctor will discuss the options with you.

Your doctor may treat you with both heparin and warfarin at the same time. Heparin acts quickly. Warfarin takes two to three days before it starts to work. Once the warfarin starts to work, the heparin is stopped.

Pregnant women usually are treated with just heparin because warfarin is dangerous during pregnancy.

Treatment for DVT using blood thinners usually lasts for six months. The following situations may change the length of treatment:

- If your blood clot occurred after a short-term risk (for example, surgery), your treatment time may be shorter.

- If you've had blood clots before, your treatment time may be longer.

- If you have certain other illnesses, such as cancer, you may need to take blood thinners for as long as you have the illness.

The most common side effect of blood thinners is bleeding. Bleeding can happen if the medicine thins your blood too much. This side effect can be life threatening.

Sometimes the bleeding is internal (inside your body). People treated with blood thinners usually have regular blood tests to measure their blood's ability to clot. These tests are called PT [prothrombin time] and PTT [partial thromboplastin time] tests.

These tests also help your doctor make sure you're taking the right amount of medicine. Call your doctor right away if you have easy bruising or bleeding. These may be signs that your medicines have thinned your blood too much.

Thrombin Inhibitors

These medicines interfere with the blood clotting process. They're used to treat blood clots in patients who can't take heparin.

Thrombolytics

Doctors prescribe these medicines to quickly dissolve large blood clots that cause severe symptoms. Because thrombolytics can cause sudden bleeding, they're used only in life-threatening situations.

Other Types of Treatment

Vena cava filter: If you can't take blood thinners or they're not working well, your doctor may recommend a vena cava filter.

The filter is inserted inside a large vein called the vena cava. The filter catches blood clots before they travel to the lungs, which prevents pulmonary embolism. However, the filter doesn't stop new blood clots from forming.

Graduated compression stockings: Graduated compression stockings can reduce leg swelling caused by a blood clot. These stockings are worn on the legs from the arch of the foot to just above or below the knee.

Compression stockings are tight at the ankle and become looser as they go up the leg. This creates gentle pressure up the leg. The pressure keeps blood from pooling and clotting.

There are three types of compression stockings. One type is support pantyhose, which offer the least amount of pressure.

The second type is over-the-counter compression hose. These stockings give a little more pressure than support pantyhose. Over-the-counter compression hose are sold in medical supply stores and pharmacies.

Prescription-strength compression hose offer the greatest amount of pressure. They also are sold in medical supply stores and pharmacies. However, a specially trained person needs to fit you for these stockings.

Talk with your doctor about how long you should wear compression stockings.

Section 41.3

Headache after Lumbar Puncture

Excerpted from "Headache: Hope Through Research," by the National Institute of Neurological Disorders and Stroke (NINDS, www.ninds.nih .gov), part of the National Institutes of Health, September 19, 2012.

Anyone can experience a headache. Nearly two out of three children will have a headache by age 15. More than 9 in 10 adults will experience a headache sometime in their life. Headache is our most common form of pain and a major reason cited for days missed at work or school as well as visits to the doctor. Without proper treatment, headaches can be severe and interfere with daily activities.

Certain types of headache run in families. Episodes of headache may ease or even disappear for a time and recur later in life. It's possible to have more than one type of headache at the same time.

Primary headaches occur independently and are not caused by another medical condition. It's uncertain what sets the process of a primary headache in motion. A cascade of events that affect blood vessels

545

and nerves inside and outside the head causes pain signals to be sent to the brain. Brain chemicals called neurotransmitters are involved in creating head pain, as are changes in nerve cell activity (called cortical spreading depression). Migraine, cluster, and tension-type headache are the more familiar types of primary headache.

Secondary headaches are symptoms of another health disorder that causes pain-sensitive nerve endings to be pressed on or pulled or pushed out of place. They may result from underlying conditions including fever, infection, medication overuse, stress or emotional conflict, high blood pressure, psychiatric disorders, head injury or trauma, stroke, tumors, and nerve disorders (particularly trigeminal neuralgia, a chronic pain condition that typically affects a major nerve on one side of the jaw or cheek).

Headaches can range in frequency and severity of pain. Some individuals may experience headaches once or twice a year, while others may experience headaches more than 15 days a month. Some headaches may recur or last for weeks at a time. Pain can range from mild to disabling and may be accompanied by symptoms such as nausea or increased sensitivity to noise or light, depending on the type of headache.

When to See a Doctor

Not all headaches require a physician's attention. But headaches can signal a more serious disorder that requires prompt medical care. Immediately call or see a physician if you or someone you're with experience any of these symptoms:

- Sudden, severe headache that may be accompanied by a stiff neck

- Severe headache accompanied by fever, nausea, or vomiting that is not related to another illness

- First or worst headache, often accompanied by confusion, weakness, double vision, or loss of consciousness

- Headache that worsens over days or weeks or has changed in pattern or behavior

- Recurring headache in children

- Headache following a head injury

- Headache and a loss of sensation or weakness in any part of the body, which could be a sign of a stroke

- Headache associated with convulsions

- Headache associated with shortness of breath

- Two or more headaches a week

- Persistent headache in someone who has been previously headache-free, particularly in someone over age 50

- New headaches in someone with a history of cancer or HIV/AIDS [human immunodeficiency virus/acquired immunodeficiency syndrome]

Headaches after Surgery: Spinal Fluid Leak

About one fourth of people who undergo a lumbar puncture (which involves a small sampling of the spinal fluid being removed for testing) develop a headache due to a leak of cerebrospinal fluid following the procedure. Since the headache occurs only when the individual stands up, the cure is to lie down until the headache runs its course—anywhere from a few hours to several days. Severe postdural headaches may be treated by injecting a small amount of the individual's own blood into the low back to stop the leak (called an epidural blood patch). Occasionally spinal fluid leaks spontaneously, causing this low pressure headache.

Section 41.4

Lung Function Tests Help Identify Lung Complications after Surgery

Excerpted from "What Are Lung Function Tests?" by the National Heart, Lung, and Blood Institute (NHLBI, www.nhlbi.nih.gov), part of the National Institutes of Health, September 17, 2012.

Lung function tests, also called pulmonary function tests, measure how well your lungs work. These tests are used to look for the cause of breathing problems, such as shortness of breath.

Lung function tests measure:

- how much air you can take into your lungs (This amount is compared with that of other people your age, height, and sex. This allows your doctor to see whether you're in the normal range.);

- how much air you can blow out of your lungs and how fast you can do it;

- how well your lungs deliver oxygen to your blood;

- the strength of your breathing muscles.

Doctors use lung function tests to help diagnose conditions such as asthma, pulmonary fibrosis (scarring of the lung tissue), and COPD (chronic obstructive pulmonary disease).

Lung function tests also are used to check the extent of damage caused by conditions such as pulmonary fibrosis and sarcoidosis. Also, these tests might be used to check how well treatments, such as asthma medicines, are working.

Types of Lung Function Tests

Breathing Tests

Spirometry: Spirometry measures how much air you breathe in and out and how fast you blow it out. This is measured two ways: Peak expiratory flow rate (PEFR) and forced expiratory volume in one second (FEV1).

PEFR is the fastest rate at which you can blow air out of your lungs. FEV1 refers to the amount of air you can blow out in one second.

During the test, a technician will ask you to take a deep breath in. Then, you'll blow as hard as you can into a tube connected to a small machine. The machine is called a spirometer.

Your doctor may have you inhale a medicine that helps open your airways. He or she will want to see whether the medicine changes or improves the test results.

Spirometry helps check for conditions that affect how much air you can breathe in, such as pulmonary fibrosis (scarring of the lung tissue). The test also helps detect diseases that affect how fast you can breathe air out, like asthma and COPD (chronic obstructive pulmonary disease).

Lung volume measurement: Body plethysmography is a test that measures how much air is present in your lungs when you take a deep breath. It also measures how much air remains in your lungs after you breathe out fully.

During the test, you sit inside a glass booth and breathe into a tube that's attached to a computer.

For other lung function tests, you might breathe in nitrogen or helium gas and then blow it out. The gas you breathe out is measured to show how much air your lungs can hold.

Lung volume measurement can help diagnose pulmonary fibrosis or a stiff or weak chest wall.

Lung diffusion capacity: This test measures how well oxygen passes from your lungs to your bloodstream. During this test, you breathe in a type of gas through a tube. You hold your breath for a brief moment and then blow out the gas.

Abnormal test results may suggest loss of lung tissue, emphysema (a type of COPD), very bad scarring of the lung tissue, or problems with blood flow through the body's arteries.

Tests to Measure Oxygen Level

Pulse oximetry and arterial blood gas tests show how much oxygen is in your blood. During pulse oximetry, a small sensor is attached to your finger or ear. The sensor uses light to estimate how much oxygen is in your blood. This test is painless and no needles are used.

For an arterial blood gas test, a blood sample is taken from an artery, usually in your wrist. The sample is sent to a laboratory, where its oxygen level is measured. You may feel some discomfort during an arterial blood gas test because a needle is used to take the blood sample.

What to Expect during Lung Function Tests

Spirometry might be done in your doctor's office or in a special lung function laboratory (lab). Lung volume measurement and lung diffusion capacity tests are done in a special lab or clinic. For these tests, you sit in a chair next to a machine that measures your breathing. For spirometry, you sit or stand next to the machine.

Before the tests, a technician places soft clips on your nose. This allows you to breathe only through a tube that's attached to the testing machine. The technician will tell you how to breathe into the tube. For example, you might be asked to breathe normally, slowly, or rapidly.

Some tests require deep breathing, which might make you feel short of breath, dizzy, or light-headed, or it might make you cough.

Spirometry

For this test, you take a deep breath and then exhale as fast and as hard as you can into the tube. With spirometry, your doctor may give you medicine to help open your airways. Your doctor will want to see whether the medicine changes or improves the test results.

Lung Volume Measurement

For body plethysmography, you sit in a clear glass booth and breathe through the tube attached to the testing machine. The changes in pressure inside the booth are measured to show how much air you can breathe into your lungs.

For other tests, you breathe in nitrogen or helium gas and then exhale. The gas that you breathe out is measured.

Lung Diffusion Capacity

During this test, you breathe in gas through the tube, hold your breath for 10 seconds, and then rapidly blow it out. The gas contains a small amount of carbon monoxide, which won't harm you.

Pulse Oximetry

Pulse oximetry is done in a doctor's office or hospital. For this test, a small sensor is attached to your finger or ear using a clip or flexible tape. The sensor is then attached to a cable that leads to a small machine called an oximeter. The oximeter shows the amount of oxygen in your blood. This test is painless and no needles are used.

Arterial Blood Gas

An arterial blood gas test is done in a lab or hospital. During this test, your doctor or technician inserts a needle into an artery, usually in your wrist, and takes a sample of blood. You may feel some discomfort when the needle is inserted. The sample is then sent to a lab where its oxygen level is measured.

After the needle is removed, you may feel mild pressure or throbbing at the needle site. Applying pressure to the area for 5 to 10 minutes should stop the bleeding. You'll be given a small bandage to place on the area.

Section 41.5

Malignant Hyperthermia: A Rare But Serious Reaction to Anesthesia

Malignant Hyperthermia (MH) Effects in Surgery

MH complications include a rise in heart rate, extreme temperature elevation, muscle breakdown, and changes in body chemistry that can lead to excessive bleeding and the failure of organs and other body systems. The reaction can occur during any part of a procedure under general anesthesia or even in the recovery room, and in any surgical setting from office and ambulatory centers to hospitals. It can be treated with dantrolene sodium if the case is identified and treatment is administered very early in the onset of the condition. Unfortunately, a few cases of malignant hyperthermia can result in death even if proper treatment is administered.

Detecting MH

A very specialized muscle biopsy test, only available at a few institutions, is the most accurate test for malignant hyperthermia susceptibility. However, DNA [deoxyribonucleic acid] testing can help provide answers for people who suspect they might be at risk. You can be assured that MH is an extremely uncommon condition, and your anesthesiologist and other surgical team members are well-trained for adverse reactions that can occur during procedures.

Patient Responsibility

To be sure you receive the highest level of care no matter what happens in the OR [operating room], it is critical that you request an anesthesiologist's presence for any procedure involving anesthesia. This ensures the person giving you anesthesia is a fully trained licensed physician, and you know you have the most highly trained professional physician at your side to manage any complications that may arise.

Prior to undergoing general anesthesia for surgery, patients concerned about malignant hyperthermia inform their anesthesiologist of any personal or family history of malignant hyperthermia, or adverse reactions to anesthetics. You also may ask if a supply of dantrolene is available in the facility where surgery will take place and whether treatment protocols are also available.

MH Patient Registry

While 95 percent of patients who experience malignant hyperthermia reactions survive it, the ASA-MHAUS [American Society of Anesthesiologists–Malignant Hyperthermia Association of the United States] partnership still needs the public's help to build a database of patients who are already aware they have the gene mutation that leads to malignant hyperthermia. Since its formation in 1981, MHAUS has been working through its growing member network of patients that are MH-susceptible and their family members, as well as anesthesiologists and health care providers to educate other members of the medical community and the public regarding the risks MH can unexpectedly pose in conjunction with some of the most commonly used anesthetics in hospital operating rooms, dental offices, and surgical centers.

Section 41.6

Shock

Excerpted from "What Is Cardiogenic Shock?" by the National
Heart, Lung, and Blood Institute (NHLBI, www.nhlbi.nih.gov), part
of the National Institutes of Health, July 1, 2011.

The medical term "shock" refers to a state in which not enough blood and oxygen reach important organs in the body, such as the brain and kidneys. Shock causes very low blood pressure and may be life threatening.

Shock can have many causes. Cardiogenic shock is only one type of shock. Other types of shock include hypovolemic shock and vasodilatory shock.

Hypovolemic shock is a condition in which the heart can't pump enough blood to the body because of severe blood loss.

In vasodilatory shock, the blood vessels suddenly relax. When the blood vessels are too relaxed, blood pressure drops and blood flow becomes very low. Without enough blood pressure, blood and oxygen don't reach the body's organs.

A bacterial infection in the bloodstream, a severe allergic reaction, or damage to the nervous system (brain and nerves) may cause vasodilatory shock.

When a person is in shock (from any cause), not enough blood and oxygen are reaching the body's organs. If shock lasts more than a few minutes, the lack of oxygen starts to damage the body's organs. If shock isn't treated quickly, it can cause permanent organ damage or death.

Some of the signs and symptoms of shock include the following:

- Confusion or lack of alertness

- Loss of consciousness

- A sudden and ongoing rapid heartbeat

- Sweating

- Pale skin

- A weak pulse

- Rapid breathing

- Decreased or no urine output

- Cool hands and feet

If you think that you or someone else is in shock, call 911 right away for emergency treatment. Prompt medical care can save your life and prevent or limit damage to your body's organs.

Outlook

In the past, almost no one survived cardiogenic shock. Now, about half of the people who go into cardiogenic shock survive. This is because of prompt recognition of symptoms and improved treatments, such as medicines and devices. These treatments can restore blood flow to the heart and help the heart pump better.

In some cases, devices that take over the pumping function of the heart are used. Implanting these devices requires major surgery.

Medical Procedures and Surgery

Medical procedures and surgery can restore blood flow to the heart and the rest of the body, repair heart damage, and help keep a patient alive while he or she recovers from shock.

Surgery also can improve the chances of long-term survival. Surgery done within six hours of the onset of shock symptoms has the greatest chance of improving survival.

The types of procedures and surgery used to treat underlying causes of cardiogenic shock include the following:

- Angioplasty and stents: Angioplasty is a procedure used to open narrowed or blocked coronary (heart) arteries and treat an ongoing heart attack. A stent is a small mesh tube that's placed in a coronary artery during angioplasty to help keep it open.

- Coronary artery bypass grafting: For this surgery, arteries or veins from other parts of the body are used to bypass (that is, go around) narrowed coronary arteries. This creates a new passage for oxygen-rich blood to reach the heart.

- Surgery to repair a break in the wall that separates the heart's chambers: This break is called a septal rupture.

- Heart transplant: This type of surgery rarely is done during an emergency situation like cardiogenic shock because of other available options. Also, doctors need to do very careful testing to make sure a patient will benefit from a heart transplant and to find a matching heart from a donor. Still, in some cases, doctors may recommend a transplant if they feel it's the best way to improve a patient's chances of long-term survival.

Surgery to repair damaged heart valves may also be used to treat underlying causes of shock.

Part Five

Recovering from Surgery

Chapter 42

Recovering from Surgery

Chapter Contents

Section 42.1

What to Expect in the Postanesthesia Care Unit (PACU)

Where do I go after surgery?

Right after surgery, you will be taken to the post anesthesia care unit (PACU) or directly to the intensive care unit where nurses will take care of you and watch you closely. A nurse will check your temperature, blood pressure, and pulse often, look at your bandages, regulate your IV [intravenous line], and give you pain medication, as you need it.

What do I need to tell the PACU nurse?

Please tell the nurse if you are having pain. The nurse will ask you to give your pain a number on a scale of 0 to 10, with 0 meaning you have no pain, and 10 you have the worst pain. The nurse will check your pain and continue to help you manage it until you are as comfortable as possible.

What do I need to do with my nausea (feeling sick to your stomach)?

Some patients feel very sick to their stomach (nausea). It is important to tell your nurse about it right away, so it can be treated with medication. If you have had problems with nausea in the past, the anesthesia care provider knows this before surgery.

What other feelings may I experience after surgery?

You may feel sleepy, dizzy, and/or forgetful from the medication given to you during your surgery.

When will I see my family after surgery?

Depending on the facility you are at will determine visitation in the PACU. Check with the nursing staff to find out if your family will be allowed to visit you.

What type of information do I need to know before going home?

If you are going home that same day, you will be given printed discharge instructions for your care at home. The nursing staff will go over all the information with you and a family member or friend. Your instructions will include:

- activity restrictions;

- diet;

- pain medication;

- follow up instructions with your surgeon;

- signs to watch for if you need to call the doctor.

You might be given a prescription depending on your doctor's orders and what kind of surgery you had done.

Section 42.2

What to Expect If You Are Going Home the Day of Surgery

Once your surgery is over and you have been moved from the post anesthesia care unit (PACU), you will either be sent to an inpatient bed or taken to the area where the nurses will get you ready to go home.

What do I need to know before going home?

Before leaving the building, you must meet certain discharge criteria. You may be asked to urinate before going home after certain surgical procedures. If you had a spinal anesthetic, you may be sent home with special instructions about what you should do if you cannot urinate within a certain time period.

Your nurse will go over your postoperative/after surgery instructions with you and your family/friend. The goal is to teach you several things about going home. These things include:

- pain medicines;
- special diet plans;
- special instructions related to your surgery;
- follow up with your surgeon;
- signs to watch for infection;
- when you should report to your surgeon.

If you have stopped taking medications before your surgery, your nurse or doctor will let you know when you can start taking them again. You may also be given a prescription from your doctor at this time.

How long will it take me to feel normal again?

Be prepared at home to continue your recovery. Plan to take it easy for a few days until you feel back to normal. Patients often feel minor effects following surgery due to anesthesia, which might include:

- being very tired;
- muscle aches;
- a sore throat;
- dizziness;
- headaches.

Sometimes patients can feel very sick to their stomach and may throw up. These side effects usually go away quickly in the first few hours after surgery, but it can take several days before they are completely gone. Due to feeling tired or having some discomfort, most patients do not feel up to their normal activities for several days.

Can I drive myself home?

Patients who have outpatient/same day surgery must have someone drive them home and stay with for 24 hours following their surgery. The medications you were given during your surgery may affect your memory and mental judgment for the next 24 hours. During that time frame, do not use alcoholic beverages and tobacco products. It is also advised for you not to make any important business or personal decisions and do not use machinery or electrical equipment.

In a day or two after surgery, a nurse may call to check to see how you are feeling. It is important that you provide the staff with a correct working phone number, so they can contact you.

Section 42.3

Reducing Depression after Heart Surgery

Excerpted from "Your Guide to Living Well with Heart Disease," from the National Heart, Lung, and Blood Institute (NHLBI, www.nhlbi.nih.gov), part of the National Institutes of Health, November 2005. Reviewed by David A. Cooke, MD, FACP, October 11, 2012.

Anyone who has had a heart attack or has undergone heart surgery knows that it can be an upsetting experience. You've just come through a major health crisis, and your usual life has been disrupted.

Afterward, it's normal to experience a wide range of feelings. You may feel some relief. But you may also feel worried, angry, or depressed. It may be reassuring to know that these reactions are very common, and that most difficult feelings pass within a few weeks. Here are some things to remember:

Take one day at a time. Try not to think too much about next week or next month. Do what you can do today. Enjoy small pleasures: A walk in your neighborhood, a conversation with a loved one, a snuggle with a pet, or a good meal.

Share your concerns. Talk with family members and friends about your feelings and concerns, and ask for support. Be sure to ask for the kind of support you need. (For example, if you want a sympathetic ear rather than advice, gently let your loved ones know.)

Be sure to give family members time to say what they feel and need, too. Supportive relationships may actually help to lengthen life after a heart attack.

Get support from veterans. Whether you've had a heart attack or gone through heart surgery, consider joining a support group for people who have shared your experience. Groups for heart patients can provide emotional support as well as help you develop new ways of handling everyday challenges. For a list of support groups in your local area, contact Mended Hearts at www.mended.hearts.org. Your local American Heart Association chapter may also offer support groups.

Keep moving. Regular physical activity not only helps to reduce the risk of future heart problems, but also helps to relieve anxiety, depression, and other difficult feelings. Any regular physical activity—even gentle walking—can help to lift your mood.

Seek help for depression. Up to 20 percent of heart disease patients battle serious depression, and many more suffer milder cases of the blues. If you find yourself feeling very sad or discouraged for more than a week or so, be sure to let your doctor know. Counseling and/or medication can often be very helpful. Seeking help is very important, not only because you deserve to enjoy life as fully as possible, but also because heart patients who are successfully treated for depression are less likely to have future serious heart problems.

Chapter 43

Hospital Discharge Planning

During your stay, your doctor and the staff will work with you to plan for your discharge. You and your caregiver (a family member or friend who may be helping you) are important members of the planning team. In the following text is a list of important things you and your caregiver should know to prepare for discharge.

What's Ahead?

- Ask where you will get care after discharge. Do you have options (like home health care)? Be sure you tell the staff what you prefer.

- If a caregiver will be helping you after discharge, write down their name and phone number.

Your Health

- Ask the staff about your health condition and what you can do to help yourself get better.

- Ask about problems to watch for and what to do about them. Write down a name and phone number to call if you have problems.

- Write down your prescription drugs, over-the-counter drugs, vitamins, and herbal supplements.

Excerpted from "Your Discharge Planning Checklist," by the Centers for Medicare and Medicaid Services (www.medicare.gov), January 2012.

- Review the list with the staff.

- Tell the staff what drugs, vitamins, or supplements you took before you were admitted. Ask if you should still take these after you leave.

- Write down a name and phone number to call if you have questions.

Recovery and Support

- Ask if you will need medical equipment (like a walker). Who will arrange for this? Write down where to call if you have questions about equipment.

- Ask if you're ready to do the activities listed in the following text. Write down the ones you need help with and tell the staff.

  - Bathing, dressing, using the bathroom, climbing stairs

  - Cooking, food shopping, house cleaning, paying bills

  - Getting to doctors' appointments, picking up prescription drugs

- Make sure you have support (like a caregiver) in place that can help you.

- Ask the staff to show you and your caregiver any other tasks that require special skills (like changing a bandage or giving a shot). Then, show them you can do these tasks. Write down a name and phone number to call if you need help.

- Ask to speak to a social worker if you're concerned about how you and your family are coping with your illness. Write down information about support groups and other resources.

- Talk to a social worker or your health plan if you have questions about what your insurance will cover and how much you will have to pay. Ask about possible ways to get help with your costs.

- Ask for written discharge instructions (that you can read and understand) and a summary of your current health status. Bring this information and your completed list of medications to your follow-up appointments.

- Write down any appointments and tests you will need in the next several weeks.

For the Caregiver

- Do you have any questions about the items on this list or on the discharge instructions? Write them down and discuss them with the staff.

- Can you give the patient the help he or she needs?

- What tasks do you need help with?

- Do you need any education or training? Talk to the staff about getting the help you need before discharge.

- Write down a name and phone number to call if you have questions.

- Get prescriptions and any special diet instructions early, so you won't have to make extra trips after discharge.

Resources

The agencies listed here have information on community services, (like home-delivered meals and rides to appointments). You can also get help making long-term care decisions. Ask the staff in your health care setting for more information.

- **Area Agencies on Aging (AAAs) and Aging and Disability Resource Centers (ADRCs):** Help older adults, people with disabilities, and their caregivers. To find the AAA/ADRC in your area, visit the Eldercare Locator at www.eldercare.gov, or call 800-677-1116.

- **Ask Medicare:** Provides information and support to caregivers of people with Medicare. Visit www.medicare.gov/caregivers.

- **Long-Term Care (LTC) Ombudsman Program:** Advocate for and promote the rights of residents in LTC facilities. Visit www .ltcombudsman.org.

- **Senior Medicare Patrol (SMP) Programs:** Work with seniors to protect themselves from the economic and health-related consequences of Medicare and Medicaid fraud, error, and abuse. To find a local SMP program, visit www.smpresource.org.

- **Centers for Independent Living (CILs):** Help people with disabilities live independently. For a state-by-state directory of CILs, visit www.ilru.org/html/publications/directory/index .html.

- **State Technology Assistance Project:** Has information on medical equipment and other assistive technology. Visit www.resna .org, or call 703-524-6686 to get the contact information in your state.

- **National Long-Term Care Clearinghouse:** Provides information and resources to plan for your long-term care needs. Visit www.longtermcare.gov.

- **National Council on Aging:** Provides information about programs that help pay for prescription drugs, utility bills, meals, health care, and more. Visit www.benefitscheckup.org.

- **State Health Insurance Assistance Programs (SHIPs):** Offer counseling on health insurance and programs for people with limited income. Also help with claims, billing, and appeals. Visit www.medicare.gov/contacts, or call 800-MEDICARE (800-633-4227) to get your SHIP's phone number. TTY users should call 877-486-2048.

- **State Medical Assistance (Medicaid) Office:** Provides information about Medicaid. To find your local office, visit www.medi care.gov/contacts, or call 800-MEDICARE and say, Medicaid.

Chapter 44

Moving to a Rehabilitation Unit or Facility

What Is Rehab?

If your family member is in the hospital for an acute illness or injury or for surgery, you may be told that the next step in care is rehab. Rehabilitation (or simply rehab) is treatment to help patients regain (get back) all or some of the movement and function they lost because of the current health problem.

Rehab itself is very different from hospital care. While your family member might still be quite ill and need medical attention, he or she will be expected to be active during the rehab process. Rehab is hard work.

You will find that things are done differently in rehab than in a hospital. You will see many active patients and therapists in the halls and treatment rooms. In general, you will find that rehab has an active, workout atmosphere that may not feel like a place for sick people.

Your family member will be expected to work as hard as possible during the rehab process, and you will have many responsibilities. For example, you will be expected to provide loose, comfortable clothing for your family member to make it easy for him or her to get dressed and to take part in therapy sessions. You will be expected to participate in meetings with the medical team. This will allow you to ask questions and understand your family member's rehab process.

"Planning for Inpatient Rehabilitation (Rehab) Services," © 2010 United Hospital Fund. All rights reserved. Reprinted with permission. For additional information, visit http://nextstepincare.org.

Here are five important points to remember:

1. The goal of rehab is to help patients be independent—doing as much for themselves as they can.

2. Rehab is done with a patient, not to a patient. Your family member must be willing and able to work with rehab services during active treatment and, later, with caregivers or by themselves at home.

3. The patient's chronic (long-term) health conditions, such as high blood pressure or cholesterol, are treated during rehab, but they are not the reason the patient is in rehab.

4. Most rehab services last weeks, not months.

5. Most insurance policies cover rehab when ordered by a doctor, but there will probably be extra costs.

Where Are Rehab Services Provided?

Patients can get rehab services at home, in a local clinic, or at an inpatient setting (either a rehab unit within a hospital, nursing home, or a separate rehab facility).

While this text looks only at inpatient rehab services, rehab services can be provided by a home health agency as a skilled service. In this case, your family member must be well enough to be at home. You may want to consider whether home care including rehab is an option for your relative. There are also outpatient rehab services. In this case, your family member must be able to travel back and forth to the clinic or hospital that provides rehab.

Inpatient Rehab Settings

Inpatient rehab can take place at any of these settings:

•   Rehab unit within a hospital or a separate inpatient rehab facility (IRF): These rehab programs are usually very intense. Patients must be able to benefit from, and receive, at least three hours of therapy five days each week. Some patients may be admitted even though they are not able to tolerate an intense program at first if the therapists believe that the patient will be able to improve quickly. If possible, talk with your family member about whether this setting is right for his or her needs. Think about his or her current illness as well as other chronic health problems. Check with your family member's doctor and physical therapist about this level of rehab.

- Rehab unit within a skilled nursing facility (SNF)—also called a nursing home: Most patients who are discharged to rehab go to a SNF (pronounced like sniff). These programs offer the same types of services as an IRF but at a less intense level. Rehab services at a SNF are not the same as long-term care in a nursing home. Indeed, most patients at a SNF are discharged home when rehab is over. Some patients do move to the regular long-term care part of a SNF, however, so you should be aware of this possibility.

- Special settings: Some types of rehab take place in special settings such as brain injury units or cardiac (heart) units. Ask hospital staff if this is an option you and your family member should consider.

Making a Choice about Settings

The hospital treatment team may suggest that your family member go to rehab after leaving the hospital. (Sometimes staff members will say "go to a nursing home" when what they really mean is going to a rehab unit in a SNF.)

Rehab settings are different from hospitals. They decide which patients they accept on the basis of whether the person can benefit from the level and kind of services they provide. So, even if you decide, for example, that your family member would like to have rehab in an IRF, the IRF may not be willing to accept him or her.

Here are some things to think about when making a choice about rehab setting:

- Amount of services: Some rehab settings are more intense and active than others. Think about your family member's current health problem as well as any chronic concerns. Talk about these with your family member's medical team to make the best choice.

- Location: The ideal is to find a rehab setting near where you live or work. This way, it is easy for you to visit. You might want to go to therapy with your family member, learn how to help your family member do the exercises, find out how to get the house ready, help plan for discharge, or offer comfort and moral support throughout the rehab process.

- Cost: Medicare, Medicaid, and most private health insurance plans may pay all or some of the rehab costs. But there are strict guidelines, and you need to pay all costs that insurance does not cover. It is important to learn as much as you can. You can do so by talking with the discharge planner or someone at the financial office in the rehab facility.

Rehab Services

Patients often work with two or more rehab services. These include:

- Physical therapy (PT): This helps patients with problems moving, balancing, walking, and performing other activities. PT can also help patients with prosthetic (artificial) arms or legs, shoe inserts, wheelchairs, walkers, and other assistive devices.

- Occupational therapy (OT): This helps patients be more independent with self-care and other daily tasks, such as eating, getting dressed, typing, and using the telephone.

- Speech therapy: This helps patients relearn language skills such as talking, reading, and writing. It can also help with swallowing problems.

- Psychological counseling (or simply counseling): This helps patients (and sometimes also their family members) adjust to major life changes caused by an illness or injury. Counseling may be offered individually (one patient at a time) or in a group.

Going from Hospital to Inpatient Rehab to Home

Going from hospital to rehab: Hospital staff should tell the rehab staff about what they did as treatment and care for your family member.

Clothing: Your family member will need to wear loose, comfortable clothes (not gowns) to participate in therapy sessions (such as physical therapy or occupational therapy). The facility does not provide such clothing, so you will have to bring them from home or buy them. It is important to put labels in the clothing and bring them to the rehab facility at the time of admission. Make sure to ask the rehab team about the facility's specific policies about clothing.

Initial assessment for restorative potential: Rehab staff will assess your family member within two days of admission. The most important finding is restorative potential. This means the level of function (ability to move or do activities) that your family member is likely to regain from rehab. Restorative potential has to do with only the current illness, and not any chronic condition, such as diabetes, arthritis, or dementia. Insurance pays for rehab only when your family member is making progress toward restorative potential.

Rehab begins: The amount of time your family member spends in rehab depends on the type of setting. Staff will assess your family member throughout the rehab process to make sure he or she is making progress toward restorative potential.

Care plan (team) meeting: This meeting takes place after rehab has started. It includes staff from nursing, social services, dietary, recreation, and rehabilitation who discuss your family member's progress. You and your family member will be asked to attend. This is a good time to ask questions and raise any concerns.

Discharge to home: Patients are discharged from rehab when the team assesses that they have reached a plateau (a time when the patient is not making any progress, but is not getting any worse). This means that the patient is not likely to make more progress. When your family member reaches a plateau, rehab staff will give you a written notice stating that Medicare or other insurance will end on a certain date (often the day after this notice is given). Speak up and let the staff know if you feel that your family member needs more time.

Rehab after discharge: Many patients continue their rehab after leaving an inpatient setting. This can happen at home or in the community as an outpatient. Many patients feel much better and improve quickly when they have returned to the comforts of home.

Factors That Affect a Patient's Rehab Progress

To repeat, rehab is hard work. Here are some factors that can affect a patient's progress:

Patient motivation (how much a patient is willing to work at rehab): People differ when it comes to motivation. It can depend on a person's illness, type of rehab, and restorative potential. A person's personality is also a factor; some people like a challenge while others do better without pressure. Sometimes it is hard to know whether to respond with a gentle or a firm approach. Praise is always good, even if progress seems slow. Caregivers can help by talking with rehab staff about how their family member has dealt with other life challenges.

Relationships with therapists: Your family member will likely work with many therapists. Of course, each has his or her own style.

Let each therapist know what style works best and ask that this information be written in the treatment plan.

Expectations: One of the hardest parts of rehab is being realistic about how much function a patient can get back. Some patients make a full recovery and get back to the same level as before. Other patients improve just a little. You and your family member may need to adjust expectations and learn new ways of doing daily tasks.

Feelings: Patients can have a lot of feelings during rehab. These can be feelings about the injury or illness itself, attitudes about rehab and restorative potential, or expectations for recovery. Feeling tired, angry, discouraged, or overwhelmed is normal and part of the rehab process. Talk with the staff if you think these feelings are so strong in your family member that they may affect the rehab progress. As a family caregiver who is watching or being part of the rehab process, you will also have many strong feelings. You may need someone to talk to as well. It may help to discuss these feelings with the social worker, or ask the staff who can help you.

How Family Caregivers Can Help

Have a good relationship with rehab staff: Talk with staff about the rehab plan. Ask how your family member is doing in treatment. Speak up if you have concerns about the care your family member is getting.

Encourage independence: The purpose of rehab is to help patients be as independent as possible. You can help by encouraging your family member to do as much as he or she can. This is a sign of love, not disrespect. It does not help to be overprotective, which can slow a patient's progress.

Balance your need to know with your family member's wish for privacy: While some patients always want caregivers with them, others prefer to have therapy sessions alone. Talk with your family member about the right balance between these options.

Figure out when and how much to visit: While of course you want to help your family member, you likely have other work or family responsibilities. Even if you can visit only in the evening, you can still talk with night staff or make an appointment to meet with staff another time.

Find ways to help: This can be friendly visits, bringing pictures from home, going to care plan meetings, talking with staff about discharge, going to rehab sessions, or working with the therapists.

Paying for Rehab Services

Insurance coverage can be confusing. Your family member may have Medicaid, Medicare, private health insurance, or some combination of these plans. Make sure you fully understand what insurance will and will not pay for. We strongly suggest that you learn more by talking with the financial office at your family member's rehab facility.

Here are some basic facts about paying for rehab:

Medicaid: Medicaid will pay for rehab if your family member meets its strict guidelines about the type and amount of service. If your family member is eligible for Medicaid but does not yet have it, staff at the rehab setting can help you apply.

Medicare: Medicare may or may not pay for rehab services from a skilled nursing facility (SNF). To qualify, your family member must:

- Need skilled nursing care seven days a week or skilled rehab services five days a week. A doctor or nurse practitioner must certify that your family member needs these services.

- Have been in a hospital for at least three consecutive days (not counting the discharge day) within the 30-day period before going to a SNF.

- Be admitted to the SNF for the same illness or injury that was treated in the hospital.

- Be assessed by rehab staff at least once a week to find out whether he or she has reached restorative potential. Medicare stops paying for rehab services when patients reach this level. Medicare uses the term benefit period to define the time for rehab services. Here are some facts:

  - A benefit period begins on the first day your family member is admitted to a hospital or a SNF and continues for up to 100 days. It ends when your family member has not received services from a hospital or SNF for 60 days in a row. Medicare will assess staff reports of your family member's progress and stop paying for rehab services when he or she has reached restorative potential. This may take less than 100 days.

  - You can appeal if Medicare says that it will no longer pay for rehab services. Understand that there is a lot of paperwork involved. To learn more about how to appeal a Medicare decision, talk with the people at the financial office at the rehab facility.

577

- Medicare puts no limits on the number of benefit periods a patient can have.

- When Medicare pays for rehab services, it pays the full cost for the first 20 days and part of the cost for the next 80. Your family member or you will have to pay a co-insurance cost during these 80 days. This fee is set by Medicare and not the rehab setting.

Medicare and Medicaid: Some patients are dually eligible; this means they have Medicaid and Medicare at the same time. When this happens, Medicaid pays for rehab services not covered by Medicare.

Private health insurance: Most health insurance plans follow the same guidelines as Medicare, but may require more frequent assessments of the patient's restorative potential. Talk with the health insurance company when your family member is admitted to rehab and throughout the course of care.

Other Costs

Even when Medicare or other insurance pays for all or most of rehab, there may still be costs that you or your family member has to pay. They may include [the following]:

- Private telephones, haircuts, and other personal care services

- Ambulance transportation: While Medicare or other insurance will pay for an ambulance to take your family member from the hospital to an inpatient rehab facility, it may not pay the costs of going elsewhere for other tests.

- Service after a patient reaches restorative potential: Some patients need more time to reach their full potential. If Medicare or other health insurance has ended, your family member may have to move to another setting. Staff will assess your family member to get a better idea of what services he or she needs. You or your family member must pay all costs that insurance does not cover. This situation is quite common, especially with older adults. The good news is that your family member is still making progress toward rehab goals.

Chapter 45

Nutrition and Exercise Concerns after Surgery

Chapter Contents

Section 45.1

Overview of Postsurgical Nutrition and Exercise Recommendations

This chapter contains text from "Physical Activity" and "Post-Surgery Diet Tips," by JoAnn Coleman, RN, MS, ACNP, AOCN. Reprinted with permission from the website of the Sol Goldman Pancreatic Cancer Research Center, http://pathology.jhu.edu/pc. © 2012. All rights reserved.

Physical Activity

Physical activity levels tend to decrease after cancer diagnosis and treatment. Even though one may feel fatigued, regular light physical activity should be encouraged.

Regular activity may:

- improve appetite;

- stimulate digestion;

- prevent constipation;

- maintain energy level;

- muscle mass;

- provide relaxation or stress reduction;

- lower levels of anxiety.

Increased levels of physical activity can improve overall quality of life. In choosing a level of activity, it is important to take into consideration the patient's physical functioning and previous levels of activity.

Physical activity should be individualized, initiated slowly, and progress gradually. A nutrition and physical activity plan should be customized for each patient to help rebuild muscle strength and correct problems with anemia or any impaired organ functioning. Adequate food intake and physical activity are crucial to patients recovering from any treatment for pancreatic cancer.

If a patient has limited mobility or is confined to bed rest, physical therapy in bed should be initiated to maintain enough strength and range of motion of joints. Physical activity can help counteract the fatigue spiral and feelings of low energy that some patients experience under those circumstances. Various medications and physical activity can help to increase appetite, and if needed, nutritional support can be provided in other ways for those who cannot eat enough. When patients are in the terminal stages of their disease, it is always necessary to listen to the wishes and decision of the patient regarding the intake of food or fluids.

Advice from a health care provider qualified in nutritional assessment can be helpful in assessing problems with eating and physical activity and in creating an individualized plan to meet specific challenges.

Post-Surgery Diet Tips

Food and Diet

How do I select a diet that is right for me? Start with the Food Guide Pyramid and American Cancer Society Cancer Prevention Guidelines. If you are having problems with particular foods, many others in the same food group can be substituted. Special problems might require consultation with a registered dietitian or nutritionist.

How many servings of fruit and vegetables should I eat every day? Although everyone should eat at least five servings of fruits and vegetables each day, it may be difficult. Nevertheless, by incorporating balanced meals with nutritional snacks, and drinking juices, eating up to 10 servings of fruits and vegetables per day is quite possible, and may be beneficial.

Can I get the same nutritional value from frozen and canned fruits and vegetables? Yes. In fact, frozen foods are often more nutritious than fresh foods because they are usually picked ripe and quickly frozen. Canning can reduce some of the nutrients, but the nutritional value of canned fruits and vegetables is often equivalent to those that are fresh.

Should I be juicing my fruits and vegetables? Juicing is not necessary, but can add variety to the diet and is a good way to consume fruits and vegetables, especially if there are difficulties with chewing or swallowing. Juicing also improves the absorption of some of the nutrients in fruits and vegetables. If you buy commercially juiced products, avoid those that have not been pasteurized.

How much water should I drink? Try to drink at least eight cups of water each day. Many symptoms of fatigue, lightheadedness, and nausea can be due to dehydration.

Should I limit my caffeine intake? Although many heart problems can be better controlled without caffeine, and sleep disturbances are less common, caffeine will have no adverse effects on your surgery.

Should I eat high-fiber foods? Yes, fiber from whole grains and high-fiber cereals can improve bowel function and help to decrease heart disease risk. Other high-fiber foods, such as beans, are good meat substitutes. Fruits and vegetables are good choices for their fiber content, as well as for the many other nutrients they contain. Fiber supplements do not contain the beneficial vitamins and other substances in fruits and vegetables.

Should I reduce my fat content? While consuming a diet that is low in fat has been shown to help reduce the risk of heart disease, the possible benefit for prevention of cancer recurrence is not yet proven. After surgery, adding moderate amounts of fats and fat-containing foods can help to improve caloric intake.

Should I avoid refined sugar? Refined sugars can cause fatigue due to fluctuating blood sugar levels, and they do not contain the same level of nutritional value as sugars naturally present in whole foods. It is therefore wise to limit intake of refined sugars (including brown sugar) in favor of more nutritious foods.

Should I become a vegetarian? It is not necessary to eliminate meat from the diet after surgery, but reducing red meat intake (and other sources of saturated fats) can reduce one's risk of heart disease, and may also reduce risk of colon and prostate cancers. Diets that include lean meats in small to moderate amounts can also be healthy.

Dietary Supplements

Should I supplement my diet with vitamins and minerals? The best source of vitamins and minerals is foods. During illness and recovery dietary intake may not be optimal, so a vitamin and mineral supplement may be needed. The best choice is a balanced multivitamin/mineral supplement containing as much as 100% of the Daily Value of most nutrients (formerly known as the RDA—Recommended Daily Allowance). Some people believe that if a little bit of a nutrient is good for you, then a lot must be better. There is no scientific evidence to support that idea. In fact, high doses of nutrients can have harmful effects. Be sure to discuss vitamin and mineral supplement use with your health care provider.

Can I get the nutritional equivalent of fruits and vegetables in a pill? No. Many hundreds of healthful compounds are found in fruits and vegetables. The small amount of dried powder contained in pills that are presented as being equivalent to fruits and vegetables includes only a small fraction of the levels contained in the whole foods.

Should I take antioxidants? It is not a good idea to take megadoses of any vitamin or mineral, including the antioxidant nutrients, at any time. High doses of antioxidants may interfere with the effectiveness of any further therapy such as chemotherapy or radiation therapy. Be sure to discuss your use of supplements with your health care provider. Fruits and vegetables are the best sources for naturally occurring antioxidants.

Should I take supplements containing beta-carotene? Supplements containing five mg or less of beta-carotene are unlikely to be harmful, as this is similar to the levels available from foods. However, higher dose supplements should be avoided because studies have shown that higher doses may actually increase the risk for certain cancers such as lung cancer.

How do I know that alternative or complementary methods are safe for me? Study all sources of information, but beware of testimonials or information that comes only from those who are selling a product. Also, be sure to tell your health care providers about the methods you wish to use, so they may advise you about any particular interaction that might occur with conventional medical therapy. It is also best to remember, if it sounds too good to be true, it likely is not true.

Diet and Symptoms

Are there foods that will help with my loss of appetite? Loss of appetite and nausea are commonly experienced after your surgery. Taste perceptions often change. Adding or increasing spices and condiments to meals may be needed temporarily to increase food appeal. Experiment with spices and flavorings often, as tastes may change. If you are having problems with food odors try cool or cold foods instead of hot to decrease aromas. Using covered pots, boiling bags, or a kitchen fan can minimize cooking odors. Taste changes are common. Try using plastic eating utensils and nonmetal cooling containers to help alleviate this problem. Try to eat small, more frequent meals and snacks. In some instances, medications can be helpful to reduce nausea. There are also medications that can help to stimulate appetite. Ask your health care provider if those might be good for you.

What can I do to reduce fatigue? Fatigue can be reduced by nutrition and physical activity. After surgery, many patients become fatigued because they do not eat enough, do not drink enough fluids, or do not exercise enough. Starting slowly with an exercise regimen, even if only for a few minutes a day can help restore energy. The frequency and duration of a simple activity like walking can be steadily increased. Do not hesitate to tell your health care providers about your fatigue.

Should I be concerned about unintentional weight loss? Weight loss often occurs after surgery. Continued weight loss should be avoided. Weight loss can be minimized by adequate dietary intake. Use of between-meal snacks that are good sources of calories, fat, and protein can help.

Is there a diet to help improve anemia? A balanced diet can help support the body's repair system for producing new blood cells. Iron supplements should be taken only after consulting with your health care provider. Extra iron is useful to correct iron deficiency, but it is not helpful for other conditions, and it can cause digestive system side effects.

Section 45.2

Nasogastric Tube Feedings at Home

What is a nasogastric (feeding) tube?

A nasogastric tube is a thin, flexible, soft tube that is passed through your child's nose (nostril), down the back of the throat, through the swallowing tube (esophagus), and into the stomach. It is taped under the nose to stay in place. A nasogastric tube is sometimes called an NG or feeding tube.

Why does my child need a NG (feeding) tube?

A nasogastric feeding tube is used to give fluids, food, and medicine when a child cannot take them by mouth. Reasons a child may need an NG include:

- problems with sucking, chewing, or swallowing;
- unable to get enough nutrition with a normal diet;
- unable to swallow needed medicines;
- to remove fluids and gas from the stomach;
- to prevent nausea and vomiting;
- to prevent pressure on stitches after surgery.

How is the NG used?

If the tube is needed for giving medicine, this is done using a syringe. For scheduled feedings, a syringe or pump may be used. For continuous feeding, formula is given using a pump. The pump controls the rate of fluid flow.

What is the feeding schedule?

[Editor's Note: Ask your doctor and write down the following information.]

585

- Feeding method:

- Formula name:

- Total amount of formula per day:

- Total amount of water per day:

- Amount of each feeding:

- Feeding schedule:

- Flush the tube with _____ mL of water before and after each feeding

- Other instructions:

  - Do not make changes in the type or amount of formula without talking to your child's provider first.

  - Provider to call:

  - Provider:

  - Phone:

  - After Hours Instructions:

How do I give formula with a feeding bag?

1. Wash your hands with soap and water for 30 seconds.

2. Position your child sitting up if possible, or on the right side with the head of bed raised 30–45 degrees.

3. Be sure the NG tube is in the stomach by looking at the placement of the tape, and measuring the distance from the nose to the tip of the tube. The tape should be in the same place as the last feeding. The measurement should be the same as the last feeding.

4. Clamp the feeding bag tubing.

5. Fill the feeding bag with formula.

6. Close the cover tightly. Hang the bag at least two feet above your child's head.

7. Open the clamp. Let the tubing fill until you see no air. Air in the tubing will not hurt your child, but will make your child's stomach feel full.

8. Clamp the tubing.

9. Connect the bag to the feeding tube.

10. Open the clamp.

11. Watch your child for any signs of nausea, vomiting, diarrhea, stomach swelling, or increased fussiness. Any one of these signs may mean that your child is not able to digest the formula at the rate it is running. If these symptoms occur, stop the feeding and contact your provider for instructions.

12. When the feeding is done, fill the bag with the prescribed amount of water. If it isn't time to take extra water, be sure to flush the tube after each feeding with at least 10 mL of tap water so that it doesn't clog.

13. Clamp or cap the tube. Disconnect the tube from your child.

14. Clean the supplies by rinsing the bag and tubing with cold water. Then, swish them in warm water and a drop of liquid dishwashing soap. Rinse thoroughly so that all of the soap is removed. Hang to dry.

How do I give formula with a syringe?

1. Wash your hands with soap and water for 30 seconds.

2. Position your child in a sitting position, or on the right side with the head raised 30–45 degrees.

3. Check placement of the NG tube using the method described in step 3 in the preceding text.

4. Remove the plunger from a 60 mL syringe. Connect the syringe to the feeding tube.

5. Hold the syringe upright and pour the formula into it.

6. Hold the syringe 10–12 inches above your child's head. Allow formula to be delivered by gravity over 20–30 minutes.

7. Keep filling the syringe as it empties until the entire amount of formula is given.

8. If the feeding should stop, you may use the plunger of the syringe to give a gentle push to get the feeding going again.

9. Give the prescribed amount of water to flush the tube.

10. Clean supplies as above (step 14).

Can I give medicines through the NG tube?

- Medicine can be given with a syringe through the feeding tube.

- It is best to use medicine in a liquid form. If you must take pills, be sure to thoroughly crush and dissolve pills in warm water so they do not clog the tube.

- Give each medicine separately. Do not mix medicines together or mix with formula.

- Never crush enteric-coated or time-release capsules. If you have questions about which medicines can be crushed, please talk to your pharmacist or health care provider.

- Flush the feeding tube with 5 mL of water after each medicine is given, and 10–20 mL of water after all medicines are given to be sure they get into the stomach.

- Do not add any medicines to formula in the feeding container.

How do I check the placement of the feeding tube?

The most important part of caring for an NG at home is checking that it is in the correct position (i.e., sitting in the stomach) before you put anything down it. The feeding tube should be marked where it exits the nose after the first placement. This mark should not change over time. Use a tape measure to measure the distance from where your child's tube exits the nostril to the end cap of the tube. Record this measurement every time you use the tube, or every 4–6 hours during a continuous feeding. If the mark moves, and the tube has slipped, call your provider before using the tube. Another way to tell if the NG tube is in the stomach is to attach a syringe to the end of the feeding tube and gently pull back. There may be fluid in the syringe and/or tubing that looks like formula, or clear green to yellow fluid. Return this fluid to the stomach. If you do not obtain fluid, it may be a sign that the tube is not in the stomach. Contact your provider before using the tube.

The securing tape should be changed every other day, or when it is loose, so that the NG tube stays secure.

Babies and children who need the tube for a long time at home will need to have the tube replaced at times. This normally means your child will need to return to a provider to have the tube replaced. Do not try to reinsert an NG tube if you have not been trained to do so. If you are going home with an NG tube, you need to have a clear plan in place before leaving the hospital. This plan should include who to contact and what to do if the tube moves or comes out. Any adult caring for your child will need education on how to care for the tube and how to feed your child. Please ask your nurse for more information.

If your child's nose is sore, move the tape to a different place on the nose. The tape may also need to be changed if it is coming loose. This is a good time to clean the skin under the tape. Be careful not to let the tube slip out.

1. Wrap or swaddle your child in a blanket, or have another person hold your child's arms so the tube cannot be pulled while you are caring for the site.

2. Wash your hands with soap and water. Dry well.

3. Prepare your supplies—tape, cotton-tipped swabs, water, soap, and lotion.

4. While carefully holding the tube, remove the old tape.

5. Use a cotton-tipped swab moistened with water and soap to clean the edges of both nostrils. Rinse thoroughly. Pat dry.

6. Look inside the nostril where the tube is to check for any redness, pain, or sores. You may put a small amount of lotion or Vaseline in the nostril to prevent irritation.

7. Secure the tube to the nose by wrapping a narrow piece of tape around the tube in each direction. Secure the other end of the tube to the cheek on the same side of the face where the tube exits.

8. If you feel your child is having pain, you note a sore area, or the tube has come out, tape the tube down. Do not use the tube. Contact the provider who is ordering the feedings to get further instruction.

What is a residual, and how do I check for it?

The residual is the amount of contents remaining in your child's stomach from the previous feeding. The residual is checked before a feeding to make sure your child is not too full before another feeding is given. To check for a residual:

1. Place an empty syringe on the end of the feeding tube.

2. Pull the plunger back to withdraw stomach contents.

3. Measure the amount of residual on the syringe. Your provider will discuss with you how much residual is appropriate for your child.

4. Return the stomach contents to your child.

5. Flush the tube with 5–10 mL of warm water to prevent clogging.

6. If the residual is more than recommended for your child, delay the feeding for 30 minutes, and then check the residual again.

What can I do while my child is being fed?

Feeding time is a special time for babies. Babies enjoy being held closely, cuddled, rocked, or talked to during tube feedings just as if they were being fed by mouth. Hold your baby, and encourage the baby to use a pacifier during feeding to practice sucking and swallowing. Toddlers will need to stay in one place, so playing a game or doing a quiet activity may be useful. Older children can sit at the table with the family and receive a tube feeding while the family eats a meal.

What should I do if the tube is blocked?

If the tube won't flush, try using warm water. Gently flush 10–15 mL of fluid through the tube. Do not use carbonated beverages, juice, or vigorous pressure to unclog the tube. If the tube still will not flush, call your nurse or doctor. Flushing the tube before and after giving medicines, after intermittent feedings, and every 4–6 hours during continuous feedings will prevent this problem.

What should I do if the tube is leaking?

If the tube is cracked or leaking, the tube will need to be replaced.

What should I do if my child is vomiting?

- Call your doctor if vomiting persists after one day. Vomiting causes a loss of body fluids, salts, and nutrients.

- Do not give a feeding if your child is vomiting.

- Check the residual. If the residual is higher than recommended, delay the feeding. Recheck the residual every 30–60 minutes until the residual is low enough to start the feeding.

- Give feedings in an upright position to decrease the chances of vomiting.

- Try smaller, more frequent feedings, being sure that the total amount of feeding for the day is the same as what is ordered.

- Try to slow the rate of the feeding.

- Have your child rest after each feeding. But, do not let him or her lie down flat during the feeding and for one hour after a feeding.

- If your child develops difficulty breathing during or immediately after a feeding, stop the feeding and call your provider. It is possible your child may have inhaled formula or stomach contents into the lungs.

- Infection may cause vomiting. Clean and rinse equipment well between feedings.

- Do not let formula in the feeding bag hang longer than eight hours.

- After the formula can is opened, the can should be stored in the refrigerator until used.

- If your child has nausea and vomiting, your provider may recommend changing the feedings temporarily. Follow your provider's instructions about feeding during illness.

What should I do if my child has diarrhea?

Diarrhea is frequent loose, watery stools. Diarrhea can be caused by giving too much feeding at once, running the feeding too quickly, unable to tolerate the type of formula, spoiled formula, or infection. Some medicines can cause diarrhea. Some children have loose stools with changes in formula, medicines, or feeding routines.

- Avoid hanging formula for longer than eight hours.

- Keep opened formula in the refrigerator for no more than 24 hours.

- Slow the feeding rate or give smaller amounts of formula more often.

- Give more water after each feeding to replace water lost in diarrhea.

- Call your provider if the diarrhea does not stop after one day.

What should I do if my child becomes dehydrated?

Dehydration is a loss of water and fluids from the body. Dehydration may occur for a variety of reasons—diarrhea, vomiting, fever, or sweating for example.

- Signs of dehydration include decreased or dark urine, crying with no tears, dry skin, fatigue, irritability, dizziness, dry mouth, weight loss, and/or headache.
- Extra water may be given after each feeding to replace water lost.
- Call your provider if you notice signs of dehydration.

What should I do if my child becomes constipated?

Constipation may be caused by certain types of formula, changes in formula, medicines, or feeding patterns, or not enough water. Give more water flushes throughout the day, especially during hot weather. If constipation becomes chronic, contact your provider.

How do I bathe my child with a NG in place?

Bathe your child as is normal for the age and developmental level, as long as the NG tube is not submerged under water.

What should I do if my child has gas, bloating, or cramping?

Be sure there is no air in the tubing before attaching the feeding tube.

Why is oral care still important?

Good mouth care is essential for overall health. Your child should have their teeth, gums, and mouth brushed at least twice a day using a soft toothbrush or sponge brush even if he/she is not eating by mouth.

What [should I] do if the tube is out of place?

If the tube is longer in the stomach, call your provider or home health nurse. Do not use the tube. You will need to have a new tube placed. If the tube is pulled out during a feeding, stop the feeding immediately, and contact your provider to have the tube replaced.

When should I call my child's provider?

- Your child has trouble breathing.

- Your child turns blue.

- You see blood around the tube, in your child's stool, or in stomach contents.

- Your child coughs, chokes, or vomits while feeding (stop the feeding if this occurs during feeding).

- Your child has a bloated or rigid belly (belly feels hard when it is gently pressed).

- Your child has diarrhea or constipation.

- Your child has a fever of 100.4 degrees Fahrenheit or higher.

Section 45.3

Nutrition Considerations after Weight-Loss Surgery

"Patient Guide to Endocrine and Nutritional Management After
Bariatric Surgery," reprinted with permission from www.hormone.org.
© Hormone Health Network, 2010. All rights reserved.

Bariatric (weight loss) surgery is a treatment option for people who are dangerously obese. But treatment does not end with the surgical procedure. All bariatric surgery patients need careful medical follow-up to reduce their chances of regaining weight and to ensure good management of other obesity-related health problems. Care after surgery is provided by primary care physicians, endocrinologists (doctors who specialize in hormone-related diseases and conditions), or gastroenterologists (doctors who specialize in diseases and conditions affecting the digestive system).

This text is based on The Endocrine Society's practice guidelines for physicians that focus on the care patients need immediately after surgery, as well as long-term management to prevent complications and weight regain.

How does bariatric surgery help weight loss?

Bariatric surgery procedures promote weight loss in one of three ways:

593

- Restriction, or limiting the amount of food you can eat before feeling full by reducing the size of the stomach

- Malabsorption, or limiting the absorption of nutrients in the intestines by bypassing part of the small intestine (removing it from the path of food through the digestive tract)

- Combination of restriction and malabsorption

What are the different bariatric procedures?

There are four operations commonly offered in the United States for weight loss.

- **Adjustable gastric banding (AGB):** In this restrictive procedure, an adjustable band is placed around the top of the stomach, creating a small pouch that holds only a little food. When the pouch is full, feelings of hunger go away and you are ready to stop eating even though you have had a small meal. Patients who have AGB lose less weight than those who have malabsorptive procedures. Weight loss depends on following a strict diet.

- **Roux-en-Y gastric bypass (RYGB):** RYGB is mainly a restrictive operation but also includes some malabsorption. Food intake is limited by stapling the stomach to create a small pouch. Absorption is somewhat limited by cutting and reattaching the small intestine so that the upper third of the small intestine is bypassed and the remaining portion is joined to the pouch.

- **Biliopancreatic diversion with duodenal switch (BPD-DS):** BPD-DS works by restriction and malabsorption. It shortens the distance between the stomach and the colon (large intestine) even more than RYGB and causes more malabsorption. Most of the stomach is removed and a tube-like stomach (called a vertical gastric sleeve) is created. The sleeve remains connected to a very short segment of the upper small intestine, which is then directly connected to a lower part.

- **Vertical sleeve gastrectomy (VSG):** VSG reduces the size of the stomach, so it restricts food intake but doesn't decrease absorption by the intestines. VSG has mainly been performed as the first part of BPD-DS. However, recent studies suggest that some patients who undergo VSG lose weight with that procedure alone.

How can weight regain be prevented or treated?

Preventing weight regain begins with realistic expectations about what bariatric surgery can do and what you have to do for yourself to lose weight and keep it off. While the surgery can help you limit the amount of food you eat, you must be ready to change lifestyle habits that led to weight gain. After surgery, you need to follow your doctor's nutritional recommendations and exercise regularly (150 minutes per week of physical activity is recommended). Participation in a support group could help you stick with new habits. It's also important to keep follow-up medical appointments to monitor the effects of surgery.

How are postoperative nutritional deficiencies managed?

Because your body absorbs fewer nutrients after bariatric surgery, especially malabsorptive procedures, you need to keep a close eye on what you eat and make sure that you are getting all the nutrients your body needs for good health. You also need to see your doctor periodically for blood tests to monitor levels of macronutrients (protein, fats, carbohydrates) and micronutrients (vitamins, minerals, trace elements).

- Every three months for the first year, you should have blood tests to measure your blood count (to check for anemia), glucose (to check blood sugar levels), and creatinine (to check kidney function).

- Every six months for the first year, you should have blood tests to see if your body is lacking any specific nutrients (nutritional deficiencies) that could cause such problems as fatigue, weakness, loss of muscle mass, heart palpitations, depression, tingling sensations, bone disease, loss of night vision, or hypocalcemia (low levels of calcium in the blood).

- After the first year, you should repeat all of these tests annually.

Protein malnutrition is the most severe macronutrient complication of malabsorptive surgical procedures. You should consume an average of 60–120 grams of protein daily during weight loss and for the long term. Experts recommend daily multivitamin-mineral and calcium plus vitamin D supplements for all weight-loss surgery patients. If you have had a malabsorptive procedure, you may need to take additional supplements, such as vitamin B12 or iron, to prevent nutritional deficiencies.

Both weight loss itself and too little calcium and vitamin D can lead to increased risk of osteoporosis (brittle bones). If you had a malabsorptive procedure, you should have your blood levels of these nutrients tested every six months and have a dual-energy X-ray absorptiometry

(DEXA) for bone density performed yearly until your bone health is stable. Based on these tests, your doctor may adjust the amount of vitamin D and calcium supplementation you take.

How are vomiting and dumping syndrome managed?

Vomiting and dumping syndrome are possible side effects of operations that reduce the size of the stomach. Vomiting occurs most commonly during the first few postoperative months, when you are adapting to a small stomach pouch. Vomiting can result from eating foods that are too tough—you need to gradually progress from liquid to soft to solid food. It may also be due to eating too quickly or too much, taking bites that are too big, or not chewing your food enough. Vomiting can also be caused by dehydration. To prevent vomiting, you need to pay attention to signs of fullness, eat slowly, and drink plenty of fluids. AGB patients may need an adjustment of the band.

Dumping syndrome refers to a group of symptoms, such as nausea, weakness, light-headedness, and abdominal cramps, that occur when the undigested contents of your stomach are dumped into your small intestine too quickly. This rapid emptying can be triggered by too much sugar or fatty foods.

Dumping symptoms tend to decrease with time and can usually be controlled with certain nutritional changes, such as:

- avoiding drinking liquids within 30 minutes of a solid-food meal;

- increasing the amount of protein you eat;

- avoiding simple carbohydrates (such as sugary foods and drinks), which are easily digested;

- increasing your intake of fiber and complex carbohydrates (such as whole grain foods), which take longer to digest.

If this approach doesn't work, then your doctor may prescribe a medication for you to take before meals to manage your symptoms.

What effect will bariatric surgery have on obesity-related health conditions?

The effect of bariatric surgery goes beyond weight loss in people who are severely obese. In most patients, obesity-related health problems disappear or greatly improve. For example, very soon after a malabsorptive procedure, type 2 diabetes can improve to the point that little or no diabetes medication is necessary.

Likewise, insulin-treated patients require much less insulin, and most can discontinue insulin therapy by six weeks after surgery.

Bariatric surgery can also improve or resolve other conditions, such as hypertension (high blood pressure), high cholesterol, non-alcoholic fatty liver disease, obstructive sleep apnea, joint disease, asthma, and infertility due to polycystic ovarian syndrome. If you were taking medications before surgery to treat conditions such as diabetes, high blood pressure, or high cholesterol, you may need to adjust your dosage right after surgery. It is important for your doctor to monitor such conditions in follow-up exams.

What can you do to help your treatment process?

Surgery isn't a quick fix to obesity and obesity-related health problems. You and your health care team will need to work together for the long term to ensure the best outcome. After surgery, follow your doctor's advice for treatment and see him or her regularly for testing and monitoring of your condition so needed changes can be made before serious complications develop. You also need to make a lifelong commitment to eating healthy meals and exercising regularly to prevent weight regain.

Chapter 46

Caring for Surgical Incisions and Drains

Chapter Contents

Section 46.1

Caring for Your Incision

"Surgical Wound Care—Open,"
© 2012 A.D.A.M., Inc. Reprinted with permission.
This document is dated June 27, 2010.

An incision is a cut through the skin that is made during surgery. It also called a surgical wound. Some incisions are small, and others are very long. The size of the incision will depend on the kind of surgery you had.

Do not wear tight clothing that rubs against the incision while it is healing.

Sometimes, a surgical wound will break open (wound dehiscence). This may happen along the entire cut or just part of it. Your doctor may decide not to close it again with sutures, or stitches.

If your doctor does not close your wound again with sutures, you will need to learn how to care for it at home, since it may take time to heal. The wound will heal from the bottom to the top. The dressings help to soak up any drainage and to keep the skin from closing before the wound underneath fills in.

Proper Handwashing

It is important to clean your hands before you change your dressings. You may use an alcohol-based cleaner like Purell, or you may wash your hands using these steps:

- Take all jewelry off your hands.

- Wet your hands, pointing them down under warm running water.

- Add soap and wash your hands for 15 to 30 seconds (sing "Happy Birthday" or the "Alphabet Song" one time through). Clean under your nails also.

- Rinse well.

- Dry with a clean towel.

Removing the Old Dressing

Your doctor will tell you how often to change your dressing. Be prepared before starting the dressing change:

- Clean your hands before touching the dressing.
- Make sure you have all the supplies you will need handy.
- Have a clean work surface for all of the equipment you will need.

Remove the old dressing:

- Carefully loosen the tape.
- Use a clean (not sterile) medical glove to grab the old dressing and pull it off.
- If the dressing sticks to the wound, get it wet and try again, unless your doctor instructed you to pull it off dry.
- Put the old dressing in a plastic bag and set it aside.
- Clean your hands again after you take off the old dressing.

Caring for the Wound

You may use a gauze pad or soft cloth to clean the skin around your wound:

- Use a normal saline solution (salt water) or mild soapy water.
- Soak the gauze or cloth in the saline solution or soapy water, and gently dab or wipe the skin with it.
- Try to remove all drainage and any dried blood or other matter that may have built up on the skin.
- Do not use skin cleansers, alcohol, peroxide, iodine, or soaps with antibacterial chemicals. These can damage the wound tissue and slow your healing.

Your doctor may also ask you to irrigate, or wash out, your wound:

- Fill a syringe with salt water or soapy water, whichever your health care provider recommends.
- Hold the syringe one to six inches away from the wound, and spray hard enough into the wound to wash away drainage and discharge.

- Use a soft, dry cloth or piece of gauze to carefully pat the wound dry.

Do not put any lotion, cream, or herbal remedies on or around your wound without asking your doctor first.

Putting on the New Dressing

Place the clean dressing on the wound as your health care provider taught you to. You may be using a wet-to-dry dressing.

Clean your hands when you are finished.

Throw away all the old dressings and other used supplies in a waterproof plastic bag. Close it tightly, then double it before putting it in the trash.

Wash any soiled laundry from the dressing change separately from other laundry. Ask your doctor if you need to add bleach to the wash water.

Use a dressing only once. Never reuse it.

When to Call the Doctor

Call your doctor if:

- You see any of these changes around the incision:
  - More redness
  - More pain
  - Swelling
  - Bleeding
  - The wound is larger or deeper
  - The wound looks dried out or dark
- The drainage coming from or around the incision:
  - Is increasing
  - Becomes thick, tan, green or yellow, or smells bad (pus)
- Your temperature is above 100 degrees Fahrenheit for more than four hours.

Section 46.2

Caring for a Surgical Drain

"How to Care for the Jackson-Pratt Drain," by the National
Institutes of Health Clinical Center (www.cc.nih.gov), July 2008.

The Jackson-Pratt (JP) drain is a special tube that prevents body fluid from collecting near the site of your surgery. The drain pulls this fluid (by suction) into a bulb. The bulb can then be emptied and the fluid inside measured.

At first, this fluid is bloody. Then, as your wound heals, the fluid changes to light pink, light yellow, or clear. The drain will stay in place until less than 30 cc (about 2 tablespoons) of fluid can be collected in a 24-hour period.

Caring for the JP drain is easy. Depending on how much fluid drains from your surgical site, you will need to empty the bulb every 8 to 12 hours. The bulb should be emptied when it is half full. Before you are discharged from the hospital, your nurse will show you how to do the following:

- Empty the collection bulb

- Record the amount of fluid collected

- Squeeze the bulb flat and plug so that the suction works again

- Keep the drain site clean and free of infection

How to Empty the Drain

1. Wash your hands well with soap and water.

2. Pull the plug out of the bulb.

3. Pour the fluid inside the bulb into a measuring cup.

4. Clean the plug with alcohol. Then squeeze the bulb flat. While the bulb is flat, put the plug back into the bulb. The bulb should stay flat after it is plugged so that the vacuum suction can restart. If you can't squeeze the bulb flat and plug it at the same time, use a hard, flat surface (such as a table) to help you press the bulb flat while you replug it.

5. Measure how much fluid you collected. Write the amount of drainage, and the date and time you collected it.

603

6. Flush the fluid down the toilet.

7. Wash your hands.

How to Care for the Skin and the Drain Site

1. Wash your hands well with soap and water.

2. Remove the dressing from around the drain. Use soap and water or 0.9 percent normal saline (on a gauze or cotton swab) to clean the drain site and the skin around it. Clean this area once a day.

3. When the drain site is clean and dry, put a new dressing around the drain. Put surgical tape on the dressing to hold it down against your skin.

4. Place the old dressing into the trash. If it is bloody, wrap it in a small plastic bag (like a sandwich bag).

5. Wash your hands.

Complications

Sometimes, a large amount of fluid may leak from around the drain site, making the gauze dressing completely wet. If this happens, use soap and water to clean the area. Verify that the bulb drain is secured and flat to provide the needed suction.

Another potential side effect is the development of a clot within the drain. This appears as a dark, stringy lining. It could prevent the drainage from flowing through the tube.

Be sure to notify your doctor if either of these complications occurs.

How to Check for Infection

Watch the skin around the drain for these signs of infection:

- Increased redness
- Increased pain
- Increased swelling

Other signs of infection include the following:

- Fever greater than 101 degrees Fahrenheit
- Cloudy yellow, tan, or foul-smelling drainage

Report any of these symptoms to your doctor as soon as possible.

Chapter 47

Caring for an Ostomy Bag after Surgery

As always, in order to obtain answers to your individually specific questions, be sure to consult with your doctor or ostomy nurse for help.

Who should I tell? What should I say about my surgery?

You should tell those who need to know, such as healthcare providers, your spouse or significant others, and people who are involved in your recuperative care.

You need not feel you have to explain your surgery to everyone who asks. Those who are just curious need to know only that you had abdominal surgery, or that you had part or all of your colon or bladder removed.

If you are considering marriage, thorough discussions with your future spouse about life with an ostomy and its effect on sex, children, and family acceptance will help alleviate misconceptions and fear on the part of the spouse.

If you have children, answer their questions simply and truthfully. A simple explanation will be enough for them. You may want to confide in your employer or a good friend at work because keeping it a complete secret may cause practical difficulties.

Will I be able to continue my daily activities once I recover from surgery?

As your strength returns, you can go back to your regular activities. Most people can return to their previous line of work; however, communicate with your healthcare team about your daily routines, so they can assist you to returning to maximum health as early as possible.

An ostomy should not limit your participation in sports. Many physicians do not allow contact sports because of possible injury to the stoma from a severe blow or because the pouching system may slip, but these problems can be overcome with special ostomy supplies. Weight lifting may result in a hernia at the stoma. Check with your doctor about such sports. There are many people who are distance runners, skiers, swimmers, and participants in many other types of athletics.

What about showering and bathing? Should I bathe with or without my pouch?

You may bathe with or without your pouching system in place. If you wish to take a shower or bath with your pouch off, you can do so. Normal exposure to air or contact with soap and water will not harm the stoma, and water does not enter the opening. Choose a time for bathing when the bowel is less active. You can also leave your pouch on while bathing.

What can I eat? Will I need to change my diet?

There may be some modifications in your diet according to the type of ostomy surgery. People with colostomy and ileostomy surgery should return to their normal diet after a period of adjustment. Introduce foods back into your diet a little at a time and monitor the effect of each food on the ostomy function. Chew your food well and drink plenty of fluids. Some less digestible or high roughage foods are more likely to create potential for blockage problems (i.e., corn, coconut, mushrooms, nuts, raw fruits, and vegetables).

There are no eating restrictions as a result of urostomy surgery. Urostomates should drink plenty of liquids each day following the healthcare team's recommendations.

Will I be able to wear the same clothes as before?

Whatever you wore before surgery, you can wear afterward with very few exceptions. Many pouching systems are made today that are unnoticeable even when wearing the most stylish, form fitting clothing for men and women.

Depending on your stoma location you might find belts uncomfortable or restrictive. Some people choose to wear higher or looser waistbands on trousers and skirts.

Cotton knit or stretch underpants or panty hose may give the support and security you need. Some men finds that jockey type shorts help support the pouch.

Women may want to choose a swimsuit that has a lining to provide a smoother profile. Stretch panties (with Lycra) can also be worn under a swimsuit to add support and smooth out any bulges or outlines. Men may prefer to wear a tank shirt and trunks if the stoma is above the belt line.

What about sex and intimacy? Will I be able to get pregnant after surgery?

Sexual relationships and intimacy are important and fulfilling aspects of your life that should continue after ostomy surgery. Your attitude is a key factor in re-establishing sexual expression and intimacy. A period of adjustment after surgery is to be expected. Sexual function in women is usually not impaired, while sexual potency of men may sometimes be affected, usually only temporarily. Discuss any problems with your physician and/or ostomy nurse.

Your ability to conceive does not change and pregnancy and delivery should be normal after ostomy surgery. However, if you are thinking about becoming pregnant, you should first check with your doctor about any other health problems.

Is travel possible?

All methods of travel are open to you. Many people with ostomies travel extensively, from camping trips to cruises to plane excursions around the world. Take along enough supplies to last the entire trip plus some extra, double what you think you may need. Checked luggage sometimes gets lost; carry an extra pouching system and other supplies on the plane with you. When traveling by car, keep your supplies in the coolest part, and avoid the trunk or back window ledge. Seat belts will not harm the stoma when adjusted comfortably.

When traveling abroad, take adequate amount of supplies, referral lists for physicians and medical centers, and some medication to control any diarrhea and stop the fluid and electrolyte loss. When going through customs or luggage inspection, a note from your doctor stating that you need to carry ostomy supplies and medications by hand may be helpful.

For more information, see www.ostomy.org/ostomy_info/travel_tips .shtml.

What about medications? Can I take vitamins?

Absorption may vary with individuals and types of medication. Certain drug problems may arise depending on the type of ostomy you have and the medications you are taking. Make sure all your health-care providers know the type of ostomy you have and the location of the stoma. This information will help your pharmacist and other health-care providers monitor your situation (i.e., time-released and enteric coated medications may pass through the system of ileostomates too quickly to be effective).

Will I always be wearing the same size and type of pouch?

The type of pouching system that was used in the hospital may need to be changed as the healing process takes place. Your stoma may shrink and may require a change in the size opening of your pouch. Your lifestyle may necessitate a change of the pouching system after a recuperative period. Make an appointment with your ostomy nurse to evaluate your management system.

Do you have any tips on emptying the pouch?

Check the pouch occasionally to see if it needs emptying before it gets too full and causes a leakage problem. Always empty prior to going out of the house and away from a convenient toilet. Most people find the easiest way to empty the pouch is to sit on the toilet with the pouch between the legs. Hold the bottom of the pouch up and remove the clamp. Slowly unroll the tail of the pouch into the toilet. Clean the outside and inside of the pouch tail with toilet paper. Replace the clamp.

How often should I change the pouch?

The adhesiveness and durability of pouching systems vary. Anywhere from three to seven days is to be expected. Itching or burning is a sign that the wafer should be changed. Changing too frequently or wearing one too long may be damaging to the skin.

What should I do if hospitalized again?

Take your ostomy supplies with you since the hospital may not have your brand in supply. If you are in doubt about any procedure, ask to talk to your doctor.

Ask to have the following information listed on your chart: 1) type of ostomy or continent diversion, 2) whether or not your rectum is intact, 3) describe in detail your management routine and list the ostomy products used. For urinary stomas, 4) do not take a urine specimen from the urostomy pouch, use a catheter inserted into the stoma.

Where can I purchase supplies?

Supplies may be ordered from a mail order company or from a medical supply or pharmacy in your town. Check the yellow pages under "Ostomy Supplies" or "Surgical Supplies" or "Hospital Supplies." (For more information, see the Ostomy Product & Suppliers page at www .ostomy.org/ostomy_info/suppliers.shtml)

Does insurance cover the cost of ostomy supplies?

Medicare Part B covers ostomy equipment. Medicare only allows a predetermined maximum quantity each month.

Medicaid is the federal/state insurance of last resort for low income persons. Check with the state Medicaid office for specifics.

Individual Health Insurance: Most plans typically will pay you 80% of the "reasonable and customary" costs after the deductible is met.

For help with insurance issues, see the Advocacy section at https:// uoaa.capwiz.com/uoaa/home.

When should I seek medical assistance?

You should call the doctor or ostomy nurse when you have:

- severe cramps lasting more than two or three hours;

- a deep cut in the stoma;

- excessive bleeding from the stoma opening (or a moderate amount in the pouch at several emptyings);

- continuous bleeding at the junction between the stoma and skin;

- severe skin irritation or deep ulcers;

- unusual change in stoma size and appearance;

- severe watery discharge lasting more than five or six hours;

- continuous nausea and vomiting; or;

- the ostomy does not have any output for four to six hours and is accompanied by cramping and nausea.

Where can I find help?

For medical assistance, seek help from your physician, surgeon, or ostomy nurse. Contact UOAA [www.ostomy.org/contact.shtml] for more information and referrals to local support groups [www.ostomy .org/supportgroups.shtml] and to request an ostomy visitor. Contact the Wound, Ostomy and Continence Nurses [www.wocn.org] national office, 800-224-9626 for information and local referrals for ostomy nurse specialists. Contact the American Cancer Society [www.cancer.org] at 800-ACS-2345 for cancer information.

Chapter 48

Driving and Travel after Surgery

Chapter Contents

Section 48.1

Postsurgical Patients at Risk for Impaired Driving

Excerpted from "Section 12: Effects of Anesthesia and Surgery," from the Physician's Guide to Assessing and Counseling Older Drivers, by the National Highway Traffic Safety Administration (NHTSA, www.nhtsa.gov), September 2003. Reviewed by David A. Cooke, MD, FACP, October 11, 2012.

Physicians should be alert to peri- and postoperative risk factors that may affect the patient's cognitive function postsurgery, placing the patient at risk for impaired driving. Risk factors include the following:

- Pre-existing cognitive impairment

- Duration of surgery

- Age (over 60 years)

- Altered mental status postsurgery

- The presence of multiple comorbidities

- Emergency surgery

If the physician is concerned that residual visual, cognitive, or motor deficits following the surgery may impair the patient's driving performance, referral to a driver rehabilitation specialist for a driver evaluation (including on-road assessment) is highly recommended.

Physicians should counsel patients who undergo surgery—both inpatient and outpatient—not to drive themselves home following the procedure. Although they may feel capable of driving, their driving skills may be affected by pain, physical restrictions, anesthesia, and/or analgesics. Physicians should also remind patients to wear their safety belts properly (over the shoulder, rather than under the arm) and position themselves at least 10 inches from the vehicle airbags whenever they are in a vehicle as a driver or passenger. The patient should sit in the vehicle seat that is most likely to accommodate these needs.

In counseling patients about their return to driving after a surgical procedure, it is useful for the physician to ask whether the patient's car has power steering and automatic transmission. Physicians can tailor their driving advice accordingly.

As patients resume driving, they should be counseled to assess their comfort level in familiar, traffic-free areas before driving in heavy traffic. If the patient feels uncomfortable driving in certain situations, he/she should avoid these situations until his/her confidence level has returned. A patient should never resume driving until he/she feels ready to do so.

Here are general recommendations for driving after surgery:

- **Abdominal, back, and chest surgery:** The patient may resume driving after demonstrating the necessary strength and range of motion for driving.

- **Anesthesia:** Because anesthetic agents and adjunctive compounds (such as benzodiazepines) may be administered in combination, the patient should not resume driving until the motor and cognitive effects from all anesthetic agents have subsided.

- **General:** Both the surgeon and anesthesiologist should advise patients against driving for at least 24 hours after a general anesthetic has been administered. Longer periods of driving cessation may be recommended depending on the procedure performed and the presence of complications.

- **Local:** If the anesthetized region is necessary for driving tasks, the patient should not drive until he/she has recovered full strength and sensation (barring pain).

- **Epidural:** The patient may resume driving after recovering full strength and sensation (barring pain) in the affected areas.

- **Spinal:** The patient may resume driving after recovering full strength and sensation (barring pain) in the affected areas.

Section 48.2

Driving and Travel after Heart Surgery

Excerpted from "Your Guide to Living Well with Heart Disease," by the
National Heart, Lung, and Blood Institute (NHLBI, www.nhlbi.nih.gov),
part of the National Institutes of Health, November 2005. Reviewed by
David A. Cooke, MD, FACP, October 11, 2012.

Driving

After heart surgery, driving can usually begin within a week for
most patients, if allowed by state law. Each state has its own regula-
tions for driving a motor vehicle following a serious illness, so contact
your state's Department of Motor Vehicles for guidelines. People with
complications or chest pain should not drive until their symptoms have
been stable for a few weeks.

Travel

Once your doctor tells you it's safe for you to travel, keep these tips
in mind:

- Keep your medications in your purse or carry-on luggage so they
  will be easily available when you need them.

- Pack light so that you can lift your luggage without strain. At
  the airport, train, or bus station, use a pull-cart to cut down on
  lifting. If possible, get help from a porter.

- Allow more time than usual to catch your flight, train, or bus.
  Who needs the extra stress?

- Walk around at least every two hours during trips. While sitting, flex your feet frequently and do other simple exercises to
  increase blood flow in your legs and prevent blood clots.

- Check with your doctor before traveling to locations at high alti-
  tudes (greater than 6,000 feet) or places where the temperature
  will be either very hot or very cold. When you first arrive, give
  yourself a chance to rest.

Remember, each person's recovery process is different. Don't try to guess when you can return to normal activities. Always ask your doctor first.

Part Six

Additional Help
and Information

Chapter 49

Glossary of Terms
Related to Surgery

advance directive: A legal document that states the treatment or care a person wishes to receive or not receive if he or she becomes unable to make medical decisions; for example, as a result of being unconscious. Some types of advance directives are living wills and do-not-resuscitate (DNR) orders.[1]

anesthesia: Drugs or substances that cause loss of feeling or awareness. Local anesthetics cause loss of feeling in a part of a person's body. General anesthetics put a person to sleep.[1]

anesthesiologist: A doctor who specializes in giving drugs or other agents to prevent or relieve pain during surgery or other procedures being done in the hospital.[2]

biopsy: The removal of body tissues for examination under a microscope or for other tests on the tissue.[1]

blood pressure: The force of circulating blood on the walls of the arteries. Blood pressure is taken using two measurements: systolic (measured when the heart beats, when blood pressure is at its highest) and diastolic (measured between heartbeats, when blood pressure is at its lowest).Blood pressure is written with the systolic blood pressure first, followed by the diastolic blood pressure, such as 120/80.[1]

Definitions in this chapter were compiled from documents published by the following government agencies: Terms marked 1 are from the Office on Women's Health (www.womenshealth.gov); terms marked 2 are from the National Cancer Institute (www.cancer.gov), and the term marked 3 is from the Centers for Disease Control and Prevention.

blood transfusion: A procedure in which a person is given an infusion of whole blood or parts of blood. The blood may be donated by another person, or it may have been taken from the patient earlier and stored until needed.[2]

computed tomography (CT) scan: A series of detailed pictures of areas inside the body taken from different angles; the pictures are created by a computer linked to an X-ray machine.[1]

cryosurgery: A procedure in which tissue is frozen to destroy abnormal cells. Liquid nitrogen or liquid carbon dioxide is used to freeze the tissue.[2]

deep vein thrombosis: The formation of a blood clot in a deep vein of the leg or lower pelvis. Symptoms may include pain, swelling, warmth, and redness in the affected area.[2]

epidural block: A tube (catheter) placed into the lower back, into a small space below the spinal cord. Small doses of medicine can be given through the tube as needed.[1]

general surgery: The branch of surgery that covers the main areas of surgical treatment. General surgeons treat diseases of the abdomen, breast, head and neck, blood vessels, and digestive tract. They also manage care of patients who have been injured or who have deformities or other conditions that need surgery.[2]

incision: A cut made in the body to perform surgery.[2]

informed consent: A process in which patients are given important information, including possible risks and benefits, about a medical procedure or treatment, a clinical trial, or genetic testing. This is to help them decide if they want to be treated, tested, or take part in the trial. Patients are also given any new information that might affect their decision to continue.[2]

laparoscopic surgery: Surgery done with the aid of a laparoscope. A laparoscope is a thin, tube-like instrument with a light and a lens for viewing. It may also have a tool to remove tissue to be checked under a microscope for signs of disease.[2]

laser surgery: A surgical procedure that uses the cutting power of a laser beam to make bloodless cuts in tissue or to remove a surface lesion such as a tumor.[2]

lung function test: A test used to measure how well the lungs work. It measures how much air the lungs can hold and how quickly air is moved into and out of the lungs. It also measures how much oxygen is used and how much carbon dioxide is given off during breathing. A lung function test can be used to diagnose a lung disease and to see how well treatment for the disease is working.[2]

magnetic resonance imaging (MRI): A procedure in which radio waves and a powerful magnet linked to a computer are used to create detailed pictures of areas inside the body. These pictures can show the difference between normal and diseased tissue.[2]

mortality: Mortality refers to the death rate, or the number of deaths in a certain group of people in a certain period of time.[2]

nasogastric tube: A tube that is inserted through the nose, down the throat and esophagus, and into the stomach. It can be used to give drugs, liquids, and liquid food, or used to remove substances from the stomach. Giving food through a nasogastric tube is a type of enteral nutrition. Also called gastric feeding tube and NG tube.[2]

nonsteroidal anti-inflammatory drugs (NSAIDs): Pain relievers such as aspirin, ibuprofen, and naproxen. These medicines are safe and effective when taken as directed, but they can cause stomach bleeding or kidney problems in some people.[1]

opioids: Also called narcotics, opioids are medicines given through a tube inserted in a vein or by injecting the medicine into a muscle. Sometimes, opioids also are given with epidural or spinal blocks.[1]

ostomy: An operation to create an opening (a stoma) from an area inside the body to the outside. Colostomy and urostomy are types of ostomies.[2]

outpatient: A patient who visits a health care facility for diagnosis or treatment without spending the night. Sometimes called a day patient.[2]

patient-controlled analgesia: A method of pain relief in which the patient controls the amount of pain medicine that is used. When pain relief is needed, the person can receive a preset dose of pain medicine by pressing a button on a computerized pump that is connected to a small tube in the body. Also called PCA.[2]

pneumonia: A severe inflammation of the lungs in which the alveoli (tiny air sacs) are filled with fluid. This may cause a decrease in the amount of oxygen that blood can absorb from air breathed into the lung. Pneumonia is usually caused by infection but may also be caused by radiation therapy, allergy, or irritation of lung tissue by inhaled substances. It may involve part or all of the lungs.[2]

rehabilitation: In medicine, a process to restore mental and/or physical abilities lost to injury or disease, in order to function in a normal or near-normal way.[2]

sepsis: The presence of bacteria or their toxins in the blood or tissues.[2]

septicemia: Disease caused by the spread of bacteria and their toxins in the bloodstream. Also called blood poisoning and toxemia.[2]

spinal block: A small dose of medicine given as a shot into the spinal fluid in the lower back.[1]

stereotactic radiosurgery: A type of external radiation therapy that uses special equipment to position the patient and precisely give a single large dose of radiation to a tumor. It is used to treat brain tumors and other brain disorders that cannot be treated by regular surgery. It is also being studied in the treatment of other types of cancer.[2]

surgical site infection: A surgical site infection is an infection that occurs after surgery in the part of the body where the surgery took place. Surgical site infections can sometimes be superficial infections involving the skin only. Other surgical site infections are more serious and can involve tissues under the skin, organs, or implanted material.[3]

ultrasound: Also called sonography, it is a painless, harmless test that uses sound waves to produce images of the organs and structures of the body on a screen.[1]

ventilator: In medicine, a machine used to help a patient breathe. Also called a respirator.[2]

Chapter 50

Directory of Organizations That Provide Information about Surgery

Government Agencies That Provide Information about Surgery

Agency for Healthcare Research and Quality
Office of Communications and Knowledge Transfer
540 Gaither Road
Suite 2000
Rockville, MD 20850
Phone: 301-427-1104
Website: www.ahrq.gov

Centers for Medicare and Medicaid Services
7500 Security Boulevard
Baltimore, MD 21244-1850
Toll-Free: 800-MEDICARE
(800-633-4227)
Toll-Free TTY: 877-486-2048
Website: www.medicare.gov

Centers for Disease Control and Prevention
1600 Clifton Road
Atlanta, GA 30333
Toll-Free: 800-CDC-INFO
(800-232-4636)
Toll-Free TTY: 888-232-6348
Phone: 404-639-3311
Website: www.cdc.gov
E-mail: cdcinfo@cdc.gov

Federal Trade Commission
600 Pennsylvania Avenue NW
Washington, DC 20580
Toll-Free: 877-FTC-HELP
(877-382-4357)
Toll-Free TTY: 866-653-4261
Phone: 202-326-2222
Website: www.ftc.gov
E-mail: webmaster@ftc.gov

Resources in this chapter were compiled from several sources deemed reliable; all contact information was verified and updated in October 2012.

Healthfinder®
National Health
Information Center
PO Box 1133
Washington, DC 20013-1133
Toll-Free: 800-336-4797
Phone: 301-565-4167
Fax: 301-984-4256
Website:
www.healthfinder.gov
E-mail: healthfinder@nhic.org

National Cancer Institute
NCI Office of Communications
and Education
Public Inquiries Office
6116 Executive Boulevard
Suite 300
Bethesda, MD 20892-8322
Toll-Free: 800-4-CANCER
(800-422-6237)
Toll-Free TTY: 800-332-8615
Website: www.cancer.gov
E-mail:
cancergovstaff@mail.nih.gov

National Center for Health Statistics
3311 Toledo Road
Hyattsville, MD 20782
Toll-Free: 800-CDC-INFO
(800-232-4636)
Website: www.cdc.gov/nchs
E-mail: cdcinfo@cdc.gov

National Eye Institute
Information Office
31 Center Drive MSC 2510
Bethesda, MD 20892-2510
Phone: 301-496-5248
Website: www.nei.nih.gov
E-mail: 2020@nei.nih.gov

National Heart, Lung, and Blood Institute
PO Box 30105
Bethesda, MD 20824-0105
Phone: 301-592-8573
Fax: 240-629-3246
Website: www.nhlbi.nih.gov
E-mail: nhlbiinfo@nhlbi.nih.gov

National Institute of Neurological Disorders and Stroke
NIH Neurological Institute
PO Box 5801
Bethesda, MD 20824
Toll-Free: 800-352-9424
Phone: 301-496-5751
TTY: 301-468-5981
Website: www.ninds.nih.gov

National Institute on Aging
Building 31, Room 5C27
31 Center Drive, MSC 2292
Bethesda, MD 20892
Toll-Free: 800-222-2225
Toll-Free TTY: 800-222-4225
Phone: 301-496-1752
Fax: 301-496-1072
Website: www.nia.nih.gov
E-mail: niaic@nia.nih.gov

National Institute of Arthritis and Musculoskeletal and Skin Diseases
1 AMS Circle
Bethesda, MD 20892-3675
Phone: 301-495-4484
Toll-Free: 877-22-NIAMS
(877-226-4267)
TTY: 301-565-2966
Fax: 301-718-6366
Website: www.niams.nih.gov
E-mail:
NIAMSinfo@mail.nih.gov

National Institute of Diabetes and Digestive and Kidney Diseases
NIDDK, NIH
Building 31, Room 9A06
31 Center Drive, MSC 2560
Bethesda, MD 20892-2560
Phone: 301-496-3583
Website: www.niddk.nih.gov

National Institutes of Health
9000 Rockville Pike
Bethesda, MD 20892
Phone: 301-496-4000
TTY: 301-402-9612
Website: www.nih.gov
E-mail: NIHinfo@od.nih.gov

National Women's Health Information Center
Office on Women's Health
200 Independence Avenue SW
Room 712E
Washington, DC 20201
Toll-Free: 800-994-9662
Toll-Free TDD: 888-220-5446
Phone: 202-690-7650
Fax: 202-205-2631
Website:
www.womenshealth.gov

U.S. Department of Health and Human Services
200 Independence Avenue SW
Washington, DC 20201
Toll-Free: 877-696-6775
Website: www.hhs.gov

U.S. Food and Drug Administration
10903 New Hampshire Avenue
Silver Spring, MD 20993
Toll-Free: 888-INFO-FDA
(888-463-6332)
Website: www.fda.gov

U.S. National Library of Medicine
8600 Rockville Pike
Bethesda, MD 20894
Toll-Free: 888-FIND-NLM
(888-346-3656)
Toll-Free TDD: 800-735-2258
Phone: 301-594-5983
Fax: 301-402-1384
Website: www.nlm.nih.gov
E-mail: custserv@nlm.nih.gov

Private Agencies That Provide Information about Surgery

Accreditation Association for Ambulatory Health Care
5250 Old Orchard Road
Suite 200
Skokie, IL 60077
Phone: 847-853-6060
Fax: 847-853-9028
Website: www.aaahc.org
E-mail: info@aaahc.org

American Academy of Dermatology
PO Box 4014
Schaumburg, IL 60168
Toll-Free: 866-503-SKIN
(866-503-7546)
Phone: 847-240-1280
Fax: 847-240-1859
Website: www.aad.org

American Academy of Facial Plastic and Reconstructive Surgery
310 South Henry Street
Alexandria, VA 22314
Phone: 703-299-9291
Fax: 703-299-8898
Website: www.aafprs.org
E-mail: info@aafprs.org

American Academy of Family Physicians
11400 Tomahawk Creek Parkway
Leawood, KS 66211-2680
Toll-Free: 800-274-2237
Phone: 913-906-6000
Fax: 913-906-6075
Website: www.aafp.org

American Academy of Ophthalmology
PO Box 7424
San Francisco, CA 94120-7424
Phone: 415-561-8500
Fax: 415-561-8533
Website: www.aao.org

American Academy of Orthopaedic Surgeons
6300 North River Road
Rosemont, IL 60018-4262
Phone: 847-823-7186
Fax: 847-823-8125
Website: www.aaos.org
E-mail: orthoinfo@aaos.org

American Academy of Otolaryngology–Head and Neck Surgery
1650 Diagonal Road
Alexandria, VA 22314-2857
Phone: 703-836-4444
Website: www.entnet.org

American Association of Endodontists
211 East Chicago Avenue
Suite 1100
Chicago, IL 60611-2691
Toll-Free: 800-872-3636
Phone: 312-266-7255
Toll-Free Fax: 866-451-9020
Fax: 312-266-9867
Website: www.aae.org
E-mail: info@aae.org

American Association of Hip and Knee Surgeons

6300 North River Road
Suite 615
Rosemont, IL 60018-4237
Phone: 847-698-1200
Fax: 847-698-0704
Website: www.aahks.org
E-mail: helpdesk@aahks.org

American Association of Nurse Anesthetists

222 South Prospect Avenue
Park Ridge, IL 60068-4001
Toll-Free: 855-526-2262
Phone: 847-692-7050
Fax: 847-692-6968
Website: www.aana.com
E-mail: info@aana.com

American Cancer Society

250 Williams Street NW
Atlanta, GA 30303
Toll-Free: 800-227-2345
Toll-Free TTY: 866-228-4327
Website: www.cancer.org

American College of Chest Physicians

3300 Dundee Road
Northbrook, IL 60062-2348
Phone: 847-498-1400
Fax: 847-498-5460
Website: www.chestnet.org

American College of Obstetricians and Gynecologists

PO Box 70620
Washington, DC 20024-9998
Toll-Free: 800-673-8444
Phone: 202-638-5577
Website: www.acog.org
E-mail: resources@acog.org

American College of Radiology

1891 Preston White Drive
Reston, VA 20191
Toll-Free: 800-227-5463
Phone: 703-648-8900
Website: www.acr.org
E-mail: info@acr.org

American College of Surgeons

633 North Saint Clair Street
Chicago, IL 60611-3211
Toll-Free: 800-621-4111
Phone: 312-202-5000
Fax: 312-202-5001
Website: www.facs.org
E-mail: postmaster@facs.org

American Dental Association

211 East Chicago Avenue
Chicago, IL 60611-2678
Phone: 312-440-2500
Website: www.ada.org

American Heart Association

7272 Greenville Avenue
Dallas, TX 75231
Toll-Free: 800-AHA-USA-1
(800-242-8721)
Website: www.heart.org

American Medical Association
515 North State Street
Chicago, IL 60654
Toll-Free: 800-621-8335
Website: www.ama-assn.org

American Optometric Association
243 North Lindbergh Boulevard
St. Louis, MO 63141
Toll-Free: 800-365-2219
Phone: 314-991-4100
Website: www.aoa.org

American Pediatric Surgical Association
111 Deer Lake Road
Suite 100
Deerfield, IL 60015
Phone: 847-480-9576
Fax: 847-480-9282
Website: www.eapsa.org
E-mail: eapsa@eapsa.org

American Psychological Association
750 First Street NE
Washington, DC 20002-4242
Toll-Free: 800-374-2721
Phone: 202-336-5500
TDD/TTY: 202-336-6123
Website: www.apa.org

American Rhinologic Society
PO Box 495
Warwick, NY 10990
Phone: 845-988-1631
Fax: 845-986-1527
Website:
www.american-rhinologic.org

American Society for Dermatologic Surgery
5550 Meadowbrook Drive
Suite 120
Rolling Meadows, IL 60008
Phone: 847-956-0900
Website: www.asds.net

American Society for Laser Medicine and Surgery
2100 Stewart Avenue
Suite 240
Wausau, WI 54401
Toll-Free: 877-258-6028
Phone: 715-845-9283
Fax: 715-848-2493
Website: www.aslms.org
E-mail: information@aslms.org

American Society for Metabolic and Bariatric Surgery
100 SW 75th Street
Suite 201
Gainesville, FL 32607
Phone: 352-331-4900
Fax: 352-331-4975
Website: www.asmbs.org
E-mail: info@asmbs.org

American Society for Radiation Oncology
8280 Willow Oaks Corporate
Drive, Suite 500
Fairfax, VA 22031
Toll-Free: 800-962-7876
Phone: 703-502-1550
Fax: 703-502-7852
Website: www.astro.org

American Society for Reproductive Medicine
1209 Montgomery Highway
Birmingham, AL 35216-2809
Phone: 205-978-5000
Fax: 205-978-5005
Website: www.asrm.org
E-mail: asrm@asrm.org

American Society for Surgery of the Hand
822 West Washington Boulevard
Chicago, IL 60607
Phone: 312-880-1900
Fax: 847-384-1435
Website: www.assh.org
E-mail: info@assh.org

American Society of Anesthesiologists
520 North Northwest Highway
Park Ridge, IL 60068-2573
Phone: 847-825-5586
Fax: 847-825-1692
Website: www.asahq.org
E-mail: communications@asahq.org

American Society of Colon and Rectal Surgeons
85 West Algonquin Road
Suite 550
Arlington Heights, IL 60005
Phone: 847-290-9184
Fax: 847-290-9203
Website: www.fascrs.org
E-mail: ascrs@fascrs.org

American Society of Ophthalmic Plastic and Reconstructive Surgery
5841 Cedar Lake Road
Suite 204
Minneapolis, MN 55416
Phone: 952-646-2038
Fax: 952-545-6073
Website: www.asoprs.org
E-mail: info@asoprs.org

American Society of PeriAnesthesia Nurses
90 Frontage Road
Cherry Hill, NJ 08034-1424
Toll-Free: 877-737-9696
Fax: 856-616-9601
Website: www.aspan.org
E-mail: aspan@aspan.org

American Society of Plastic Surgeons
444 East Algonquin Road
Arlington Heights, IL 60005
Phone: 847-228-9900
Website: www.plasticsurgery.org

American Society of Transplantation
15000 Commerce Parkway
Suite C
Mount Laurel, NJ 08054
Phone: 856-439-9986
Fax: 856-439-9982
Website: www.a-s-t.org

American Thoracic Society
25 Broadway, 18th Floor
New York, NY 10004
Phone: 212-315-8600
Fax: 212-315-6498
Website: www.thoracic.org
E-mail: atsinfo@thoracic.org

American Thyroid Association
6066 Leesburg Pike, Suite 550
Falls Church, VA 22041
Phone: 703-998-8890
Fax: 703-998-8893
Website: www.thyroid.org
E-mail: thyroid@thyroid.org

Amputee Coalition of America
9303 Center Street, Suite 100
Manassas, VA 20110
Toll-Free: 888-267-5669
TTY: 865-525-4512
Website:
www.amputee-coalition.org

Arthritis Foundation
PO Box 7669
Atlanta, GA 30357-0669
Toll-Free: 800-283-7800
Website: www.arthritis.org

Cleveland Clinic
9500 Euclid Avenue
Cleveland, OH 44195
Toll-Free: 800-223-2273
Toll-Free: 866-588-2264 (Info Line)
Phone: 216-444-4508
Phone: 216-636-5860 (Info Line)
TTY: 216-444-0261
Website: my.clevelandclinic.org

Eye Surgery Education Council
Phone: 703-788-5761
Website:
www.eyesurgeryeducation.org

General Surgery News
McMahon Publishing
545 West 45th Street
8th Floor
New York, NY 10036
Phone: 212-957-5300, ext. 362
Website:
www.generalsurgerynews.com

The Joint Commission
One Renaissance Boulevard
Oakbrook Terrace, IL 60181
Phone: 630-792-5800
Fax: 630-792-5005
Website:
www.jointcommission.org

KidsHealth/TeensHealth
The Nemours Foundation
1600 Rockland Road
Wilmington, DE 19803
Phone: 302-651-4046
Website: www.kidshealth.org
Website: www.teenshealth.org
E-mail: info@kidshealth.org

Mayo Foundation for Medical Education and Research
Website: www.mayoclinic.com/
health-information

National Hospice and Palliative Care Organization
1731 King Street
Suite 100
Alexandria, VA 22314
Toll-Free: 800-658-8898
Phone: 703-837-1500
Fax: 703-837-1233
Website: www.nhpco.org
E-mail: nhpco_info@nhpco.org

Planned Parenthood Federation of America, Inc.
434 West 33rd Street
New York, NY 10001
Toll-Free: 800-230-PLAN
(800-230-7526)
Phone: 212-541-7800
Fax: 212-245-1845
Website:
www.plannedparenthood.org

Society of Critical Care Medicine
Headquarters
500 Midway Drive
Mount Prospect, IL 60056
Phone: 847-827-6869
Fax: 847-827-6886
Website: www.sccm.org
E-mail: info@sccm.org

Society of Interventional Radiology
3975 Fair Ridge Drive
Suite 400 North
Fairfax, VA 22033
Toll-Free: 800-488-7284
Phone: 703-691-1805
Fax: 703-691-1855
Website: www.sirweb.org

Society of Nuclear Medicine
1850 Samuel Morse Drive
Reston, VA 20190
Phone: 703-708-9000
Fax: 703-708-9015
Website: www.snm.org
E-mail: feedback@snm.org

Society of Thoracic Surgeons
633 North Saint Clair Street
Floor 23
Chicago, IL 60611
Phone: 312-202-5800
Fax: 312-202-5801
Website: www.sts.org

Texas Heart Institute
6770 Bertner Avenue
Houston, TX 77030
Toll-Free: 800-292-2221
Phone: 832-355-4011
Website:
www.texasheartinstitute.org

United Network for Organ Sharing
PO Box 2484
Richmond, VA 23218
Toll-Free: 888-894-6361
Phone: 804-782-4800
Fax: 804-782-4817
Website: www.unos.org

United Ostomy Associations of America, Inc.
PO Box 512
Northfield, MN 55057-0512
Toll-Free: 800-826-0826
Website: www.ostomy.org
E-mail: info@ostomy.org

Index

Index

Page numbers followed by 'n' indicate a footnote. Page numbers in *italics* indicate a table or illustration.

Health Reference Series